T0344657

Improving Mental Health Care

Improving Mental Health Care

The Global Challenge

EDITED BY

Graham Thornicroft

Professor
Health Service and Population Research Department
Institute of Psychiatry
King's College London
London

Mirella Ruggeri

Professor
Section of Psychiatry
Department of Public Health and Community Medicine
University of Verona
Verona

David Goldberg

Professor Emeritus
Institute of Psychiatry
King's College London
London

WILEY-BLACKWELL

A John Wiley & Sons, Ltd., Publication

Library of Congress Cataloging-in-Publication Data

Improving mental health care : the global challenge / edited by Graham Thornicroft, Mirella Ruggeri, David Goldberg.
    p. ; cm.
  Includes bibliographical references and index.
  ISBN 978-1-118-33797-4 (hardback : alk. paper) – ISBN 978-1-118-33798-1 (obook online product) – ISBN 978-1-118-33799-8 (eMobi) – ISBN 978-1-118-33800-1 (ePub) – ISBN 978-1-118-33801-8 (ePDF)
  I. Thornicroft, Graham. II. Ruggeri, Mirella. III. Goldberg, David P.
  [DNLM: 1. Mental Health Services. 2. Community Mental Health Services. 3. Delivery of Health Care. 4. Mental Disorders–therapy. 5. Socioeconomic Factors. 6. World Health. WM 30.1]
  RA790.5
  362.2′2–dc23
2013003251

A catalogue record for this book is available from the British Library.

Dedication

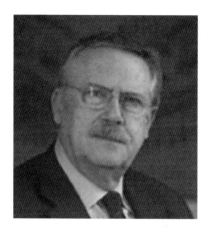

This book is appearing at the time Michele Tansella is due to retire. His colleagues both in Italy and elsewhere have marked the occasion by considering the enormous contribution he has made to mental health services in community settings. He has made the services in South Verona known to mental health professionals across the world and has been immensely influential in influencing the development of community care internationally.

The volume that has resulted has aimed to provide clear guidance on how mental health services can be provided in both high- and low-income countries, bearing in mind both the manpower and resource available in each. It is still sadly the case that most beds for patients with mental disorders are situated in mental hospitals in low-income countries: this book describes the way in which services can progress beyond this, so that community-based services can be developed. The book describes these developments and emphasises the important part that primary care services must provide in all countries, regardless of their income, in providing mental health services that are truly comprehensive.

New services need new research methods and new planning decisions. These topics are fully covered and there are also two chapters (Chapters 3 and 24) on the good and bad points in community services that have developed in high-income countries. New services need to take account of conditions that exist in any particular country, but wherever they are developed services need to be readily accessible and provided in environments which are non-institutional.

Michele Tansella arrived in Verona from the Istituto Mario Negri in Milano in 1969, then soon left to spend six months at the Institute of Psychiatry in London. At that time, he had little to learn about community mental health services at the Maudsley Hospital but a great deal to learn about epidemiology and the systematic collection and analysis of data. He also widened his circle of professional colleagues and has brought many of the authors of the present chapters to visit the Verona service and publish comparative studies. During an earlier visit to the Institute, he met his wife Christa, who has assisted him at every stage in building up a united and happy Department, publishing many joint papers [1, 2]. Michele returned to Verona in early 1970 and collaborated with the team charged with the responsibility of setting up new mental health services in South Verona.

Michele quickly made his mark, insisting from the start on the meticulous collection of data about every aspect of the developing service [3]. In those early years, he advocated the changes introduced to Italian psychiatry by Law 180 which eventually prevented new admissions to mental hospitals, in favour of services offered in less formal community settings [4, 5]. The first formal description of the South Verona service in a high-impact journal was published in 1985 [6], followed by the first description of the all-important case register [7] dealing with the epidemiology of schizophrenia in a community setting. Since that time, he has published many informative accounts of the local services [8].

Over the next few years Michele trained many future Italian academic psychiatrists, building up a formidable team of psychiatric researchers. Since these early years, he has published 286 papers in international peer-reviewed journals, as well as numerous books and chapters. A most important development was his book with Graham Thornicroft called *The Mental Health Matrix*, which sets out a detailed plan for providing mental health services to a community. The book was translated into four languages [9] and more recently brought up to date [10] in *Better Mental Health Care* (now translated into eight languages).

Since 1992, Michele has edited *Epidemiologia e Psichiatria Sociale* (now retitled *Epidemiology and Psychiatric Sciences*), which has been important in providing Italian psychiatrists with a forum for exchanging views and data. The journal has continuously increased its international reputation; in 2011, it was ranked 22nd of the 117 Journals quoted by the *Journal Citation Reports* within the category 'Psychiatry'. Since 1997, Michele has edited *Social Psychiatry and Psychiatric Epidemiology* and is a member of the board of several international journals. Between 2006 and September 2012, he served two consecutive terms as Dean of the University of Verona's medical school.

Under Michele's leadership, Verona was designated by the World Health Organization as "Collaborating Centre for Research and Training in Mental Health" on February 1987, confirmed in 2001, 2005, 2009 and still active. By

2005, his team of 23 tenured staff had produced 2000 citations in high-impact journals, and this figure climbed to 12 400 in 2011. In that year, there were 58 papers published by the team, including high-impact journals such as *Lancet*, *BMJ*, *American Journal of Psychiatry* and *Biological Psychiatry*.

These bare facts give little impression of the man. Michele is warm, witty and excellent company. He is fiercely proud of what has been achieved in South Verona and has been a major influence on the development of services for people with mental illness across the world.

References

[1] Zimmermann-Tansella C, Tansella M, Lader M. (1976) The effects of chlordesmethyldiazepam on behavioral performance and subjective judgment in normal subjects. *Journal of Clinical Pharmacology* **10**: 481–488.

[2] Zimmermann-Tansella C, Tansella M, Lader M. (1979) Psychological performance in anxious patients treated with diazepam. *Progress in Neuro-Psychopharmacology* **3** (4): 361–368.

[3] Tansella M. (1974) An institution-based register in a psychiatric university clinic. *Psychiatria Clinica* **7** (2): 84–88.

[4] Tansella M. (1985) Misunderstanding the Italian Experience. *British Journal of Psychiatry* **147**: 450–452.

[5] Tansella M. (1986) Community psychiatry without mental hospitals – the Italian Experience – a review. *Journal of the Royal Society of Medicine* **79**: 664–669.

[6] Siciliani O, Bellantuono C, Williams P et al. (1985) Self-reported use of psychotropic drugs and alcohol abuse in South-Verona. *Psychological Medicine* **15** (4): 821–826.

[7] Tansella M. (ed.) (1991) *Community-Based Psychiatry. Long-Term Patterns of Care in South-Verona*. Psychological Medicine Monograph Supplement 19. Cambridge: Cambridge University Press, pp. 1–54.

[8] Tansella M, Amaddeo F, Burti L et al. (2006) Evaluating a community-based mental health service focusing on severe mental illness. The Verona experience. *Acta Psychiatrica Scandinavica* **429** (Suppl.): 90–94.

[9] Thornicroft G, Tansella M. (1999) *The Mental Health Matrix. A Manual to Improve Services*. Cambridge: Cambridge University Press, pp. 1–291.

[10] Thornicroft G, Tansella M. (2009) *Better Mental Health Care*. Cambridge: Cambridge University Press, pp. 1–184.

Contents

Contributors

Ruben Alvarado
Faculty of Medicine,
Salvador Allende School of Public Health,
University of Chile,
Santiago,
Chile

Francesco Amaddeo
Department of Public Health and Community Medicine,
Section of Psychiatry,
University of Verona,
Verona,
Italy

Matteo Balestrieri
Department of Experimental and Clinical Medical Sciences,
University of Udine,
Udine,
Italy

Corrado Barbui
Department of Public Health and Community Medicine,
Section of Psychiatry,
University of Verona,
Verona,
Italy

Paul Bebbington
Mental Health Sciences Unit,
Faculty of Brain Sciences, UCL,
London,
UK

Thomas Becker
Department of Psychiatry II,
Ulm University,
Bezirkskrankenhaus Günzburg,
Germany

Marcella Bellani
Department of Public Health and Community Medicine,
Section of Psychiatry and Section of Clinical Psychology,
Inter-University Center for Behavioural Neurosciences (ICBN),
University of Verona,
Verona,
Italy

Loretta Berti
Department of Public Health and Community Medicine,
Section of Psychiatry,
University of Verona,
Verona,
Italy

Victoria Bird
Health Service and Population Research Department,
Institute of Psychiatry,
King's College London,
London,
UK

Department of Public Health and Community Medicine,
Section of Psychiatry,
University of Verona,
Verona,
Italy

Chiara Bonetto
Department of Public Health and Community Medicine,
Section of Psychiatry,
University of Verona,
Verona,
Italy

Elena Bonfioli
Department of Public Health and Community Medicine,
Section of Psychiatry,
University of Verona,
Verona,
Italy

Paolo Brambilla
Department of Experimental & Clinical Medical Sciences (DISM),
Inter-University Center for Behavioural Neurosciences (ICBN),
University of Udine,
Udine,
Italy

Department of Psychiatry and Behavioral Sciences,
University of Texas Medical School at Houston,
USA

Lorenzo Burti
Department of Public Health and Community Medicine,
Section of Psychiatry,
University of Verona,
Verona,
Italy

Andrea Cipriani
Department of Public Health and Community Medicine,
Section of Psychiatry,
University of Verona,
Verona,
Italy

Benedicto Crespo-Facorro
Department of Psychiatry,
Psychiatric Research Unit of Cantabria,
University Hospital "Marqués de Valdecilla",
IFIMAV, CIBERSAM,
Santander,
Cantabria,
Spain

Doriana Cristofalo
Department of Public Health and Community Medicine,
Section of Psychiatry,
University of Verona,
Verona,
Italy

Katia De Santi
Department of Public Health and Community Medicine,
Section of Psychiatry,
University of Verona,
Verona,
Italy

Lidia Del Piccolo
Department of Public Health and Community Medicine,
Section of Clinical Psychology,
University of Verona,
Verona,
Italy

Giuseppe Deledda
Department of Public Health and Community Medicine,
Section of Clinical Psychology,
University of Verona,
Verona,
Italy

Valeria Donisi
Department of Public Health and Community Medicine,
Section of Psychiatry,
University of Verona,
Verona,
Italy

Graham Dunn
Institute of Population Health,
Centre for Biostatistics,
University of Manchester,
Manchester,
UK

Nicola Dusi
Department of Public Health and Community Medicine,
Section of Psychiatry and Section of Clinical Psychology,
Inter-University Center for Behavioural Neurosciences (ICBN),
University of Verona,
Verona,
Italy

Irene Fiorini
Department of Public Health and Community Medicine,
Section of Psychiatry,
University of Verona,
Verona,
Italy

David Fowler
Division of Health Policy and Practice,
School of Medicine,
University of East Anglia,
Norwich,
UK

Carlos Garcia-Alonso
Department of Management and Quantitative Methods,
Loyola University Andalusia,
Cordoba,
Spain

Karina Gibert
Knowledge Engineering and Machine Learning Group,
Department of Statistics and Operations Research,
Universitat Politècnica de Catalunya,
Barcelona,
Spain

Nadja van Ginneken
Nutrition and Public Health Intervention Research Department,
London School of Hygiene and Tropical Medicine,
London,
UK

Sangath,
Goa,
India

David Goldberg
Health Service and Population Research Department,
Institute of Psychiatry,
King's College London,
London,
UK

Claudia Goss
Department of Public Health and Community Medicine,
Section of Clinical Psychology,
University of Verona,
Verona,
Italy

Justin Granstein
Weill Cornell Medical College,
Cornell University,
New York,
NY,
USA

Laura Grigoletti
Department of Public Health and Community Medicine,
Section of Psychiatry,
University of Verona,
Verona,
Italy

Hiske Hees
Department of Psychiatry,
Academic Medical Center,
University of Amsterdam,
Amsterdam,
The Netherlands

Assen Jablensky
School of Psychiatry and Clinical Neurosciences,
The University of Western Australia,
Australia

Martin Knapp
Personal Social Services Research Unit,
London School of Economics and Political Science,
London, UK

Centre for the Economics of Mental and Physical Health,
Institute of Psychiatry,
King's College London,
London,
UK

Maarten Koeter
Department of Psychiatry,
Academic Medical Center,
University of Amsterdam,
Amsterdam,
The Netherlands

Lian van der Krieke
University Center for Psychiatry,
University Medical Center Groningen,
University of Groningen,
Groningen,
The Netherlands

Elizabeth Kuipers
Department of Psychology,
Institute of Psychiatry,
King's College London,
London, UK

Antonio Lasalvia
Department of Public Health and Community Medicine,
Section of Psychiatry,
University of Verona,
Verona,
Italy

Clair Le Boutillier
Health Service and Population Research Department,
Institute of Psychiatry,
King's College London,
London,
UK

Mary Leamy
Health Service and Population Research Department,
Institute of Psychiatry,
King's College London,
London,
UK

Mariangela Mazzi
Department of Public Health and Community Medicine,
Section of Clinical Psychology,
University of Verona,
Verona,
Italy

Alberto Minoletti
Faculty of Medicine,
Salvador Allende School of Public Health,
University of Chile,
Santiago,
Chile

Povl Munk-Jørgensen
Department of Organic Psychiatric
Disorders and Emergency Ward,
Aarhus University Hospital,
Risskov,
Denmark

Michela Nosè
Department of Public Health and Community Medicine,
Section of Psychiatry,
University of Verona,
Verona,
Italy

Niels Okkels
Organic Psychiatric Disorder Research Unit,
Aarhus University Hospital,
Risskov,
Denmark

Bernd Puschner
Department of Psychiatry II,
Ulm University,
Bezirkskrankenhaus Günzburg,
Germany

Michela Rimondini
Department of Public Health and Community Medicine,
Section of Clinical Psychology,
University of Verona,
Verona,
Italy

Graciela Rojas
Department of Psychiatry,
Clinical Hospital,
University of Chile,
Santiago,
Chile

Diana Rose
Service User Research Enterprise (SURE),
Health Services and Population Research,
Institute of Psychiatry,
King's College London,
London, UK

Alberto Rossi
Department of Public Health and Community Medicine,
Section of Psychiatry,
University of Verona,
Verona,
Italy

Mirella Ruggeri
Department of Public Health and Community Medicine,
Section of Psychiatry,
University of Verona,
Verona,
Italy

Luis Salvador-Carulla
Centre for Disability Research and Policy, Faculty of Health Sciences,
University of Sydney,
Australia

Spanish Research Network on Mental Health Prevention and Promotion
(Spanish IAPP Network)

Benedetto Saraceno
University Nova of Lisbon,
WHO Collaborating Center,
University of Geneva,
Geneva,
Switzerland

Norman Sartorius
Association for the Improvement of Mental Health Programmes,
Geneva,
Switzerland

Shekhar Saxena
Department of Mental Health and Substance Abuse,
World Health Organization,
Geneva,
Switzerland

Aart Schene
Department of Psychiatry,
Academic Medical Center,
University of Amsterdam,
Amsterdam,
The Netherlands

Mike Slade
Health Service and Population Research Department,
Institute of Psychiatry,
King's College London,
London,
UK

Ezra Susser
Department of Epidemiology,
Mailman School of Public Health,
Columbia University,
New York,
NY,
USA

Department of Psychiatry,
College of Physicians and Surgeons,
Columbia University and New York State Psychiatric Institute,
New York,
NY,
USA

Department of Psychiatry,
University of Göttingen,
Göttingen,
Germany

Sjoerd Sytema
University Center for Psychiatry,
University Medical Center Groningen,
University of Groningen,
Groningen,
The Netherlands

Graham Thornicroft
Health Service and Population Research Department,
Institute of Psychiatry,
King's College London,
London,
UK

Sarah Tosato
Department of Public Health and Community Medicine,
Section of Psychiatry,
University of Verona,
Verona,
Italy

Peter Tyrer
Department of Medicine,
Centre for Mental Health,
Imperial College,
London,
UK

Elie Valencia
Faculty of Medicine,
Salvador Allende School of Public Health,
University of Chile,
Santiago,
Chile

Department of Epidemiology,
Mailman School of Public Health,
Columbia University,
New York,
NY,
USA

José Luis Vázquez-Barquero
Department of Psychiatry,
Psychiatric Research Unit of Cantabria,
University Hospital "Marqués de Valdecilla",
IFIMAV, CIBERSAM,
Santander,
Spain

Javier Vázquez-Bourgon
Department of Psychiatry, Psychiatric Research Unit of Cantabria,
University Hospital "Marqués de Valdecilla",
IFIMAV, CIBERSAM,
Santander,
Spain

Gabe de Vries
Department of Occupational Therapy,
Arkin,
Amsterdam,
The Netherlands

Christa Zimmermann
Department of Public Health and Community Medicine,
Section of Clinical Psychology,
University of Verona,
Verona,
Italy

SECTION 1
The global challenge

CHAPTER 1

The nature and scale of the global mental health challenge

Mirella Ruggeri[1], Graham Thornicroft[2] and David Goldberg[2]

[1] Department of Public Health and Community Medicine, Section of Psychiatry, University of Verona, Verona, Italy

[2] Health Service and Population Research Department, Institute of Psychiatry, King's College London, London, UK

Introduction

In the last 20 years, there has been an unprecedented surge of research aimed at identifying improvements in psychiatric treatments and mental health care. This builds upon the earlier foundation of psychiatric epidemiology, which considers the occurrence and distribution of mental disorders across time and place. Yet, increasingly this work has evolved from describing these realities to going even further to understand which interventions deliver real advances in care. However, until relatively recently almost all such studies took place in high-income (HI) countries, even though most of the world's population live in low- and middle-income countries (LAMICs).

The nature of the challenge

The definition of 'Global mental health' appeared for the first time in an Editorial by Eugene Brody published in 1982 on the *American Journal of Psychiatry* [1]. However, the roots of this discipline can be found much earlier, in the field of cross-cultural epidemiology of severe mental disorders. Originally, these studies had the aim of determining the relevance of a biomedical perspective and, later on, to compare psychopathology in different contexts, as a basis for classification and clinical decision-making. This research effort found that mental disorders affect people in all cultures and societies. Since then, a growing body of cross-national research has shown that neuropsychiatric disorders constitute 13% of the world health burden, and demonstrated their substantial impact on disability, on direct and indirect societal costs [2] and the strong association of mental disorders with both societal disadvantage and physical health problems [3].

Improving Mental Health Care: The Global Challenge, First Edition.
Edited by Graham Thornicroft, Mirella Ruggeri and David Goldberg.
© 2013 John Wiley & Sons, Ltd. Published 2013 by John Wiley & Sons, Ltd.

A clear-cut discrepancy in both the resources and treatments availability for mental health between HI countries and LAMICs emerged, with resource allocation for mental health disproportionately low in the latter. This *resource–needs gap* [4, 5] goes in parallel with a *mental health treatment gap*: of all adults affected by mental illnesses, the proportion who are treated is around 30.5% in the United States and 27% across Europe, while more than 90% of individuals with serious mental illness in less-developed countries do not receive treatment for those problems [6, 7]. This stands as disconcerting evidence of a major failure in global health delivery [8–10].

To propose a framework to address the treatment gap, Thornicroft and Tansella have extended their balanced care model (BCM), originally aimed at mental health service planning based on a pragmatic balance of hospital and community care [11], to refer also to a balance between all of the service components that are present in any system, whether this is in a low-, medium- or high-resource setting, and identified three sequential steps relevant to different resource settings [12].

According to this model, in low-resource settings, the crucial resource allocation decisions will be how to balance any investment in primary and community care sites against expenditure in psychiatric hospitals. Following the *World Health Report 2001* recommendations [13], in these countries, an optimal balance between resources and response to population needs can be given by promoting mental health service delivery within the primary care system. Different forms of collaboration between psychiatric and primary care setting should be pursued, stemming from the less to the most expensive and elaborate ones. In rural areas in many low-income countries, the nearest mental health service may be very far away, and it is necessary for the primary care service to take the lead in providing basic mental health care. In places where it is practicable to refer some patients to the mental health service, then some form of stepped care should be adopted (see Chapter 7). The provision of mental health training to primary care staff is therefore of the greatest importance. Several studies have shown that these kind of mental health services based in primary care are less stigmatising, more accessible, efficacious and cost-effective [10, 14–17].

In medium-resource settings, the BCM approach proposes that services are provided in all of the five main categories of care: outpatient clinics, community mental health teams, acute inpatient services, community residential care and work/occupation.

In high-resource settings, these complex choices apply to an even greater extent, as there are even more specialized mental health teams and agencies present, resulting in a greater number of possibilities for resource investment to achieve a more balanced mix of services, as long as there is a strong emphasis upon primary health care, and attention is paid to the training needs of primary care staff. In these countries, primary care should be the priority setting especially for patients with a combination of anxious, depressive and somatic symptoms, while major disorders could benefit from more specialised and dedicated interventions [18].

A research gap between HI countries and LAMICs has also clearly been identified, showing that 94% of research takes place in countries that cover 10% of the population. This treatment deficit cannot be resolved by extending presently available services alone. The adaptation of treatments will thus be an essential accomplishment, as well as the development of service-delivery models with greater local relevance and the provision of a robust empirical base supporting their local effectiveness and feasibility [19, 20]. Innovative approaches to mental health services are thus required, including interventions that encompass both clinical and social domains of action. Finally, in-country research and training are necessary, and clinical infrastructure and capacity must be built [21].

The landmark series of papers on global mental health published in the *Lancet* between 2007 and 2012 [8, 22–31] has been influential in contributing to a social movement for global mental health, and the number and quality of studies to evaluate mental health treatment and care in the developing world is now steadily improving.

As a further contribute, this book brings together many of the world's leading practitioners and researchers active in the fields related to improving mental health care. The primary aim of the book is to present clear information arising from scientific research for a concerned readership about care and treatment for people with mental illness in community settings in relation to the global challenge to improving mental health care. The book consists of 24 chapters, with experts in each chapter area invited to give structured accounts of knowledge in that field, extensively referenced, to include critical appraisals of the strength of the evidence and the robustness of the conclusions that can be drawn.

Under the overall umbrella of the global challenge to improving mental health care and to understanding how to provide more and better mental health care worldwide, up-to-date knowledge in the following fields is included in these chapters: clinical trials, epidemiology, global mental health, health economics, health services research, implementation science, needs assessment, physical and mental co-morbidities, practitioner–patient communication, primary health care, outcome measures, pharmaco-epidemiology, public understanding of science, the recovery paradigm, spatial analyses, stigma and discrimination, and workplace aspects of mental health.

The scale of the challenge

If the *why* of the global mental health challenge has become self-evident in the last two decades, the *what* needs to be done and the *how* this approach should be scaled up are issues that deserve greater conceptual framing and operational implementation [32–34].

Using the Delphi method, the *Grand Challenges in Global Mental Health Initiative Study* – funded by the US National Institute of Mental Health, supported by the

Global Alliance for Chronic Diseases – has identified priorities for research in the next ten years that will make an impact on the lives of people living with mental, neurological and substance abuse (MNS) disorders [35]. A 'grand challenge' was defined as 'a specific barrier that, if removed, would help to solve an important health problem. If successfully implemented, the intervention(s) it could lead to would have a high likelihood of feasibility for scaling up and impact'. Twenty-five grand challenges were identified, which capture several broad themes, which can be summarised under four main issues.

First, the results emphasise the need for research that uses a life-course approach; this approach acknowledges that many disorders manifest in early life, thus efforts to build mental capital could mitigate the risk of disorders.

Second, the challenges recognise that the suffering caused by MNS disorders extends beyond the patient to family members and communities, thus, health-system-wide changes are crucial, together with attention to social exclusion and discrimination.

Third, the challenges underline the fact that all care and treatment interventions – psychosocial or pharmacological, simple or complex – should have an evidence base to provide programme planners, clinicians and policy-makers with effective care packages.

Fourth, the panel's responses underscore important relationships between environmental exposures and MNS disorders: extreme poverty, war and natural disasters affect large areas of the world, and we still do not fully understand the mechanisms by which mental disorders might be averted or precipitated in those settings.

It is thus clear that more investment in research into the nature and treatment of mental disorders is needed, and that this research must be carried out in both HI countries and LAMICs. The *mental health Gap Action Programme* (mhGAP) pro-moted by the WHO with the mandate of producing evidence-based guidelines for managing MNS disorders identified eight groups of 'priority conditions' due to their major global public health impact: depression; schizophrenia and other psychotic disorders (including bipolar disorder); suicide prevention; epilepsy; dementia; disorders due to use of alcohol and illicit drugs; and mental disorders in children [36, 37]. The first product of this programme, launched in 2010, is a 100-page manual – the World Health Organization mhGAP intervention guide for mental, neurological and substance use disorders in non-specialised health settings: mental health – Gap Action Programme (mhGAP-IG) [38] – which contains case findings and treatment guidelines, whose main focus was what can be done in routine mental health care by non-specialist health workers. This manual is based on the assumption that task sharing – that is, a rational distribu-tion of tasks among health professionals teams – might be a powerful answer to the scarcity of human personnel resources which is a barrier to the delivery of efficacious treatments in the LAMICs, but is also an emerging challenge in the HI countries in times of economical crisis [39, 40].

Evidence shows that lay people or community health workers can be trained to deliver psychological and psychosocial interventions for people with depressive and anxiety disorders, schizophrenia and dementia [17]. In a 'collaborative' model of care, a mental health specialist's task should be to train these people appropriately and provide continuing supervision, quality assurance, and support. In the new world of global mental health, where an increasing proportion of mental health care is shared with non-specialist health workers, psychiatrists and other mental health practitioners will need to be proficient in skills for training and supervising non-specialist health workers, be engaged in monitoring and evaluation for quality assurance of mental health-care programmes and acquire the management skills essential for leading teams of health workers [21].

But the challenge to scaling up mental health treatments should also deal with the violation of human rights and pervasive stigma against those who are suffering from mental disorders, for which mental health staff should serve as advocate [41–43] and catalysts for the entire community, and fight the often rather weak commitment of politicians, administrators and the other community stakeholders in the understanding of the benefits that could take place worldwide if a global mental health approach is pursued [44].

And, finally, a major barrier relates to the imperfections in our current state of knowledge about the nature of mental disorders and the armamentarium of effective treatments. What is needed is a more finely tuned understanding of the interplay between biological, psychological, relational and environmental factors [45], and also of those political, economic and cultural barriers that have for so long impeded global mental health care and that have caused a serious disadvantage to people suffering from mental illness worldwide.

From evidence to practice

Few initiatives in the health field have received the level of attention being given to 'evidence-based practice'. Growing concerns in recent years for under-utilization of evidence-based practice in health-care systems have been raised. Most of the problems derive from the barriers that prevent a continuous flow from efficacy to effectiveness.

Efficacy refers to the use of experimental standards for establishing causal relationships between interventions and positive outcomes. *Effectiveness* relates to outcomes that can be achieved in real-world practice in representative cohorts of patients, and a broader set of implementation issues involving patient's representativeness, professional consensus, generalisability, feasibility and costs.

Bridging the gap between efficacy and effectiveness implies first of all a concrete intention to test the advantages and the disadvantages of an intervention's implementation in the frame of the routine care. There is the need for investing resources in the development and use of implementation strategies and methods that are grounded in research and elaborated through accumulated experience and sensitisation on its beneficial effects as well as to develop ongoing, long-term partnerships with researchers.

The action of health service researchers should be firmly grounded in the promotion of studies that can increase knowledge about this process and offer practical guidance for both policy-makers and service providers. In particular, core intervention components of evidence-based practices should be clearly identified, field-based approaches should be used to assess the effectiveness of implementation procedures that have been put into practice, proper outcome measures to monitor these practices should be developed and operationalisation of these processes should be clarified [46].

There is also a need for studying organizational as well as broader socio-political factors that influence and sustain innovation implementation [47–49]. To this extent, an increase in the awareness that the models used in comparatively better resourced settings have little chance of addressing the huge treatment gaps in LAMICs is needed. It is also necessary to promote actions that increase awareness that investing resources to improving service delivery is essential but in itself not sufficient: a continuing commitment to implementation of evidence-based practice is vital for long-term patient benefit.

Various factors shape the process and outcomes of innovation implementation: the 'multi-level' complexities involving not only financial resources and the effectiveness of interventions but also training process and fidelity, staff clinical skills and motivation, organisations and systems characteristics, organisational climate, managerial support, long-term managerial determination and high-level policy support [50].

'Routine practice' is the culmination of such successful implementation and service consolidation. Progression through each stage is usually not rigidly linear. Indeed, there are cyclical phases of progress with setbacks involved; these dynamics represent the most vulnerable 'points of impact' for many of these change factors.

Innovations that pass these stages successfully tend to become standard 'practice' and should bring improvements to patient care. If this is accomplished, it is important that ongoing monitoring of effectiveness indicators be established and that continued attention be given to organisational functioning and continuing assessments of the costs of care.

To increase the probability that this process can penetrate in mental health service research and care, long-term investment in training and capacity development is necessary. Capacity building, in turn, requires leadership, resources and sustained commitments, if global expertise and experience are to respond effectively to local priorities and needs.

The implementation of innovative care must face problems that are different whether this task is undertaken in HI countries or in LAMICs; however, the experience developed in these two contexts can occur to allow transferrable learning with the potential to generate research questions that are more attuned to some crucial, yet unanswered, questions posed by the global mental health challenge [51–53].

Conclusions

We have clustered the chapters in this volume into the three unified sections of the book: those that deal with the specificity of mental health care in the LAMICs, those more focused on the effectiveness of interventions at the level of primary care and/or specialised services, and those which propose innovative methodologies to fully capture the complexities of mental health research. The contributions of the authors are influenced by the book's commitment to producing evidence that can be useful to pursuing the goals mentioned in this chapter, converting them into practice, and in so doing assessing how best to achieve such translation. Lively examples of the complex interactions of policy-makers, service user and carer advocacy, research findings and service provider practices are provided. The underlying thrust of the contributions can be stated plainly: *to understanding how to provide more and better mental health care worldwide.*

References

[1] Brody EB. (1982) Are we for mental health as well as against mental illness? The significance for psychiatry of a global mental health coalition. *American Journal of Psychiatry* **139**: 1588–1589.

[2] Baumgartner JN, Susser E. (2012) Social integration in global mental health: what is it and how can it be measured? *Epidemiology and Psychiatric Sciences* **25**: 1–9.

[3] Bauer AM, Fielke K, Brayley J et al. (2010) Tackling the global mental health challenge: a psychosomatic medicine/consultation-liaison psychiatry perspective. *Psychosomatics* **51**: 185–193.

[4] Hu TW. (2003) Financing global mental health services and the role of WHO. *Journal of Mental Health Policy and Economics* **6**: 145–147.

[5] Gault LM. (2008) Resources for global mental health: too little for too long. *Journal of American Academy of Child and Adolescent Psychiatry* **47**: 841–842.

[6] Kohn R, Saxena S, Levav I et al. (2004) Treatment gap in mental health care. *Bulletin of the World Health Organization* **82**: 858–866.

[7] Thornicroft G. (2007) Most people with mental illness are not treated. *Lancet* **370**: 807–808.

[8] Kleinman A. (2009) Global mental health: a failure of humanity. *Lancet* **374**: 603–604.

[9] Barbui C, Dua T, Van OM et al. (2010) Challenges in developing evidence-based recommendations using the GRADE approach: the case of mental, neurological, and substance use disorders. *PLoS Medicine* **7**: 8.

[10] Dua T, Barbui C, Clark N et al. (2011) Evidence based guidelines for mental, neurological and substance use disorders in low- and middle-income countries: summary of WHO recommendations. *PLoS Medicine* **8**: 1–11.

[11] Thornicroft G, Tansella M. (2004) Components of a modern mental health service: a pragmatica balance of community and hospital care: overview of systematic evidence. *British Journal of Psychiatry* **185**: 283–290.

[12] Thornicroft G, Tansella M. (2012) The balanced care model for global mental health. *Psychological Medicine* **11**: 1–15.

[13] World Health Organization. (2001) *World Health Report 2001: Mental Health: New Understanding, New Hope.* Geneva: WHO Press.

[14] Chisholm D, Lund C, Saxena S. (2007) Cost of scaling up mental healthcare in low- and middle-income countries. *British Journal of Psychiatry* **191**: 528–535.

[15] Kigozi F. (2007) Integrating mental health into primary health care – Uganda's experience. *South African Psychiatry Review* **10**: 17–19.

[16] Jenkins R, Kiima D, Njenga F et al. (2010) Integration of mental health into primary care in Kenya. *World Psychiatry* **9**: 118–120.

[17] Patel V, Weiss HA, Chowdhary N et al. (2010) Effectiveness of an intervention led by lay health counsellors for depressive and anxiety disorders in primary care in Goa, India (MANAS): a cluster randomised controlled trial. *Lancet* **376**: 2086–2095.

[18] Thornicroft G, Tansella M. (2009) *Better Mental Health Care.* Cambridge: Cambridge University Press.

[19] Becker AE, Kleinman A. (2012) An agenda for closing resource gaps in global mental health: innovation, capacity building, and partnerships. *Harvard Review of Psychiatry* **20**: 3–5.

[20] Tol WA, Patel V, Tomlinson M et al. (2012) Relevance or excellence? Setting research priorities for mental health and psychosocial support in humanitarian settings. *Harvard Review of Psychiatry* **20**: 25–36.

[21] Thornicroft G, Cooper S, Bortel TV et al. (2012) Capacity building in global mental health research. *Harvard Review of Psychiatry* **20**: 13–24.

[22] Lancet Global Mental Health Group, Chisholm D, Flisher AJ, et al. (2007) Scale up services for mental disorders: a call for action. *Lancet* **370**: 1241–1252.

[23] Lancet Global Mental Health Group. (2008) A movement for global mental health is launched. *Lancet* **372**: 1274.

[24] Lancet Global Mental Health Group. (2009) Movement for global mental health gains momentum. *Lancet* **374**: 587.

[25] Prince M, Patel V, Saxena S et al. (2007) No health without mental health. *Lancet* **370**: 859–877.

[26] Saxena S, Thornicroft G, Knapp M et al. (2007) Resources for mental health: scarcity, inequity, and inefficiency. *Lancet* **370**: 878–889.

[27] Patel V, Garrison P, de Jesus Mari J et al. (2008) Advisory group of the Movement for Global Mental Health. The Lancet's series on global mental health: 1 year on. *Lancet* **372**: 1354–1357.

[28] Eaton J, McCay L, Semrau M et al. (2011) Scale up of services for mental health in low-income and middle-income countries. *Lancet* **378**: 1592–1603.

[29] Lee PT, Henderson M, Patel V. (2010) A UN summit on global mental health. *Lancet* **376**: 516.

[30] Patel V, Boyce N, Collins PY et al. (2011) A renewed agenda for global mental health. *Lancet* **378**: 1441–1442.

[31] Hock RS, Or F, Kolappa K et al. (2012) A new resolution for global mental health. *Lancet* **379**: 1367–1368.

[32] Tomlinson M, Rudan I, Saxena S et al. (2009) Setting priorities for global mental health research. *Bulletin of the World Health Organization* **87**: 438–446.

[33] Patel V, Prince M. (2010) Global mental health: a new global health field comes of age. *Journal of the American Medical Association* **303**: 1976–1977.

[34] Patel V. (2012) Global mental health: from science to action. *Harvard Review of Psychiatry* **20**: 6–12.

[35] Collins PY, Patel V, Joestl SS et al. (2011) Scientific Advisory Board and the Executive Committee of the Grand Challenges on Global Mental Health: grand challenges in global mental health. *Nature* **475**: 27–30.

[36] Saraceno B. (2007) Advancing the global mental health agenda. *International Journal of Public Health* **52**: 140–141.

[37] Saraceno B, Dua T. (2009) Global mental health: the role of psychiatry. *European Archives of Psychiatry and Clinical Neuroscience* **259** (Suppl. 2): 109–117.

[38] World Health Organization. (2010) *Intervention Guide for Mental, Neurological and Substance Use Disorders in Non-specialized Health Settings: mental health GAP Action Programme (mhGAP-IG).* Geneva: WHO.

[39] Myers NL. (2010) Culture, stress and recovery from schizophrenia: lessons from the field for global mental health. *Culture, Medicine and Psychiatry* **34**: 500–528.

[40] Fernando GA. (2012) The roads less traveled: mapping some pathways on the global mental health research roadmap. *Transcultural Psychiatry* **49**: 396–417.

[41] Thornicroft G. (2006) *Shunned: Discrimination Against People with Mental Illness.* Oxford: Oxford University Press.

[42] United Nations. (2006) *Convention on the Rights of Persons with Disabilities.* New York: United Nations.

[43] Callard F, Sartorius N, Arboleda-Florez J et al. (2012) *Mental Illness, Discrimination and the Law: Fighting for Social Justice.* Oxford: Wiley-Blackwell.

[44] Jenkins R, Baingana F, Ahmad R et al. (2011) Social, economic, human rights and political challenges to global mental health. *Mental Health in Family Medicine* **8**: 87–96.

[45] Ruggeri M, Tansella M. (2009) The interaction between genetics and epidemiology: the puzzle and its pieces. *Epidemiology and Psychiatric Sciences* **18**: 77–80.

[46] Ruggeri M, Bonetto C, Lasalvia A et al. (2012) A multi-element psychosocial intervention for early psychosis (GET UP PIANO TRIAL) conducted in a catchment area of 10 million inhabitants: study protocol for a pragmatic cluster randomized controlled trial. *Trials* **13**: 73.

[47] Simpson D, Flynn PM. (2007) Moving innovations into treatment: a stage-based approach to program change. *Journal of Substance Abuse Treatment* **33**: 111–120.

[48] Lasalvia A, Bonetto C, Bertani M et al. (2009) Influence of perceived organisational factors on job burnout: survey of community mental health staff. *British Journal of Psychiatry* **195**: 537–544.

[49] Thornicroft G, Lempp H, Tansella M. (2011) The place of implementation science in the translational medicine continuum. *Psychological Medicine* **41**: 2015–2021.

[50] Ruggeri M, Tansella M. (2011) New perspectives in the psychotherapy of psychoses at onset: evidence, effectiveness, flexibility, and fidelity. *Epidemiology and Psychiatric Sciences* **20**: 107–111.

[51] Summerfield D. (2008) How scientifically valid is the knowledge base of global mental health? *BMJ* **336**: 992–994.

[52] Cutcliffe JR. (2011) Global mental health in an interconnected, reciprocal world. *Archives of Psychiatric Nursing* **25**: 307–310.

[53] Limb M. (2012) US focus on new psychiatric disorders is distracting attention from tackling global mental health problems. *BMJ* **344**: e2071.

CHAPTER 2

Scaling up mental health care in resource-poor settings

Shekhar Saxena[1], Benedetto Saraceno[2] and Justin Granstein[3]

[1] Department of Mental Health and Substance Abuse, World Health Organization, Geneva, Switzerland
[2] University Nova of Lisbon, WHO Collaborating Center, University of Geneva, Geneva, Switzerland
[3] Weill Cornell Medical College, Cornell University, New York, NY, USA

Introduction

Mental health is paramount to personal well-being, building relationships and making contributions to society. Mental, neurological and substance use (MNS) disorders are major contributors to premature mortality and morbidity. The stigma, discrimination and human rights violations directed towards people with these disorders compound the difficulties in accessing care, increase socioeconomic vulnerability and hinder efforts to rise out of poverty. Nearly 14% of the global burden of disease is attributable to MNS disorders; likewise, almost 30% of the total non-communicable disease (NCD) burden is due to these disorders. Nearly 75% of all disability-adjusted life years (DALYs) lost due to neuropsychiatric disorders are in low- and lower-middle-income countries. The total number of DALYs lost in low-income countries alone due to neuropsychiatric disorders is 2.3 times that seen in high-income countries.

Regarding long-term disability specifically, 31% of the years lived with disability are attributable to neuropsychiatric disorders. Unipolar depressive disorders account for one-third of those attributed to neuropsychiatric disorders [1]. The World Health Organization (WHO) has, from its inception, recognised the need for action to reduce the burden of MNS disorders worldwide, and for enhancing the capacity of member states to respond to this rising challenge. In 2001, the issue of mental health was highlighted to the general public, national and international institutions and organisations, the public health community and other stakeholders. Through the World Health Day, World Health Assembly and *World Health Report 2001* (*Mental Health: New Understanding, New Hope*), WHO and its member states pledged their full and unrestricted commitment to this vital public health issue.

Improving Mental Health Care: The Global Challenge, First Edition.
Edited by Graham Thornicroft, Mirella Ruggeri and David Goldberg.
© 2013 John Wiley & Sons, Ltd. Published 2013 by John Wiley & Sons, Ltd.

Table 2.1 Burden of mental disorders and budget for mental health.

	Burden of mental disorder[a] (%)	Proportion of budget for mental health[b] (%)
Low-income countries	7.88	0.53
Lower-middle-income countries	14.50	1.90
Upper-middle-income countries	19.56	2.38
High-income countries	21.37	5.10
All countries	11.48	2.82

[a] Proportion of disability-adjusted life years (DALYs), defined as the sum of the years of life lost due to premature mortality in the population and the years lost due to disability for incident cases of mental disorders [1].
[b] Median values for proportion of total health budget allocated to mental health [3].

The last decade has seen an increasing awareness of the large gap between the prevalence of MNS disorders and the availability of treatment for them. A consensus has emerged that improved access to mental health care for people with these disorders, especially in the poorer parts of the world, is the highest priority for global health. This exciting development follows an unprecedented era of increasing efforts to address global health inequalities, largely as part of the UN's Millennium Development Goals (MDGs) initiative. HIV/AIDS, tuberculosis, malaria and maternal and child health (specifically addressed in the MDGs) have seen a huge increase in targeted resources: development assistance for health grew from $5.6 billion in 1990 to $21.8 billion in 2007, and there has been a similar escalation in activity related to other priorities in education and social development [2]. The investment of the global health community has been traditionally directed to infectious diseases; only recently have NCDs and MNS disorders received some attention. The likely culprit behind such a lack of attention is the fact that NCDs and MNS disorders have long been considered diseases of affluence because they reflect ill-health resulting from improved living standards. Today, however, it is well known that countries with economies in transition and many middle-income countries face a double burden as the increasing prevalence of NCDs and MNS disorders coexists with infectious diseases.

However, the resources provided to tackle the huge burden of MNS disorders remain grossly insufficient. Almost one-third of countries still do not have a specific budget for mental health [3]. Of the countries that do have a designated mental health budget, 21% spend less than 1% of their total health budgets on mental health. Table 2.1 [1, 3] compares the burden of mental disorders with the budget assigned to mental health; it shows that countries allocate disproportionately small percentages of their budgets to mental health compared to the distribution of their disease burdens.

The scarcity of committed resources is even more serious for human resources; Figure 2.1 presents the distribution of human resources for mental health across

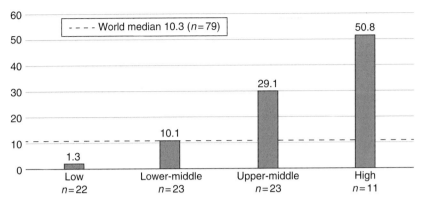

Figure 2.1 Total number of human resources (per 100 000 population) working in the mental health sector by World Bank income group (Reproduced from *Mental Health Atlas 2011* ([3], p. 55)).

different income categories. This scarcity is exacerbated by inefficiency and inequitable distribution of resources. For example, many middle-income countries that have made substantial investments in large mental hospitals are reluctant to replace them with community-based and inpatient facilities in general hospitals, despite evidence that mental hospitals provide inadequate care and that community-based services are more effective.

WHO has described scaling up as 'deliberate efforts to increase the impact of health service innovations successfully tested in pilot or experimental projects so as to benefit more people and to foster policy and programme development on a lasting basis' [4]. Developing these key themes further, in this chapter we take scaling up to mean 'deliberate efforts to increase the availability, coverage and sustainability of effective health care interventions to confer benefit on people needing treatment and care for MNS disorders'.

Progress in scaling up services can be best measured by comparing change in effective coverage, for example, the proportion of the population having a mental disorder that is receiving appropriate treatment. This concept combines response to need with the quality of interventions delivered. Information relating to scaling up mental health services, however, is not widely published in the governmental or scientific literatures, and research from low- and middle-income countries (LAMICs) is particularly poorly represented. There are, therefore, little available baseline prevalence data in LAMICs, and even if standardised prevalence rates were used, service impact data are not available to estimate coverage at any particular point in time, let alone for changes over a period of time.

Recognising the alarming extent of these issues, the *Lancet Series on Global Mental Health* in 2007 sounded a call for action to scale up mental health care in the world. WHO responded and launched its mental health Gap Action Programme (mhGAP) the following year. This chapter provides an introduction to mental health system assessment and WHO's efforts to scale up mental health care.

Assessment of needs, resources and constraints

WHO Atlas study reports that in 2005, more than 24% of countries did not have any system for collecting and reporting mental health information. Many other countries have reporting systems but they often are of limited scope and quality. This lack of good information is an important impediment to the development of mental health policies, plans and services [3].

To combat these basic and strategic weaknesses, WHO developed the World Health Organization Assessment Instrument for Mental Health Systems (WHO-AIMS). This tool enables countries to perform a comprehensive, information-based assessment of their mental health system, as well as the services and support offered to people with mental disorders that are provided outside the psychiatric services sector (e.g. mental health in primary care, links with other key sectors) [5]. Moreover, WHO-AIMS allows countries to monitor progress in implementing policy reforms, the provision of community services and the involvement of consumers, families and other stakeholders in mental health promotion, prevention, maintenance and rehabilitation.

The ten recommendations of the *World Health Report 2001* served as the foundation for the instrument, as they still represent WHO's vision for mental health [6].

The *World Health Report 2001* recommendations are:
1 Provide treatment in primary care
2 Make psychotropic drugs available
3 Give care in the community
4 Educate the public
5 Involve communities, families and consumers
6 Establish national policies, programmes and legislation
7 Develop human resources
8 Link with other sectors
9 Monitor community mental health
10 Support more research

In order to operationalise the recommendations, many indicators were generated and grouped together into domains and facets. Experts and other respondents from resource-poor countries were consulted to ensure clarity, content validity and feasibility of the generated items. Based on this feedback, a pilot version of the instrument was released and tested in 12 LAMICs. Following further consultations with other international experts, the final version was released for use in country assessments in February 2005, consisting of the following six domains [4]:

1 *Policy and legislative framework* – Covers key components of mental health governance, including mental health policies, plans and legislation. Financing of mental health services and monitoring and training on human rights are also addressed.

2 *Mental health services* – The organisational context of service provision as well as service delivery within mental health facilities; equity of access to mental health care is also addressed.

3 *Mental health in primary care* – Service delivery within the primary health-care system (both physician-based and non-physician-based clinics, as well as interactions with complementary practitioners (e.g. traditional healers)).

4 *Human resources* – The availability of human resources in mental health as well as training of mental health professionals; the presence and activities of user and family associations and NGOs are also covered.

5 *Public information and links with other sectors* – Public awareness and educational campaigns on mental health as well as collaborative links with key health (e.g. primary health care) and other sectors (social welfare).

6 *Monitoring and research* – Mental health information systems and research conducted on mental health.

These 6 domains address the 10 recommendations of the *World Health Report 2001* through 28 facets comprising 155 items. The instrument consists largely of input and process indicators, given that in many LAMICs outcome data are extremely difficult to collect. WHO-AIMS assessments are carried out by a local team headed by an in-country 'focal point' which in most cases is identified and approved by that country's ministry of health. Technical support for the project is provided by WHO staff at the country, regional and head-quarters levels.

To date, WHO-AIMS assessments have been conducted in over 80 LAMICs. An analysis of the first 42 countries to complete an assessment indicated that 62% of the countries used the information gathered through WHO-AIMS to either develop or revise a mental health policy or plan, 55% used the assessment for some other planning purpose, 74% of countries presented the results of the assessment in a national workshop attended by key stakeholders, 24% published the results of the assessment in a scientific journal and 29% of countries used WHO-AIMS to improve their mental health information system [7]. Notably, while the data provide baseline information that can be used to develop plans to strengthen or scale up services, the process of data collection itself brings together key stakeholders within the countries, placing them in a stronger position to collaborate and press ahead with needed reforms.

Synthesising the information gathered through WHO-AIMS enables countries to better gauge the major challenges they face in providing care for their citizens with mental disorders. This deeper understanding of the type and depth of constraints that affect a country's health system at different levels – be it community care, service delivery, health policy or environment – allows countries to take stock of available resources, prioritise needs and strengthen mental health care.

Scaling up care

The term 'scaling up' was first widely used as part of the reaction to the global HIV/AIDS pandemic. This response was made possible by a number of factors: the availability of an effective intervention (anti-retroviral drugs), a strong advocacy movement that succeeded in influencing political motivation to mobilise resources and the field's prioritisation in the global development agenda (including the MDGs). Scaling up has also been used to refer both to the objective of increasing access to evidence-based, sustainable services as well as to the attainment process itself, including mobilising political will, developing human resources, increasing the availability of essential medicines, and monitoring and evaluating interventions.

WHO endeavours to provide health planners, policymakers and donors with a set of clear and coherent activities for scaling up care for MNS disorders. A result of this commitment is the mhGAP, which provides a framework for combating these disorders, while simultaneously taking into account the various constraints which exist in different countries. The two overarching objectives are (a) reinforcing the financial and human resources commitments of governments, international organisations and other stakeholders for care of MNS disorders and (b) achieving much higher coverage rates with key interventions in the countries with low- and lower-middle incomes that have a large proportion of the global burden of MNS disorders [8].

The programme is grounded in the best available scientific and epidemiological evidence on priority conditions, such as depression, schizophrenia and other psychotic disorders, suicide, epilepsy, dementia, disorders due to use of alcohol and illicit drugs and mental disorders in children. These disorders are common in all countries where their prevalence has been examined, causing substantial interference with the abilities of children to learn and of adults to function in their families, at work and in broader society. The economic burden imposed by these disorders can be crippling, including loss of employment, with the attendant loss of family income; the need for caregiving, with further potential loss of wages; the cost of medicines; and the need for other medical and social services. These costs are particularly devastating for poor individuals and communities [9].

Considerable information concerning the efficacy of various interventions for reducing the burden of MNS disorders is now available. Although it is useful to determine which interventions are effective (and cost-effective) for a particular set of disorders, this is not the end of the scaling up process. Other criteria must be considered when determining which interventions to deliver, including the severity of different disorders (in terms of suffering and disability), the potential for reduction of poverty in people with different disorders and the protection of the human rights of those with severe MNS disorders.

mhGAP framework for scaling up care

The mhGAP is intended as a guide for action, designed to be consultative and participatory, adaptable to national needs and resources, and to build on existing services.

Political commitment

Success in implementation of the programme rests, first and foremost, on achievement of political commitment at the highest level. One way to achieve this prerequisite is to establish a core group of key stakeholders who have multidisciplinary expertise to guide the process. Such key stakeholders include policy advisors, programme managers from relevant areas (such as essential medicines and human resources), communication experts and experts from community development and health systems. The programme requires inputs from psychiatric, neurological and primary care health professionals; social scientists; health economists; key multilateral and bilateral partners; and non-governmental organisations (NGOs). Finally, service users are the most important stakeholders and their input is essential.

Development of a policy and legislative infrastructure

Once political will has been affirmed and policy advisors have the needs assessment results in hand, policy development can begin. Mental health legislation is essential to address MNS disorders, by codifying and consolidating the fundamental principles, values, aims and objectives of mental health policies and programmes. It provides a legal framework to prevent violations, to promote human rights and to address critical issues that affect the lives of people with mental disorders.

Policies need to be grounded in the principles of respect for human rights and the fulfillment, promotion and protection of those rights. When clearly conceptualised, a policy can coordinate essential services and activities to ensure that treatment and care are most efficiently delivered to those in need. The Mental Health Policy and Service Guidance Package that has been developed by WHO consists of a series of practical, interrelated modules designed to address issues related to the reform of mental health systems. This Guidance Package can be used as a framework to assist countries in creating policies and plans, and then putting them into practice.

Development and delivery of the intervention package

Scaling up efforts are facilitated by the development of a package of interventions that needs to be delivered by the health-care system. The mhGAP

Intervention Guide (mhGAP-IG) [10] is at the centre of such a package; it has been developed through an intensive process of evidence review. Systematic reviews were conducted to develop evidence-based recommendations. The process involved a WHO Guideline Development Group of international experts, which closely collaborated with WHO Secretariat. The recommendations were then converted into clearly presented stepwise interventions, again with the collaboration of an international group of experts. The mhGAP-IG was then circulated among a wider range of reviewers across the world to include all the diverse contributions.

The mhGAP-IG was developed for use in non-specialised health-care settings. It is aimed at health-care providers working at first- and second-level facilities. They include general physicians, family physicians, nurses and clinical officers. Other non-specialist health-care providers can use the mhGAP-IG with necessary adaptation. Although mhGAP-IG is to be implemented primarily by non-specialists, specialists may also find it useful in their work. Additionally, specialists have an essential and substantial role in training, support and supervision of non-specialists and other health-care workers. Full implementation ideally requires coordinated action by public health experts and managers, and dedicated specialists with a public health orientation.

The mhGAP calls for mental health to be integrated into primary health care. Management and treatment of MNS disorders in primary care should enable the largest number of people to get easier and faster access to services; many already seek help at this level. This integration of additional roles into existing health systems means they will need additional support to deliver these new interventions; mhGAP has identified the drugs, equipment and supplies required at each level of service delivery, but mechanisms that ensure their sustained supply need to be developed individually. Appropriate referral pathways and feedback mechanisms between all levels of service delivery remain critical and will need to be strengthened.

Poor knowledge of mental illnesses among primary health-care staff and scarcity of mental health specialists for liaison and supervision have been identified as key concerns [11–13]. Task sharing has proved to be an effective strategy in other areas of health, such as immunisation uptake and management of tuberculosis and HIV. There is growing evidence that lay people and health workers can also provide care that is traditionally delivered by psychiatrists. The difficulty of giving increased responsibilities to busy primary health-care staff is often cited as a potential barrier; however, a possible solution is found in the integration of mental health care with services for people with long-term (chronic) conditions [14–16], since services for individuals with chronic conditions share many of the characteristics of services for people with mental and neurological disorders [5].

Delivery of a package of interventions will require fostering community mobilisation and participation, as well as activities that aim to raise awareness and improve the uptake of interventions and the use of services. Concurrent efforts should also be made to combat stigma surrounding mental health help-seeking, and discrimination against those with mental health disorders.

Planning for implementation of the intervention package also needs to incorporate populations with special needs (e.g. different cultural and ethnic groups or other vulnerable groups such as indigenous populations). The approach used for delivery of services must also be gender-sensitive. Gender differences create inequities between men and women in health status. Additionally, gender differences result in differential access to and use of health information, care and services (e.g. a woman might not be able to access health services because norms in her community prevent her from travelling alone to a clinic).

Strengthening human resources

Development and upgrading of human resources are the backbone of organisational capacity building and one of the primary challenges of scaling up services. Human resources with adequate and appropriate training are essential for scaling up all health interventions, but are especially important for MNS disorders, since care for these conditions relies heavily on health personnel rather than on technology or equipment. Most countries with low and middle incomes have few trained human resources available, and the problem has been exacerbated by the migration of trained professionals to other countries [17]. Additionally, infrastructure and facilities for continuing education and training of health workers in many low-income countries are often lacking.

For each intervention, a specific category of health personnel is identified to take responsibility for patient care at each level of service delivery. For example, primary health-care professionals may be able to identify and treat most cases of psychoses with first-line anti-psychotic medicines, whereas cases with bipolar disorders requiring maintenance treatment will need to be referred to a specialist. Access to health services can be improved by involving multiple cadres at various levels of the health system. As described earlier, where doctors and nurses are in short supply, some of the priority interventions can be delivered by community health workers – after specific training and with the necessary supervision. For many priority conditions, delivery should be implemented with a stepped-care model, which consists of clearly defined roles for each level of care from primary to highly specialised care. This requires relevant training for each level of health professional.

Mobilisation of financial resources

Most countries with low and middle incomes do not assign adequate financial resources for care of MNS disorders. Mobilisation of the necessary financial resources for scaling up is therefore an important task. Accurate costing is a necessary first step, to set realistic budgets and to estimate resource gaps, before resources can be mobilised. Different types of cost estimates will be required for different purposes. WHO has developed a costing tool to estimate the financial costs of reaching a defined coverage level with a set of integrated interventions.

Although the estimated investments are not large in absolute terms, they likely represent a substantial departure from the budget allocations currently accorded to mental health. If the total health budget remained unchanged for ten years, delivery of the specified package for mental health care at target coverage would account for 50% of total health spending in Ethiopia, and 8.5% of the total in Thailand. Thus, health budgets need to be increased, especially in low-income countries. In such settings, additional money (from domestic sources, international donors, or both) is therefore needed; in other countries, the challenge will be reallocation of existing resources and capital [18].

Prior work [19] suggests that the extra cost of scaling up mental health services over a ten-year period in order to provide extensive coverage of a core package covering bipolar disorder, schizophrenia and depression is not large in absolute terms (an additional investment of around $0.20 per capita per year for low-income countries and $0.30 for lower-middle-income countries, leading to a total financial outlay of up to $2 per person in low-income countries and $3–4 in lower-middle-income countries by 2015). Such a level of investment is neither large nor startling, especially when compared to estimated funding requirements for tackling other major contributors to the global disease burden. For example, the full estimated costs of scaling up a neonatal health care package to 90% coverage have been put at $5–10 per capita [20], whereas the cost of providing universal access to basic health services has been estimated to exceed $30 per person per year [21].

For sustainability, the marginal costs of strengthening the services for MNS disorders should be minimised by building on existing strategies and plans. Funding from governments will be required to deliver services for MNS disorders, and this will require that stakeholders argue their case determinedly. If strategies for MNS disorders can be integrated with the governmental development plans for other sectors, sustained investment and resources for this area can be secured.

Monitoring and evaluation

The saying 'what gets measured gets done' summarises the importance of monitoring and evaluation for mental health planning and emphasises that service measurement must not end with the initial assessment. In order to address the urgent need for improvement in the provision of mental health care in LAMICs, regular monitoring, outcome surveillance and policy re-evaluation are necessary.

The mhGAP framework also stresses the importance of monitoring and evaluation of the programme planning and implementation efforts. Selection of inputs and processes, outcomes and impact indicators, together with identification of tools and methods for measurement, are an integral part of the process. Each country will need to decide which indicators to measure and for what purpose, when and where to measure them, how to measure them and which data sources to use. Suggested indicators for measurement include programme inputs and activities, programme outputs, outcomes and impact/health status. Ultimately, all countries will share this surveillance data with a 'global observatory' to enhance international exchange and cooperation in efforts to scale up mental health service delivery.

Building partnerships

Fundamental to mhGAP is the establishment of productive partnerships – for example, to reinforce existing relationships, attract and energise new partners, accelerate efforts and increase investments to reduce the burden of MNS disorders. Scaling up mental health care is a social, political and institutional process that engages many contributors, interest groups and organisations. Governments, health professionals for MNS disorders, civil society, communities and families, with support from the international community, are all jointly responsible for successfully undertaking this scaling up process. The way forward is to build innovative partnerships and alliances, with a strong commitment from all partners to respond to this urgent public health need.

Conclusion

The paramount priority in the area of global mental health at this time is to provide treatment and care to people with mental disorders and support to their families. WHO's mhGAP attempts to do this by increasing the capacity of the existing health-care system to deliver evidence-based care within the community using the primary health-care system.

As demonstrated by the May 2012 World Health Assembly resolution on mental health [22], the international community has responded to the urgent needs in global mental health. The global health-care community acknowledges not only the importance of addressing the mental health concerns of populations but also that much work remains to be done in order to scale up mental health services to adequate levels. The mhGAP provides a crucial roadmap for reducing the global burden of MNS disorders in the years ahead.

References

[1] The Global Burden of Disease (GBD). (2012) World Health Organization. Available from: http://www.who.int/healthinfo/global_burden_disease/en/index.html. Accessed on 31 December 2012.

[2] Ravishankar N, Gubbins P, Cooley RJ et al. (2009) Financing of global health: tracking development assistance for health from 1990 to 2007. *Lancet* **373**: 2113–2124.

[3] World Health Organization. (2011) *Mental Health Atlas 2011*. Geneva: WHO Press.

[4] Eaton J, McCay L, Semrau M et al. (2011) Scale up of services for mental health in low-income and middle-income countries. *Lancet* **378** (9802): 1592–1603.

[5] World Health Organization. (2005) World Health Organization Assessment Instrument for Mental Health Systems (WHO-AIMS 2.2). Geneva: WHO Press.

[6] World Health Organization. (2001) *World Health Report 2001: Mental Health: New Understanding, New Hope*. Geneva: WHO Press.

[7] World Health Organization. (2009) *Mental Health Systems in Selected Low- and Middle-Income Countries: A WHO-AIMS Cross-National Analysis*. Geneva: WHO Press.

[8] World Health Organization. (2008) *Mental Health Gap Action Programme: Scaling Up Care for Mental, Neurological, and Substance Use Disorders*. Geneva: WHO Press.

[9] World Health Organization. (2010) *Mental Health and Development: Targeting People with Mental Health Conditions as a Vulnerable Group*. Geneva: WHO Press.

[10] World Health Organization. (2010) *mhGAP-Intervention Guide for Mental, Neurological, and Substance Use Disorders in Non-Specialized Settings*. Geneva: WHO Press. Available from: http://www.who.int/mental_health/evidence/mhGAP_intervention_guide/en/index. html. Accessed on 31 December 2012.

[11] Ssebunnya J, Kigozi F, Ndyanabangi S. (2010) Integration of mental health into primary healthcare in a rural district in Ugranda, MHaPP Research Programme Consortium. *African Journal of Psychiatry* **13**: 128–131.

[12] Patel V, Thornicroft G. (2009) Packages of care for mental, neurological, and substance use disorders in low- and middle-income countries. *PLoS Medicine* **6** (10): e1000160.

[13] On'okoko MO, Jenkins R, Ma Miezi SM et al. (2010) Mental health in the Democratic Republic of Congo: a post-crisis country challenge. *International Psychiatry* **7** (2): 41–42.

[14] Patel V. (2009) Integrating mental health care with chronic diseases in low-resource settings. *International Journal of Public Health* **54** (1): 1–3.

[15] Mwape L, Sikwese A, Kapungwe A et al. (2010) Integrating mental health into primary health care in Zambia: a care provider's perspective. *International Journal of Mental Health Systems* **4**: 21.

[16] Beaglehole R, Epping-Jordan J, Patel V et al. (2008) Improving the prevention and management of chronic disease in low-income and middle-income countries: a priority for primary health care. *Lancet* **372** (9642): 940–949.

[17] Saraceno B, van Ommeren M, Batniji R et al. (2007) Barriers to improvement of mental health services in low-income and middle-income countries. *Lancet* **370** (9593): 1164–1174.

[18] Chisholm D, Flisher AJ, Lund C et al. (2007) Scale up services for mental disorders: a call for action. *Lancet* **370** (9594): 1241–1252.

[19] Chisholm D, Lund C, Saxena S. (2007) The cost of scaling up mental health care in low- and middle-income countries. *British Journal of Psychiatry* **191**: 528–535.

[20] Knippenberg R, Lawn JE, Darmstadt GL et al. (2005) Systematic scaling up of neonatal care in countries. *Lancet* **365** (9464): 1087–1098.

[21] Commission on Macroeconomics and Health. (2001) *Macroeconomics and Health: Investing in Health for Economic Development.* Geneva: WHO Press.

[22] World Health Organization. (2012) The global burden of mental disorders and the need for a comprehensive, coordinated response from health and social sectors at the country level. World Health Assembly Resolution WHA 65.4. Geneva: World Health Organization. Available from: http://apps.who.int/gb/e/e_wha65.html. Accessed on 31 December 2012.

CHAPTER 3

The swings and roundabouts of community mental health: The UK fairground

Peter Tyrer

Centre for Mental Health, Department of Medicine, Imperial College, London, UK

I write this chapter in a state of some puzzlement. Many people in the United Kingdom are going round the world trying to teach the principles of community mental health care to practitioners in low- and middle-income countries while at the same time finding in our country that the initiatives I am talking about elsewhere no longer have any benefits, or, in the more accurate parlance of today, are not cost-effective. Why should this be, and are there any lessons we need to learn before we carry out any new reforms?

To get the issues into perspective, it is useful to take a historical approach. To avoid confusion, I will confine my account to the services that I know best, and in which until very recently I was a frontline practitioner, often a useful corrective when theory has the danger of taking over from practice. My account will span the history of community psychiatry in the United Kingdom and, because I have been a close part of the action associated with it, I add my personal comments about the merits and disadvantages of each form of community care as I have seen them in practice.

Brief history of community psychiatry before 1950

In 1996, a perceptive paper was published by Sumathipala and Hanwella in *Psychiatric Bulletin* on the history of community psychiatric care [1]. They postulated a spiral model of psychiatric care which over the course of centuries oscillated between the care (or at least 'placement' when no care was provided) of the mentally ill in the community and in hospital. Thus, in the period between 1250 and 1750, the only hospital in England for the mentally ill was the Bethlem Hospital founded in 1247. As a consequence, almost all people with mental

---

Improving Mental Health Care: The Global Challenge, First Edition.
Edited by Graham Thornicroft, Mirella Ruggeri and David Goldberg.
© 2013 John Wiley & Sons, Ltd. Published 2013 by John Wiley & Sons, Ltd.

illness lived in the community but without any formal care. After the Vagrancy Act of 1774 made the first distinction between lunatics and paupers, several private 'madhouses' were founded and other mental hospitals were opened such as the lunatic ward at Guy's Hospital in 1728 and St Luke's Hospital in 1751. The spiral of care had shifted slightly from 'no care in the community' towards hospital or institutional care.

Then there was a period of rapid growth with the building of many new mental hospitals in the early nineteenth century. This was associated with a more humane approach to the care of mentally ill in institutions championed by Edward Parker Charlesworth in Lincoln and Conolly in Hanwell, so that care in mental institutions replaced incarceration, and this accelerated after 1845, when the Lunatics Act required each county to build an asylum. The early asylums were forward thinking places where enthusiasts for reform were also keen on promoting new treatments. But this was replaced gradually with stasis, with overcrowding and fewer staff and concentration more on risk management and custodial approaches. The Lunacy Act of 1890 imposed restrictions on the discharge of patients from hospital, and these persisted well into the twentieth century.

The pendulum then swung back towards optimism after World War I, and there was a return to community care in the form of outpatient care. The Maudsley Hospital opened in 1923 and, with its combined outpatient treatment and voluntary inpatient treatment, helped to bring the asylums back into the medical care system. This rekindled enthusiasm for a new form of community care was summarised in a paper by Ian Skottowe, one of the pioneers of community psychiatry, in 1931 [2]:

1 It brings psychiatry and general medicine closer together;
2 It provides unparalleled clinical experience for students if they care to attend it, for this is the sort of thing they are going to come across in general practice;
3 It establishes closer relationship between mental hospital patients and their physicians by paving the way for their admission and by providing a follow-up or after-care service;
4 It provides a consulting service for all classes and, in this respect, particularly with difficult relatives, it is a great help to the general practitioner;
5 It provides treatment for cases not ill enough to justify their admission to a mental hospital, and yet who will not recover without some form of treatment;
6 It paves the way for enlightenment of the lay mind on the subject of mental illness.

Despite these developments, the inpatient population continued to grow until a peak in 1954. Its continued reduction since has often been put down to the introduction of antipsychotic drugs, the 'chlorpromazine revolution', but this has been disputed as it all coincided with a new thrust in social psychiatry [3]. We are now still in this phase of community expansion although there are beginning to be loud voices harkening towards retrenchment [4].

What Sumathipala and Hanwella maintain in their account is that each of the reincarnations of community psychiatry has left care in a better position than the previous one, and so the spiral model has been one of overall improvement.

Phase 1: Outpatient care

The period between 1950 and 1975 can be regarded as a continuation of the outpatient phase of community psychiatry. It was reinforced to some extent by the introduction of the day hospital by Joshua Bierer in the 1940s, introduced as part of a personal drive to increase patients' autonomy [5]. Day hospitals did not get fully established until the 1970s, and they tended to concentrate initially on the care of patients with minor mental disorder seen for complex psychotherapies, and their outcomes were no different from outpatient care in both the short and longer term [6, 7].

The outpatient clinic (shown in Figure 3.1) was a useful but staggered form of community care. It allowed patients to be seen outside hospital in large numbers; it was a valuable form of after-care, and it was a useful bridge between the mental hospital and the general practitioner. It did not always have the same catchment area as the hospital – hence its position straddling the hexagon in

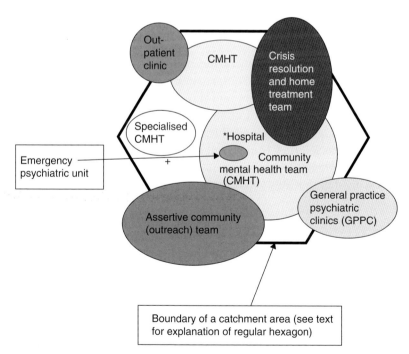

Figure 3.1 Schematic diagram of the variety of community psychiatric provision in the United Kingdom (1952–2012).

Figure 3.1 – and most of the patients seen were those with less serious mental illness, so the level of continuity between inpatient and community care was not as strong as it might have appeared. It also was essentially a medical phenomenon; although occasionally nurses were involved in some clinics, doctors at all levels of training saw the patients and reported back to doctors at their parent hospitals.

Personal comment

This phase was my first introduction to community psychiatry, initially at St John's Hospital in Buckinghamshire in 1968, where I carried out clinics in High Wycombe 20 miles away from the main hospital, and then at Knowle Hospital in Hampshire (where Dr Skottowe subsequently worked), when I saw patients at several clinics up to 30 miles away. I found the work stimulating and interesting, and follow-up of inpatients in a different setting very educational. It was also a great advantage seeing patients away from a mental hospital, but I quickly realised that the amount one could do as a single-handed doctor with an outpatient was limited, and it was often frustrating not being able to share discussions with colleagues at the times of seeing the patients. But it offered the possibility of much more contact with patients in larger numbers, and, by comparison, the day hospital alternative was much more limiting, with much smaller numbers and a nagging doubt that this form of care was not cost-effective.

Phase 2: Extending into primary care

In the late 1970s, there was a general feeling that mental hospitals were not the best focus for treatment, and the outpatient model was extended in many parts of the country by moving clinics into primary care, and by 1983 one in five patients was seen in these settings [8]. It is hard to believe this nowadays, when most emphasis is on major mental illness, but it was an enthusiastic time when many psychiatrists felt they could reach out further into the community, and at that time there were no established multidisciplinary teams.

It was suggested that this extension could form an ideal community service organised on the principles of bee organisation and so called the hive system [9]. This envisaged hexagonal interlocking catchment areas (hence the hexagon in Figure 3.1) with the psychiatrist equivalent to the worker bee, buzzing between the areas of high psychopathological density and the hospital (hive) and ensuring that resources were directed to areas of greatest need. The data on this model are almost entirely UK-based; there is little evidence for it elsewhere in the world.

Personal comment

I worked in Nottingham between 1979 and 1988 and used this model. This was the most satisfying period of my working life in clinical practice. Although it was very busy (I was doing 19 clinics every month in addition to my ward reviews), I relished the clinical autonomy I had and also the opportunity to find out the problems of general practitioners in looking after mentally ill patients. Many of these contacts were very brief [10], but they were a very efficient way of keeping touch and transferring information. These clinics were also successful in reducing hospital admissions [11] despite an overall 10% increase in new patient contacts.

Phase 3: The community mental health team

It is difficult to know where the notion of the community mental health team (CMHT) started in the United Kingdom. It was certainly not an extension of the assertive community team [18] as it was built up in stages between 1970 and 1990. It may have had some influence from case management, as although this began in the United States in the 1980s, it was embraced with enthusiasm [12], but it took place in a community care vacuum only very slightly filled by asser-tive community treatment teams (see following text), and when it crossed the Atlantic to the United Kingdom it became distorted by the service-provider split recommended by the Prime Minister's market guru, the late Sir Roy Griffiths, which led to social services operating as 'purchasers' of mental health care and the psychiatric services as 'providers' (The Care Programme Approach) [13]. The independent monitoring function of care management was intended to improve the matching of client need to services, to ensure value for money and to iden-tify deficiencies in services that could be addressed, but this was nonsensical, as a good psychiatric service already had social workers in its ranks and, once removed and separated from the service, became as unpopular and unhelpful as a junior teacher in one discipline (e.g. physical education) being given the task of monitoring the whole school in place of the headmaster.

When the two were separated in this way, care management was seen to be less successful than its provider equivalent, assertive community teams, who got on with their work without the intervention of a purchaser [14]. But in the United Kingdom, we, more or less silently, developed a new approach that was an excellent example of British pragmatism, CMHTs. These were multi-disciplinary groups of professionals who served the psychiatric needs of the population in a defined area, not because they were told to do by government decree but because they found it to be a sensible way of using resources and had already been muddling through with this general approach for some years.

But government noticed and caught up. CMHTs were linked to the Care Programme Approach, and initially it was suggested that a social worker or nurse should play the major part in managed care and decide on admission to hospital if it was needed, and this was understandable as there was good research evidence that community nurses were effective in providing home treatment [15]. However, the mistake was to give this role to a single profession within a multidisciplinary team without any flexibility, and when this approach was tested in a research trial, it was found to lead to a dramatic increase in bed usage (greater than 60%) even though there was less dropout from care [16]. Once it was established that each patient needed a named care coordinator who was authorised to be the link between the patient and other teams, the functioning of the CMHT became better established. As a by-product of the CMHT movement, better ways of getting the most handicapped patients out of hospital in permanent placements that could become their home were initiated [17] but were generally ignored as rehabilitation seemed to have become yesterday's word.

The well-structured CMHT is an efficient and cost-effective method of providing community care. It has never had its own champion or guru to boast about its assets, but the review evidence is that it promotes good care with low dropout, reduces hospital admissions, increases satisfaction and may also prevent early death [17, 18].

Personal comment

I was a member of a specialised CMHT, the Early Intervention Service, between 1988 and 1994. The team was the first community team to be established in the Paddington area of west London. It was one of the first parts of a replaced service which originally had outpatient clinics in central London but beds 30 miles away in Surrey and then transferred 60 of these beds to the central London site. The Early Intervention Service comprised an industrious and enterprising multidisciplinary group whose common characteristic was that they were disaffected by existing services and felt stifled by them. They blossomed in a new environment and were coordinated on a long leash by first a psychologist and then a social worker. The team created the right environment for community teams to be established in all parts of the catchment area in 1994, and so the Early Intervention Service self-immolated at this time, but not after it had made a significant impact on local services, including the full support of the Chief Executive Officer and Board of the North West (subsequently Central North West) London Mental Health Trust that hosted it, and also contributed to the research literature by showing that the service markedly reduced the use of beds [19, 20]. I felt a valued member of the team and enjoyed the work greatly, the only regret being that for an unnecessarily large part of my time I was involved in trying to persuade my consultant colleagues that their practice had to change if community psychiatry was going to be successful in the area. This persuasion was only partly successful and proper change was only effected after retirement of the key staff and replacement by keen and enthusiastic younger colleagues, who have continued to provide what I would regard as an excellent service.

Phase 4: Assertive outreach treatment

The principles of assertive outreach, or assertive community treatment, are the most prominent export of community care from the United States, first introduced in 1974 by Stein and Test and then formally evaluated [21]. ('Assertive outreach' was the term used in the United Kingdom from the beginning of this new approach in 1998 for reasons that have never been clear to me.) However, from the beginning it was clear that there were major misconceptions that led planners of psychiatric services to make the wrong decisions. One of the attractions of assertive outreach for managers of psychiatric services was the exciting early evidence that these services reduced inpatient admissions and could therefore be at least self-financing, or better, save money to spend elsewhere in the services through reduction of inpatient costs. This was certainly suggested by the initial randomised controlled trials of assertive community treatment [22] and by replications in Australia [23, 24]. This was the climate in which assertive community treatment (and its synonyms such as assertive outreach and intensive case management) was born, and in the United Kingdom was embraced by what became known as the North Birmingham model.

As a former resident of Birmingham, a city that has never had the best of publicity, it is somewhat peculiar to note why one of its dingiest parts, noted for absolutely nothing else, attracted such public attention. The reason was simple. The psychiatric planners of North Birmingham inherited a very poorly regarded run-down psychiatric hospital (Highcroft Hospital) and wanted a crash course in community psychiatry to reform mental health services. So, they wisely invested in pioneers in new community approaches, and they duly were appointed and brought prestige, new ideas and enthusiasm. Assertive outreach services, home treatment and crisis house initiatives followed afoot, and before long everything that was new and exciting appeared to be going on in this tiny and previously forgotten part of the United Kingdom. This attracted the attention of national policy makers and the North Birmingham model became embraced as the way forward for community mental health. A new Labour government was elected in 1997, and its Chancellor of the Exchequer, Gordon Brown, injected new money into the National Health Service (NHS) and this included the mental health services. A National Framework for Mental Health was proposed, and this included the setting up of 192 assertive outreach services across England and Wales.

The new enthusiasts did not take notice of research evidence and were proud to ignore it as unnecessary. One of its strongest supporters in North Birmingham, Professor Sashidharan, had a clear response to my question about research when I was evaluating his service in 2000, 'we are the pioneers, Peter, you are the researchers. We are ahead of you, let us get on with it and you come along and do your research afterwards'. He subsequently reiterated these views in published form [25]. The trouble was that the evidence that assertive outreach and home treatment services were the way forward had come from studies in Australia and the United States at a time when community psychiatric teams did not exist, and so what could be described as the 'hospital–outpatient model' was the only comparator [21–23], and this also applied to the first UK study carried out in 1990–1991 [26]. When research trials were carried out in the United Kingdom in the 1990s when the comparison service was not a hospital–outpatient model but a community psychiatric team one, the results were very different. No benefit in terms of hospital bed use, service satisfaction, symptom reduction or functioning was found, and this was a consistent finding in five major studies [27–31]. Costs, not surprisingly, were higher in the assertive outreach services so they could not be regarded as cost-effective [30, 32–34]. What was even sadder was that most of these data were available by the time the big expansion in assertive outreach took place. I and other colleagues who wanted to point out that our hypotheses had been proven wrong were 'disinvited' to the launch of this initiative.

Why should these data from the United Kingdom be different from those elsewhere? Are there other reasons why assertive outreach has, to all intents and purposes, failed in the United Kingdom, at least as far as bed reduction is concerned? There has been considerable argument about this, and these have principally fallen into two camps: (a) the 'fidelity argument' that assertive treatment has not been given with adequate fidelity and therefore the benefits have not been replicated, and (b) the 'improved comparison' argument, described earlier, suggests that because a good community team provides most of the attributes of an assertive outreach team when the two are compared directly, there is little difference between them. The proponents of the two sides have powerful and angry spokesmen, and there have been accusations that the evidence base of systematic reviews has 'possibly been used and misused and misrepresented in a highly charged atmosphere of professional media debate' [35]. However, the dust is now settling, and it is becoming clearer why the two camps feel that the truth is on their side.

Both arguments are true. Many teams that practise intensive or assertive treatment do not in fact do so, according to standard measures of fidelity [36] when their activities are examined closely [37]. The proponents of community assertive treatment suggests that a caseload should be between 8 and 12 per key worker, that teams should be operating an 'all team approach' (i.e. every member of the team knows every patient on the caseload), that teams should provide 24-hour cover and that the teams should be genuine multidisciplinary teams with a philosophy of active involvement in all parts of the patients' lives (popularly called 'activities of daily living'). Not many assertive community teams, sometimes called intensive case management teams, provide all of these attributes, but it would be surprising if they did in a modern community mental health service. For a small team to provide its own 24-hour cover when there is cover elsewhere in the catchment area seems an unnecessary duplication of resources, and similarly, the need for every single member of the team to know every patient has some advantages but should not be regarded as an absolute *sine qua non* of a viable team.

Nevertheless, there are some outcomes that are superior with assertive teams. Studies have generally shown greater engagement (particularly in those with less intellectual resources [38]) and greater satisfaction with care [31], and these should not be ignored. But these gains are very much smaller than the ones achieved by the first assertive community teams, in which bed reduction, costs, symptom reduction as well as satisfaction were all highly positive [21]. To understand this, it is useful to think of a botanical analogy.

It is possible to draw a parallel between the success of assertive community treatment in primitive services and its relative lack of success in better ones by looking at the biological phenomenon of plant succession. In alien habitats, such as deserts, seashores, mudflats and marshes, only a minority of specially adapted plants are able to gain a foothold and thrive. However, as a consequence of their success, the soil conditions become much more conducive to the growth of other plants, and these gradually take root and compete with the original specialised species. Before long, these are so successful that the specialised plants are squeezed out altogether and no longer thrive in the conditions that they helped to generate.

Assertive community treatment is a similar specialised plant. It thrives in adverse conditions when no community care exists or only the rudiments of community services are present. The more primitive the conditions are for community care, the greater the benefits of assertive community treatment. However, as it develops, the more likely it is for other community services to develop and also thrive [39]. As these become established and extend across the nation, assertive community treatment is squeezed out.

Personal comment

I worked in two assertive outreach teams between 1994 and 2009, and this represented the longest period of community mental health practice in my career. One of these (Community Rehabilitation and Assertive Focus Team (CRAFT)) was involved in the large UK700 study of intensive treatment (largely equivalent to assertive outreach) that showed no difference between the two forms of management in reducing hospital admissions in a well-organised trial [29]. However, this was a four-centre trial, and all other centres apart from the one where our team was based in west London showed an increase in admissions in patients randomised to intensive treatment. If the west London data had been analysed alone – which would clearly have been inappropriate – there would have been a 28% reduction in bed usage with intensive case management compared with standard management ($P<0.01$). The reasons for this difference are far from clear, but the west London patients had a lot more associated pathology than others, and there was a very active programme of careful home placement of patients in the intensive team. The great advantage of working in an assertive outreach team is that you get to know the patients a great deal better than in an ordinary CMHT, and so much better prediction and planning can take place. The negative aspects include the problem of the 'all-team' philosophy that can get in the way of a good individual therapeutic relationship – you cannot develop this if you see the patient only on one occasion in every three.

Phase 5: Crisis resolution and home treatment teams

The principles of crisis teams were established many years ago by Caplan [40]. By intervening early in a problem, you are more likely to get it resolved than if you intervene late, and it is often possible to effect a greater degree of change by intervention at a time of crisis than at other times when behavioural patterns have become more entrenched. But in the United Kingdom, these basic principles have been trumped by a stronger imperative to keep the patient out of hospital by intervening at the time of crisis, and since the demise of assertive outreach the route to the new Jerusalem of a virtual bedless psychiatry has been diverted to the crisis team. Despite the apparent differences, there has been some confusion at times between the functions of assertive outreach and crisis resolution teams (CRTs), as when an assertive outreach team successfully prevents someone being admitted in a time of crisis, it is obviously functioning in the same way, and services that have been cited as those of assertive outreach are really acting as crisis teams if they function at the point of possible admission.

Crisis teams are difficult to evaluate as the ideal time to allocate a patient in a good study is at the time of crisis, but this has not been achieved. Only one randomised controlled trial has been carried out into the effectiveness of a CRT [34, 41], and this, like many previous studies, randomised patients at the point that admission was being considered, not necessarily at a time of crisis. It may be considered too cynical, but my experience in recent years, because of the shortage of inpatient beds in many areas, is that the crisis in such situations exists more in the service than in the patient. 'We haven't got a bed, let's hope the crisis team can keep them out'. The trial by Johnson et al. was effective in reducing inpatient usage over a subsequent eight-week period and also suggested a marginal increase in satisfaction in those allocated to the crisis team, and there was a cost saving over this short period because of less use of beds [34], but this is hardly a finding of great import as the clear *raison d'être* of the service is to keep patients out of hospital.

Other trials are awaited. A recent review – a narrative one only as there is insufficient information to carry out a systematic one – concluded that 'the balance of evidence suggests that CRTs can reduce hospital beds and costs with similar symptomatic outcome and service user satisfaction, but there is no evidence that CRTs are the only way to do so' [42]. In the longer term, there is some evidence that compulsory admissions and suicides are increased subsequently in patients referred to crisis teams [43], and this emphasises the need for longer-term follow-up studies. An admission prevented today may be a decision regretted tomorrow.

A separate element of care, the home treatment team, now often combined with CRTs, has been systematically investigated and not shown to have any special intrinsic advantages in a *Cochrane Systematic Reviews* [44], but there is nonetheless some slight evidence that visiting at home may reduce admissions to hospital [45].

Personal comment

I left my last assertive outreach team in 2009 and only had brief contact with the new crisis resolution service that had been set up just previously. I did find it unnecessary to have to refer the patients that we wanted to admit, even if only for a very short time for a special reason, to the crisis and home treatment service, when the assessment by a completely different team was in our view quite unnecessary. (The very good consultant in charge of the crisis team agreed with me on this, but it was mandatory.) The subsequent change from the assertive outreach looking after its own patients to care by an inpatient consultant team added to this disruption. The new system of care in the United Kingdom now incorporates different consultants for community care, crisis intervention, acute inpatient and rehabilitation (now inaccurately and misleadingly called 'recovery'). In practice, this means that a patient in a mental crisis can be under the care of four different consultants within the space of a few weeks, and this is at a time when they are feeling at their most vulnerable and in need of constancy. The NHS has always embraced the concept of continuity of care [46], and it is fair to ask what has happened to continuity now, and how can this nonsensical fragmentation be of value to anyone apart from hair-splitting bureaucrats?

A synthesis

It is not easy to bring all these services and my experiences into a common framework, but there is a coherent message from these naturalistic experiments. It is first necessary to decide on the common principles that underlie good community psychiatry. These are as follows:

1 It is generally better for patients to be treated outside hospital, provided appropriate facilities are available.
2 If a hospital bed is necessary, it should be available when required and should be as close as possible to the patient's home.
3 Continuity of care may not always be possible but should be strived for as a matter of principle.

4 Individual or team-based treatment both have merits, and their choice should be determined in collaboration with the patient and his or her carers.

Most practitioners would find little fault with these fundamental tenets, but at different times in the history of community psychiatry in the United Kingdom, just one or two of these have been given prominence. The first of these lay behind the pioneering work of the early enthusiasts who first recognised the negative aspects of institutional care and wanted to get rid of the 'snake pits' (i.e. mental hospitals). Of course, this policy has been hijacked by successive governments, with the word 'cheaper' being substituted for 'better'. At times this has assumed evangelical fervour, and one of the earliest enthusiasts, John Hoult, often insisted that 'every psychiatric admission was a failure', which of course cannot be true – the hospital is part of the community care service [47]. The second of these, also an integral part of the hive system, emphasised the notion of the catchment area with the parent hospital within easy reach of all homes where patients lived. The third lay behind the notion of area-based teams within a catchment area, covering roughly equal populations and having wards within hospitals that also covered these same 'mini-areas' so that when patients were admitted they could be looked after by at least some of the staff who also worked in the same community teams. The most recent changes in the United Kingdom have gone backwards as their instigators have become obsessed by avoidance of admission at all costs, and this is likely to prove to be not only counterproductive in terms of clinical outcome but also more expensive. The principles of assertive outreach are good ones but need to be applied within the CMHT, not separately from it [48], and the flexible use of assertive community treatment with shifting of patients from assertive to normal care within the same team depending on need, called Function Assertive Community Treatment [49] (the FACT model), may be a good way forward. (I would much prefer the F in FACT to be Flexible rather than Function (which is not an adjective anyway) but that is for others to decide.) This flexibility allows the range of treatments from personal individual ones at times of relative calm to intensive multidisciplinary ones at times of crisis and greater need.

What is abundantly clear from the swings and roundabouts of the last 50 years is that government-initiated reforms, almost all introduced before evidence is available, are not helpful for psychiatric care. They disrupt patterns of care that are already working and set up phony new models of treatment that can easily give a wrong impression of success. Why a wrong impression? This becomes very clear when you are working in a service and a reform is introduced. The new service is promoted heavily, often with an increase of resources and shiny new premises, and many staff, now a little bored with a 'standard' service that has lost its shine, are encouraged to apply for a post within the new scheme. There is competition for these new posts, the best of the staff from the existing services are appointed, leading to a loss of the most valuable expertise in the older services, and any comparisons between the old and new models favour the new approach.

But it is not the new model that makes the results superior; it is just that the staff are better skilled and more motivated. It is the people who deliver the service that count, not some abstruse model that forces them to work better, and this needs to be repeated to the managers of services over and over again.

References

[1] Sumathipala A, Hanwella R. (1996) The evolution of psychiatric care – a spiral model. *Psychiatric Bulletin* **20**: 561–563.

[2] Skottowe I. (1931) The utility of the psychiatric out-patient clinic. *British Journal of Psychiatry* **77**: 311–320.

[3] Shepherd M. (1994) Neurolepsis and the psychopharmacological revolution: myth and reality. *History of Psychiatry* **5**: 89–96.

[4] Coid J. (1994) Failure in community care: psychiatry's dilemma. *BMJ* **308**: 805–806.

[5] Bierer J, Haldane FP. (1941) A self-governed patients' social club in a public mental hospital. *British Journal of Psychiatry* **87**: 419–426.

[6] Tyrer P, Remington M. (1979) Controlled comparison of day hospital and out-patient treatment for neurotic disorders. *Lancet* **313**: 1014–1016.

[7] Tyrer P, Remington M, Alexander J. (1987) The outcome of neurotic disorders after out-patient and day hospital care. *British Journal of Psychiatry* **151**: 57–62.

[8] Strathdee G, Williams P. (1983) A survey of psychiatrists in primary care: the silent growth of a new service. *Journal of the Royal College of General Practitioners* **34**: 615–618.

[9] Tyrer P. (1985) The hive system: a model for a psychiatric service. *British Journal of Psychiatry* **146**: 571–575.

[10] Darling C, Tyrer P. (1990) Brief encounters in general practice: an audit of liaison in general practice psychiatric clinics. *Psychiatric Bulletin* **14**: 592–594.

[11] Tyrer P, Seivewright N, Wollerton S. (1984) General practice psychiatric clinics – impact on psychiatric services. *British Journal of Psychiatry* **145**: 15–19.

[12] Franklin J, Solovitz B, Mason M et al. (1987) An evaluation of case management. *American Journal of Public Health* **77**: 674–678.

[13] Kingdon D. (1994) Care programme approach: recent government policy and legislation. *Psychiatric Bulletin* **18**: 68–70.

[14] Marshall M, Lockwood A, Gray A et al. (1998) Assertive community treatment for people with severe mental disorders. In: Adams CG, Duggan L, de Jesus Mari J et al. (eds.), *Schizophrenia Module of the Cochrane Database Systematic Reviews*. Oxford: Update Software.

[15] Burns T, Beadsmoore A, Bhat, AV et al. (1993) A controlled trial of home-based acute psychiatric services. I. Clinical and social outcome. *British Journal of Psychiatry* **163**: 49–54.

[16] Tyrer P, Morgan J, Van Horn E et al. (1995) Randomised controlled study of close monitoring of vulnerable psychiatric patients. *Lancet* **345**: 756–759.

[17] Goldberg DP, Bridges K, Cooper W et al. (1985) Douglas House: a new type of hostel ward for chronic psychotic patients. *British Journal of Psychiatry* **147**: 383–388.

[18] Malone D, Newton-Howes G, Simmonds S et al. (2007) Community Mental Health Teams (CMHTs) for people with severe mental illnesses and disordered personality. *Cochrane Database of Systematic Reviews* **3**: CD000270.

[19] Onyett S, Tyrer P, Connolly J et al. (1990) The early intervention service: the first eighteen months of an Inner London demonstration project. *Psychiatric Bulletin* **14**: 267–269.

[20] Merson S, Tyrer P, Onyett S et al. (1992) Early intervention in psychiatric emergencies: a controlled clinical trial. *Lancet* **339**: 1311–1314.

[21] Stein LI, Test MA. (1980) Alternative to mental hospital treatment. 1. Conceptual model, treatment program and clinical evaluation. *Archives of General Psychiatry* **36**: 1073–1079.

[22] Weisbrod BA, Test MA, Stein LI. (1980) Alternatives to mental hospital treatment: II. Economic benefit-cost analysis. *Archives of General Psychiatry* **37**: 400–405.

[23] Hoult J, Reynolds I. (1985) Schizophrenia: a comparative trial of community-oriented and hospital oriented psychiatric care. *Acta Psychiatrica Scandinavica* **69**: 359–372.

[24] Hoult J. (1986) Community care of the acutely mentally ill. *British Journal of Psychiatry* **149**: 137–144.

[25] Sashidharan SP. (2002) Commentary: rethinking research in community mental health – service change first, research later? *Psychiatric Bulletin* **26**: 408.

[26] Muijen M, Marks IM, Connolly J et al. (1992) Home based care and standard hospital care for patients with severe mental illness: a randomised controlled trial. *BMJ* **304**: 749–754.

[27] Holloway F, Carson J. (1998) Intensive case management for the severely mentally ill: controlled trial. *British Journal of Psychiatry* **172**: 19–22.

[28] Thornicroft G, Wykes T, Holloway F et al. (1998) From efficacy to effectiveness in community mental health services. PRiSM Psychosis Study 10. *British Journal of Psychiatry* **173**: 423–427.

[29] Burns T, Creed F, Fahy T et al. (1999) Intensive versus standard case management for severe psychotic illness: a randomised trial. *Lancet* **353**: 2185–2189.

[30] Harrison-Read P, Lucas B, Tyrer P et al. (2002) Heavy users of acute psychiatric beds: randomised controlled trial of enhanced community management in an outer London borough. *Psychological Medicine* **32**: 413–426.

[31] Killaspy H, Bebbington P, Blizard R et al. (2006) The REACT study: randomised evaluation of assertive community treatment in north London. *BMJ* **332**: 815–820.

[32] McCrone P, Thornicroft G, Phelan M et al. (1998) Utilisation and costs of community services on disability and symptoms. PRiSM Psychosis Study 5. *British Journal of Psychiatry* **173**: 391–398.

[33] McCrone P, Killaspy H, Bebbington P et al. (2009) The REACT study: cost-effectiveness analysis of assertive community treatment in north London. *Psychiatric Services* **60**: 908–913.

[34] McCrone P, Johnson S, Nolan F et al. (2009) Economic evaluation of a crisis resolution service: a randomised controlled trial. *Epidemiologia e Psichiatria Sociale* **18** (1): 54–58.

[35] Rosen A, Teesson M. (2001) Does case management work: the evidence and abuse of evidence-based medicine. *Australian and New Zealand Journal of Psychiatry* **35**: 731–746.

[36] Bond GR, Salyers MP. (2004) Prediction of outcome from the Dartmouth assertive community treatment fidelity scale. *CNS Spectrums* **9**: 937–942.

[37] Weaver T, Tyrer P, Ritchie J et al. (2003) Assessing the value of assertive outreach. Qualitative study of process and outcome in the UK700 trial. *British Journal of Psychiatry* **183**: 437–445.

[38] Hassiotis A, Ukoumunne OC, Byford S et al. (2001) Intellectual functioning and outcome of patients with severe psychotic illness randomised to intensive case management: report from the UK700 case management trial. *British Journal of Psychiatry* **178**: 166–171.

[39] Tyrer P. (1999) What is the future of assertive community treatment? *Epidemiologia e Psichiatrica Sociale* **8**: 16–18.

[40] Caplan G. (1964) *Principles of Preventative Psychiatry*. New York: Basic Books.

[41] Johnson S, Nolan F, Pilling S et al. (2005) Randomised controlled trial of acute mental health care by a crisis resolution team: the north Islington crisis study. *BMJ* **331**: 599.

[42] Hubbeling D, Bertram R. (2012) Crisis resolution teams in the UK and elsewhere. *Journal of Mental Health* **21**: 285–295.

[43] Tyrer P, Gordon F, Nourmand S et al. (2010) Controlled comparison of two crisis resolution and home treatment teams. *Psychiatrist* **34**: 50–54.

[44] Catty J, Burns T, Knapp M et al. (2002) Home treatment for mental health problems; a systematic review. *Psychological Medicine* **32**: 383–401.

[45] Burns T, Catty J, Wright C. (2006) De-constructing home-based care for mental illness: can one identify the effective ingredients? *Acta Psychiatrica Scandinavica* **113** (Suppl. 429): 33–35.

[46] Crawford MJ, de Jonge E, Freeman GK, Weaver T. (2004) Providing continuity of care for people with severe mental illness – a narrative review. *Social Psychiatry and Psychiatric Epidemiology* **39**: 265–272.

[47] Thornicroft G, Tansella M. (2004) Components of a modern mental health service: a pragmatic balance of community and hospital care: overview of systematic evidence. *British Journal of Psychiatry* **185**: 283–290.

[48] Tyrer P. (2007) The future of specialist community teams in the care of those with severe mental illness. *Epidemiologia e Psichiatria Sociale* **16**: 225–230.

[49] Drukker M, van Os J, Sytema S et al. (2011) Function assertive community treatment (FACT) and psychiatric service use in patients diagnosed with severe mental illness. *Epidemiology and Psychiatric Sciences* **20**: 273–278.

CHAPTER 4

Mental health services and recovery

Mike Slade, Mary Leamy, Victoria Bird and Clair Le Boutillier

Health Service and Population Research Department, Institute of Psychiatry, King's College London, London, UK

What is recovery?

The term 'recovery' has become widely used in mental health systems internationally. It is a term with at least two meanings: clinical recovery meaning recovery *from* mental illness, and personal recovery meaning recovery *with* a mental illness [1]. To note, other distinguishing terms have also been used, including clinical recovery versus social recovery [2], scientific versus consumer models of recovery [3] and service-based recovery versus user-based recovery [4].

Both meanings are underpinned by a set of values and create role expectations for mental health professionals. The distinction between the two meanings reflects a debate about the core purpose of mental health systems. We begin by differentiating these two meanings.

Clinical recovery

Clinical recovery has emerged from professional-led research and practice, and has four key features:

1 It is an outcome or a state, generally dichotomous.
2 It is observable – in clinical parlance, it is objective, not subjective.
3 It is rated by the expert clinician, not the patient.
4 The definition of recovery is invariant across individuals.

Various definitions of recovery have been proposed by mental health professionals. A widely used definition is that recovery comprises full symptom remission, full- or part-time work or education, independent living without supervision by informal carers and having friends with whom activities can be shared, all sustained for a period of two years [5]. This approach to defining clinical recovery in a way that is externally observable has allowed epidemiological research into recovery rates. Table 4.1 shows all 20-year or longer follow-up studies of outcome

---

Improving Mental Health Care: The Global Challenge, First Edition.
Edited by Graham Thornicroft, Mirella Ruggeri and David Goldberg.
© 2013 John Wiley & Sons, Ltd. Published 2013 by John Wiley & Sons, Ltd.

Table 4.1 Recovery rates in long-term follow-up studies of psychosis.

Lead researcher	Location	Year	n	Mean length of follow-up (years)	% recovered or significantly improved
Huber [6]	Bonn	1975	502	22	57
Ciompi [7]	Lausanne	1976	289	37	53
Bleuler [8]	Zurich	1978	208	23	53–68
Tsuang [9]	Iowa	1979	186	35	46
Harding [10]	Vermont	1987	269	32	62–68
Ogawa [11]	Japan	1987	140	23	57
Marneros [12]	Cologne	1989	249	25	58
DeSisto [13]	Maine	1995	269	35	49
Harrison [14]	18-site	2001	776	25	56

(meeting criteria for clinical recovery) for people with a diagnosis of psychosis (generally schizophrenia).

These empirical data challenge the applicability of a chronic disease model to mental illness, with its embedded assumption that conditions like schizophrenia are necessarily lifelong and have a deteriorating course. Rather, hope is an evidence-based attitude!

However, deep assumptions about normality are embedded in this understanding of recovery: 'This kind of definition begs several questions that need to be addressed to come up with an understanding of recovery as outcome: How many goals must be achieved to be considered recovered? For that matter, how much life success is considered "normal"?' [15], p. 5.

A new understanding of recovery has emerged from the mental health service user/survivor movement. People personally affected by mental illness have become increasingly vocal in communicating both what their life is like with the mental illness and what helps in moving beyond the role of a patient with mental illness. Early accounts were written by individual pioneers [16–19], and provide ecologically valid pointers to what recovery looks and feels like from the inside. Once individual stories were more visible, compilations and syntheses of these accounts began to emerge from around the (especially Anglophone) world, for example, Australia [20], New Zealand [21–23], Scotland [24, 25], the United States [26, 27] and England [28, 29]. It is on this form of evidence – idiographic knowledge about subjective experience rather than nomothetic knowledge about observational and experimental findings from groups – that personal recovery is based.

Personal recovery

Personal recovery has a different focus from clinical recovery, for example, in emphasising the centrality of hope, identity, meaning and personal responsibility [20]. Many specific definitions of recovery have been proposed by those who are experiencing it:

> Recovery refers to the lived or real life experience of people as they accept and overcome the challenge of the disability…they experience themselves as recovering a new sense of self and of purpose within and beyond the limits of disability [18, p. 11].
>
> For me, recovery means that I'm not in hospital and I'm not sitting in supported accommodation somewhere with someone looking after me. Since I've recovered, I've found that in spite of my illness I can still contribute and have an input into what goes on in my life, input that is not necessarily tied up with medication, my mental illness or other illnesses [25, p. 61].

The most widely cited definition, which underpins most recovery policy internationally, is by Bill Anthony:

> Recovery is a deeply personal, unique process of changing one's attitudes, values, feelings, goals, skills, and/or roles. It is a way of living a satisfying, hopeful, and contributing life even within the limitations caused by illness. Recovery involves the development of new meaning and purpose in one's life as one grows beyond the catastrophic effects of mental illness [30, p. 14].

For those who value succinctness, the definition used in our local mental health service is:

> Recovery involves living as well as possible [31, p. 6].

To illustrate the distinction between these two meanings, Table 4.2 differentiates between the types of language used in systems oriented around clinical recovery and personal recovery [1].

The dominance of personal recovery

Personal recovery has come to dominate mental health policy in the Anglophone world, underpinning, for example, national strategies in Australia [32], Canada [33], England [34], Ireland [35] and the United States [36], among others. Beyond the English-speaking world, a 2012 issue of the *International Review of Psychiatry* focused on recovery [37], with contributions from nine countries including Israel [38] and Hong Kong [39].

Scholarly overviews are now available of the linkage with civil rights movements [40], the implications for professional identity [41] and supporting recovery through rehabilitation services [42, 43]. Empirically based guides to clinical practice have been published both in the United States [44] and the United Kingdom [1], the latter containing 26 case studies from around the world illustrating recovery-oriented services.

It is now possible to synthesise the evidence about how mental health services can support recovery, in order to inform empirically based strategies. In order to

Table 4.2 Differences between language used in clinical recovery and personal recovery.

Clinical recovery	Personal recovery
Values and power arrangements	
(Apparently) value-free	Value-centred
Professional accountability	Personal responsibility
Control oriented	Oriented to choice
Power over people	Awakens people's power
Basic concepts	
Scientific	Humanistic
Pathography	Biography
Psychopathology	Distressing experience
Diagnosis	Personal meaning
Treatment	Growth and discovery
Doctors and patients	Experts by training and experts by experience
Knowledge base	
Randomised controlled trials	Guiding narratives
Systematic reviews	Modelled on heroes
Decontextualised	Within a social context
Working practices	
Recognition	Understanding
Focus on the disorder	Focus on the person
Illness-based	Strengths-based
Based on reducing adverse events	Based on hopes and dreams
Individual adapts to the programme	Provider adapts to the individual
Rewards passivity and compliance	Fosters empowerment
Expert care coordinators	Self-management
Goals of the service	
Anti-disease	Pro-health
Bringing under control	Self-control
Compliance	Choice
Return to normal	Transformation

maximise the conceptual coherence of efforts to support recovery, an organising framework for types of pro-recovery practice is needed. This is developed in the section 'How recovery can be supported by mental health services'.

How recovery can be supported by mental health services

Although guidance on recovery-oriented practice exists, there remains a lack of clarity regarding best practice [45]. An empirically based recovery practice framework was therefore developed to address this knowledge gap [46]. The practice framework was developed by analysing 30 documents from six countries

(Denmark, England, New Zealand, Republic of Ireland, Scotland, United States) detailing international practice guidance on supporting recovery. Inductive thematic analysis was used to systematically identify and synthesise the range and diversity of the key concepts of recovery-oriented practice identified in the reviewed documents. Data extracts from each document were selected by two raters on the basis of the following criteria: described characteristics of recovery-oriented practice, provided definitions of recovery-oriented practice, or offered standards or indicators of recovery-oriented practice from which a succinct summary could be extracted. Initial semantic-level analysis was then undertaken by four analysts. Equal attention was paid to each data extract to identify initial codes, and individual extracts were coded under one or several themes to fully capture their meaning. An initial coding frame was developed; all extracts were double-coded by at least two raters, and a third rater resolved any differences. Interpretive analysis was then undertaken to organise the themes into practice domains. Thematic maps were used to organise the themes by clustering all codes according to connections in the data and by considering the patterns and relationships between themes. Additional codes, refinements to the specifics of themes and thematic patterns continued until theoretical saturation was achieved. Four overarching levels of practice emerged from the synthesis: promoting citizenship, organisational commitment, supporting personally defined recovery and working relationship. Each practice domain is as important as the next, and there is no hierarchical order.

The framework shows that citizenship can be promoted across the health system, so people with mental illness are supported to live as equal citizens. Themes of seeing beyond the service user, human needs, social inclusion and meaningful occupation are grouped in the promoting citizenship practice domain. It also highlights that organisational support for recovery involves demonstrating that services are responsive to the needs of people living with mental illness and not primarily to the needs of services. Themes of recovery vision, workplace support structures, quality improvement, care pathway and workforce planning sit within the organisational commitment practice domain.

The framework points to the importance of individual practitioners viewing recovery support as central to practice and not as an additional task. Themes of individuality, informed choice, peer support, strengths focus and holistic approach are contained in the supporting personally defined recovery practice domain. It also identifies the importance of forming partnership relationships where people accessing services are empowered to lead the intervention process and to shape their own future. Themes of partnership working and hope are the focus of the working relationship practice domain.

The framework provides direction to individual professionals about supporting recovery in their own practice, and to services when considering implementation of a recovery orientation across the organisation. Although the understanding of recovery and recovery-oriented practice is still developing, the framework shows that services and professionals can play a pivotal role in supporting the implementation of recovery-oriented practice across all four practice domains.

Having established an empirically based recovery practice framework, a second conceptual contribution is to review the available evidence for interventions to support recovery.

The evidence for personal recovery

One implication of the traction gained by recovery is that ideas are appropriately becoming subject to scientific scrutiny and empirical investigation, using the methods of evidence-based medicine [47]. To provide a conceptual framework within which to understand how personal recovery is operationalised, a systematic review was undertaken to collate and synthesise published frameworks and models of recovery [48]. A total of 97 papers from 13 different countries which offered new conceptualisations of recovery were identified, based on 366 reviewed papers. The types of papers included qualitative studies, narrative literature reviews, book chapters, consultation documents reporting the use of consensus methods, opinion pieces, editorials, quantitative studies as well as papers which combined different methods. Empirical studies recruited participants from a range of settings including community mental health teams and facilities, self-help groups, consumer-operated mental health services and supported housing facilities. The majority of studies used inclusion criteria that covered any diagnosis of severe mental illness.

Data were extracted by one rater with a random subsample of 88 papers independently rated by a second, and disagreements resolved by a third rater. Included papers were quality assessed by independent raters. Analysis involved three stages. In Stage 1, a preliminary synthesis was developed using tabulation, translating data through thematic analysis of good-quality primary data and vote counting of emergent themes. An initial coding framework was developed and used to thematically analyse a subsample of qualitative research studies with the highest quality rating. The main overarching themes and related subthemes occurring across the tabulated data were identified, using inductive, open coding techniques. Additional codes were created by all analysts where needed, and these new codes were regularly merged with the master copy, and then this copy was shared with other analysts, so all new codes were applied to the entire subsample. Once the themes had been created, vote counting was used to identify the frequency with which themes appeared in all of the 97 included papers. This process produced the preliminary conceptual framework. In Stage 2, the relationships within and between studies were explored. Papers were identified from the full review which reported data from people from Black and minority ethnic (BME) backgrounds. These papers were thematically analysed separately, and the emergent themes compared with the preliminary conceptual framework. The aim of the subgroup analysis was to specifically identify any additional themes as well as any difference in emphasis placed on areas of the preliminary framework. In Stage 3, the robustness of the synthesis was assessed, in two ways. First, qualitative studies which were rated as moderate quality were thematically analysed until category saturation was achieved. The resulting themes were then compared with the preliminary conceptual framework developed in Stages 1 and 2. Second, the preliminary conceptual framework was sent to an expert consultation panel ($n=54$), and the preliminary conceptual framework was modified in response to comments.

The modified narrative synthesis of these papers showed that recovery can be thought of (a) as a journey which varies from one person to another, (b) as interlinking sets of processes, and (c) can also be understood through the application of social cognition models of how the recovery journey itself varies over time and within individuals. The narrative synthesis identified 13 characteristics of the recovery journey (e.g. Recovery is an active process, Individual and unique process, Non-linear process, Recovery as a struggle, Recovery is a life-changing experience, Recovery without cure), 5 overarching recovery processes comprising Connectedness, Hope and optimism about the future, Identity, Meaning in life and Empowerment (giving the acronym CHIME) and 13 stage models of recovery. The synthesis is applicable across Western cultures [49].

The CHIME framework identifies five key recovery processes. To fully support recovery, evidence syntheses are needed, which collate the evidence for interventions improving these five domains.

By contrast, the current evidence base which informs clinical guidelines is organised around the evidence for existing interventions, which predominantly target symptomatology and social functioning. For example, in England the National Institute for Health and Clinical Excellence produces clinical guidelines for a range of disorders, including the schizophrenia guideline updated in 2009 [50]. The clinical evidence summary chapter comprises 141 tables, organised by intervention: psychopharmacological interventions ($n=73$), family interventions ($n=14$), psychoeducation ($n=11$), Cognitive Behavioural Therapy ($n=10$), social skills training ($n=7$), service models (early intervention, ACT, crisis intervention) ($n=7$), counselling ($n=6$), psychodynamic interventions ($n=4$), arts therapy ($n=4$), Cognitive Remediation Therapy ($n=3$) and adherence therapy ($n=2$). The question of what services should be provided is a central question for planning, commissioning and evaluating services. However, the information needed to inform clinical decision-making at the level of individual services users is different, and would more helpfully be organised in relation to interventions which might improve hope, increase empowerment, etc. Evidence syntheses organised by intervention meet the service need (and is, of course, a reasonable activity), but they may not produce the information most helpful in supporting recovery.

As a related observation, most of the evidence presented in these tables relates to symptomatology, side effects and social functioning – in other words, the priorities of clinical recovery. Yet there is an emerging empirical evidence base for interventions targeting the recovery processes identified in the CHIME framework. We now briefly and selectively review some of the evidence base for interventions targeted at each process.

Connectedness

Despite the many policies [51] and books [52] highlighting the importance of social inclusion, empirical research into interventions which improve connectedness is limited [53]. The strongest evidence base relates to employment and meaningful activities [54], with Individual Placement and Support model [55] showing particular promise. There is some evidence for interventions to support relationships with others, including for example the beneficial impact of meeting other people with personal experience of mental illness – either through their employment as peer support workers within the mental health system [56] or (with weaker evidence) through mutual self-help groups [1]. A number of national anti-stigma campaigns have been undertaken internationally, using three broad approaches: educational lectures and information, video-based media and social contact with individuals with lived experience. A review of such interventions indicated that direct social contact with people with mental illness was the most effective method of changing attitudes towards mental health problems [57], and the first empirical evidence of a shift in societal attitudes following a national campaign is emerging [58].

Hope and optimism

A systematic review of candidate interventions for fostering hope identified promising interventions including collaborative illness management strategies, fostering positive relationships, peer support, and support to set and attain realistic personally valued goals [59]. A specific approach is Wellness Recovery Action Planning (WRAP), which is an evidence-based strategy used internationally to promote wellness and recovery through the development of coping strategies [60]. WRAP stands out as an intervention which has been widely evaluated using both randomised and non-randomised designs. Positive outcomes include increased hopefulness [61–63], among others.

Identity

Interventions to support the development and maintenance of a positive identity are lacking. Approaches which are worth developing as intervention technologies include life-story work and narrative therapy. Life-story work aims to help individuals develop their personal narrative. It has been shown to be effective in people with dementia [64], and has been modified for use by people with a diagnosis of psychosis [65], with an evaluation underway [66]. A key challenge for future research will be developing interventions which are sensitive to non-individualistic expressions of identity – an emphasis on collectivist identity is one way in which the experience of recovery differs for individuals from BME communities [48]. Finally, symptom severity is linked to the integrity of the person's narrative [67], so evidence-based interventions with a symptomatic focus may also contribute.

Meaning and purpose

Meaning and purpose in life finds expression in many ways, but one key aspect is through spirituality and religion. Unfortunately, these domains are not only de-prioritised but often actively excluded from clinical discourse. For example, an intervention involving spiritual assessment by psychiatrists showed benefits for service users but low acceptance by participating psychiatrists [68]. Other professional groups are more amenable to spirituality discussions [69], and the approach is starting to be incorporated into psychological therapies [70]. More generally, there is a need to use knowledge derived from other areas of research, including mental capital [71] and positive psychology [72], in the development of pro-recovery interventions for use in mental health services [73].

Empowerment

Several interventions have been developed which target personal responsibility and control, including advance directives [74], joint crisis plans [75] and shared decision-making [76]. A specific well-evaluated and widely used approach is the strengths model of case management, which focuses on the relationships between staff and consumers, prioritises strengths over deficits, is consumer led and actively promotes resource acquisition through advocacy [77]. Evaluations have included randomised controlled trials and quasi-experimental designs, showing a range of positive outcomes including reduced hospitalisation, increased social support, goal setting and goal attainment. Positive psychology interventions, such as positive psychotherapy [78], also identify and amplify an individual's capabilities and resources through the therapeutic process, with the aim of developing positive mental health including resilience and uplifting emotional experiences. These interventions can be provided online, and benefits have been shown for depressive symptomatology [79], reduced service use [80] and self-rated happiness [81]. However, routine assessment and focus on strengths is not yet widespread in mental health services [82].

The aforementioned selective review of evidence relating to the CHIME framework, if undertaken with sufficient resources to be systematic, might point to a different way of developing mental health services. Key changes would be a more explicit emphasis on outcome-focused care, and the mainstream availability of interventions which more directly target recovery outcomes (i.e. the CHIME framework), such as peer support workers, WRAP, the strengths model, life mapping and positive psychotherapy.

The REFOCUS intervention

A key knowledge gap relates to the development of manualised interventions which have a coherent conceptual foundation. Using the scientific building blocks described in the sections 'How recovery can be supported by mental health services' and 'The evidence for personal recovery', the REFOCUS Programme addresses this knowledge gap. The programme involves an inter-linked series of studies funded in England through the Programme Grants for Applied Research scheme of the National Institute for Health Research (Reference RP-PG-0707-10040). Further information about the programme of work is at researchintorecovery.com/refocus. One component of the work is the development and randomised controlled trial evaluation of a manualised intervention to support recovery.

The REFOCUS intervention is a manualised, pro-recovery, 12-month intervention which has been developed for use within adult community mental health teams [65]. In relation to the recovery practice framework described in the section 'How recovery can be supported by mental health services', it targets two domains: supporting personally defined recovery and working relationships. In other words, the focus is on the interventions provided by staff, and the interpersonal context in which those interventions are provided. It is summarised to staff as 'what you do and how you do it'. The intervention dovetails with another national initiative underway across England which targets the domain of organisational commitment [83].

The overall aim is to increase the focus of community adult mental health teams on supporting personal recovery. The intervention is delivered in addition to standard care and has been designed to be delivered by all members of staff who provide clinical input into the team, representing a variety of positions, levels and expertise. The intervention content is informed by the systematic review of recovery processes described in the section 'The evidence for personal recovery', and comprises two components: Recovery-promoting relationships and Working practices. Whilst the goal of the intervention is to change individual level practice, there is an underlying assumption that only team-level implementation will make individual change happen. Therefore, the intervention is provided to the whole team. The intervention is not specifically focused upon changing team culture; however, there is necessarily an element of needing to change how teams work by providing team-level training and reflection opportunities for the team to feel it 'owns' recovery.

The working relationship between staff and people who use the service is central to personal recovery. Developing and supporting this relationship involves a number of different activities. For teams, it involves training and reflection sessions to develop a shared understanding of personal recovery within the team, and planning and carrying out a partnership project with people who use the service. For individual workers, it involves exploring their own values and developing skills in coaching and using a coaching stance. It also is important to raise expectations held by people who use the service that their values, strengths and goals will be prioritised.

The intervention involves three working practices. First, to ensure that care planning is based around the person's values and treatment preferences, the intervention involves individuals who use the service discussing their values and treatment preferences with staff, who then record these values and treatment preferences on the clinical information system. Service users differ in how they wish to communicate this information, so staff are trained in three approaches to supporting this working practice: conversational, narrative and visual.

The second working practice involves assessing strengths, to ensure care planning is focused on amplifying a person's strengths and ability to access community supports. The intervention involves individuals who use services identifying their strengths with staff, who then record these strengths on the clinical information system. A systematic review of strengths assessments for use in mental health services was undertaken, in which the Strengths Assessment Worksheet (SAW) [77] was identified as the most widely used and evaluated. Staff are trained to undertake a strengths assessment using the SAW.

The third working practice involves supporting goal-striving, to ensure care planning is oriented around personally valued goals and that staff support active goal-striving by the service user. The intervention involves people who use the service identifying their personally valued goals with staff, staff support-ing the person in their striving towards their goals, and staff recording personally valued goals on the clinical information system.

These working practices will only be implemented in the context of relation-ships explicitly focused on supporting recovery. Therefore, the intervention also includes approaches to fostering pro-recovery relationships between front-line clinical workers and the service users with whom they work. Components of the intervention which target relationships are:

1 Information sessions with service users, to raise their expectations of having these conversations and resulting actions with staff (90 minutes)
2 Information sessions with staff, to orientate them to the intervention (60 minutes)
3 Training for staff in personal recovery, delivered by trainers with both professional expertise and lived experience, to provide the necessary knowledge, promote values self-awareness, and model partnership working (three half-day training sessions)
4 Training for staff in using coaching as an interpersonal style in their work with service users, and as a vehicle for implementing the three working practices (one full-day and three half-day training sessions)
5 Front-line staff reflection sessions, to provide a safe and facilitated space in which to reflect on and maximise the impact of the intervention on their work (six 1-hour sessions)

6 Team manager reflection sessions, to provide an opportunity for team leaders to identify and address organisational obstacles to implementation (five 1-hour sessions)

7 Use of a supervision reflection form, to encourage self-reflection and discussion in supervision of role challenges experienced

8 Telephone booster sessions for specific coaching and working practices supervision (two 1-hour sessions)

9 A partnership project, in which each team is encouraged to apply for up to UK£500 (€600) to undertake a project involving staff and service users as equal participants, such as a community development project

The intervention is based on an explicit model, and fully described in the manual [65], which can be downloaded for free at researchintorecovery.com/refocus. It is currently being evaluated in a cluster randomised controlled trial (ISRCTN02507940) being carried out in London and Gloucestershire in England [66].

Future developments

In this chapter, it has been argued that supporting personal recovery should be the goal of mental health services and systems internationally. The limitation of this argument relates to the limitations of our knowledge base.

First, it is unclear to what extent ideas of recovery, which have predominantly emerged from Western and English-speaking countries, easily translate into other cultures. Understandings of recovery and well-being exist of course in non-Western cultures. For example, the identity of indigenous Australian people is interwoven with the physical world [84]. Spiritual identity is shared with the land, a description of reality which clearly incorporates a concept of identity quite different from Western psychological, sociological and philosophical understandings. Similarly, Native American conceptions of health involve a relational or cyclical world view, balancing context, mind, body and spirit [85]. Māori and Pacific Islanders in New Zealand also have a cultural identity influenced by Whānau Ora – the diverse families embedded in the culture [23]. Using these cultural understandings to develop new frameworks for conceptualising and supporting recovery will be needed [49].

Second, there is little evidence to decide whether ideas of recovery relate to low-income countries which have a less well-developed health infrastructure. Those countries which have, for example, Mental Health Commissions (e.g. Canada, Ireland, New Zealand) or national mental health strategies (e.g. Australia, England, the United States) – through which the policy direction towards recovery are expressed – are high-income countries. Personal recovery does not yet feature prominently in global mental health initiatives, with priority indicators more oriented around health infrastructure (investment, workforce, service configurations, etc.) [86]. Similarly, the 'Grand challenges in global mental health' initiative focused on strategies for prevention and treatment of mental disorders internationally [87].

Third, there are not yet agreed approaches to measuring recovery support from services. A systematic review of recovery support measures identified 13 measures, of which 6 fitted inclusion criteria [88]. Measures were excluded because they had no published psychometric evaluation, assessing the relationship only, needing trained assessors, not providing quantitative data, or being unpublished or unavailable. Of the six included measures, none spanned the five domains of the CHIME framework (suggesting a limited conceptualisation of recovery support) and all had only limited psychometric evaluation, most notably with none having data on test–retest reliability. It was therefore not possible to recommend any measure for routine use by services. In response, a new measure called INSPIRE is being developed – further information is available at researchintorecovery.com/inspire.

Overall, the contribution of scientific research to supporting recovery is clear [89], and the evidence base is emerging. Future research to develop interventions to support key recovery processes will inform new interventions. However, 'interventions' to promote connectedness may look more like community development and anti-discrimination initiatives than health-care interventions, and mental health professionals may need to develop skills as social activists [73]. The largest contribution by mental health services to supporting recovery may come from enabling the empowerment of service users to experience the full entitlements of citizenship.

References

[1] Slade M. (2009) *Personal Recovery and Mental Illness. A Guide for Mental Health Professionals.* Cambridge: Cambridge University Press.

[2] Secker J, Membrey H, Grove B et al. (2002) Recovering from illness or recovering your life? Implications of clinical versus social models of recovery from mental health problems for employment support services. *Disability & Society* **17** (4): 403–418.

[3] Bellack A. (2006) Scientific and consumer models of recovery in schizophrenia: concordance, contrasts, and implications. *Schizophrenia Bulletin* **32**: 432–442.

[4] Schrank B, Slade M. (2007) Recovery in psychiatry. *Psychiatric Bulletin* **31**: 321–325.

[5] Libermann RP, Kopelowicz A. (2002) Recovery from schizophrenia: a challenge for the 21st century. *International Review of Psychiatry* **14**: 242–255.

[6] Huber G, Gross G, Schuttler R. (1975) A long-term follow-up study of schizophrenia: psychiatric course and prognosis. *Acta Psychiatrica Scandinavica* **52**: 49–57.

[7] Ciompi L, Muller C. (1976) *The Life-Course and Aging of Schizophrenics: A Long-Term Follow-Up Study into Old Age.* Berlin: Springer.

[8] Bleuler M. (1978) *The Schizophrenic Disorders.* New Haven: Yale University Press.

[9] Tsuang MT, Woolson RF, Fleming J. (1979) Long-term outcome of major psychosis. *Archives of General Psychiatry* **36**: 1295–1301.

[10] Harding CM, Brooks G, Ashikage T et al. (1987) The Vermont longitudinal study of persons with severe mental illness II: long-term outcome of subjects who retrospectively met DSM-III criteria for schizophrenia. *American Journal of Psychiatry* **144**: 727–735.

[11] Ogawa K, Miya M, Watarai A et al. (1987) A long-term follow-up study of schizophrenia in Japan, with special reference to the course of social adjustment. *British Journal of Psychiatry* **151**: 758–765.

[12] Marneros A, Deister A, Rohde A et al. (1989) Long-term outcome of schizoaffective and schizophrenic disorders, a comparative study, I: definitions, methods, psychopathological and social outcome. *European Archives of Psychiatry and Clinical Neuroscience* **238**: 118–125.

[13] DeSisto MJ, Harding CM, McCormick RV et al. (1995) The Maine and Vermont three-decades studies of serious mental illness: II. Longitudinal course. *British Journal of Psychiatry* **167**: 338–342.

[14] Harrison G, Hopper K, Craig T et al. (2001) Recovery from psychotic illness: a 15- and 25-year international follow-up study. *British Journal of Psychiatry* **178**: 506–517.

[15] Ralph RO, Corrigan PW. (2005) *Recovery in Mental Illness. Broadening Our Understanding of Wellness.* Washington, DC: American Psychological Association.

[16] Coleman R. (1999) *Recovery – An Alien Concept.* Gloucester: Hansell.

[17] Davidson L, Strauss J. (1992) Sense of self in recovery from severe mental illness. *British Journal of Medical Psychology* **65**: 131–145.

[18] Deegan P. (1988) Recovery: the lived experience of rehabilitation. *Psychosocial Rehabilitation Journal* **11**: 11–19.

[19] Ridgway P. (2001) Restorying psychiatric disability: learning from first person narratives. *Psychiatric Rehabilitation Journal* **24** (4): 335–343.

[20] Andresen R, Oades L, Caputi P. (2003) The experience of recovery from schizophrenia: towards an empirically-validated stage model. *Australian and New Zealand Journal of Psychiatry* **37**: 586–594.

[21] Barnett H, Lapsley H. (2006) *Journeys of Despair, Journeys of Hope. Young Adults Talk About Severe Mental Distress, Mental Health Services and Recovery.* Wellington: Mental Health Commission.

[22] Goldsack S, Reet M, Lapsley H et al. (2005) *Experiencing a Recovery-Oriented Acute Mental Health Service: Home Based Treatment from the Perspectives of Services Users, Their Families and Mental Health Professionals.* Wellington: Mental Health Commission.

[23] Lapsley H, Nikora LW, Black R. (2002) *Kia Mauri Tau! Narratives of Recovery from Disabling Mental Health Problems.* Wellington: Mental Health Commission.

[24] Scottish Recovery Network. (2007) *Routes to Recovery. Collected Wisdom from the SRN Narrative Research Project.* Glasgow: Scottish Recovery Network.

[25] Perkins R, Repper J. (2003) *Social Inclusion and Recovery.* London: Bailliere Tindall.

[26] Davidson L, Sells D, Sangster S et al. (2005) Qualitative studies of recovery: what can we learn from the person? In: Ralph RO, Corrigan PW (eds.), *Recovery in Mental Illness Broadening Our Understanding of Wellness.* Washington, DC: American Psychological Association, pp. 147–170.

[27] Spaniol L, Koehler M. (1994) *The Experience of Recovery.* Boston: Center for Psychiatric Rehabilitation.

[28] Carson J, Holloway F, Wolfson P et al. (2008) *Recovery Journeys: Stories of Coping with Mental Health Problems.* London: South London and Maudsley NHS Foundation Trust.

[29] McIntosh Z. (2005) *From Goldfish Bowl to Ocean: Personal Accounts of Mental Illness and Beyond.* London: Chipmunkapublishing.

[30] Anthony WA. (1993) Recovery from mental illness: the guiding vision of the mental health system in the 1990s. *Innovations and Research* **2**: 17–24.

[31] South London and Maudsley NHS Foundation Trust. (2010) *Social Inclusion and Recovery (SIR) Strategy 2010–2015.* London: SLAM.

[32] Department of Health and Ageing. (2009) *Fourth National Mental Health Plan: An Agenda for Collaborative Government Action in Mental Health 2009–2014*. Canberra: Commonwealth of Australia.

[33] Mental Health Commission of Canada. (2012) *Changing Directions, Changing Lives: The Mental Health Strategy for Canada*. Calgary: Mental Health Commission of Canada.

[34] HM Government. (2011) *No Health Without Mental Health. A Cross-Government Mental Health Outcomes Strategy for People of All Ages*. London: Department of Health.

[35] Department of Health Social Services and Public Safety (Northern Ireland). (2010) *Service Framework for Mental Health and Wellbeing*. Belfast: DHSSPS (NI).

[36] New Freedom Commission on Mental Health. (2003) *Achieving the Promise: Transforming Mental Health Care in America. Final Report*. Rockville: U.S. Department of Health and Human Services.

[37] Slade M, Adams N, O'Hagan M. (2012) Recovery: past progress and future challenges. *International Review of Psychiatry* **24**: 1–4.

[38] Roe D, Bril-Barniv S, Kravetz S. (2012) Recovery in Israel: a legislative recovery response to the needs-rights paradox. *International Review of Psychiatry* **24** (1): 48–55.

[39] Tse S, Cheung E, Kan A et al. (2012) Recovery in Hong Kong: service user participation in mental health services. *International Review of Psychiatry* **24**: 40–47.

[40] Davidson L, Rakfeldt J, Strauss J. (2010) *The Roots of the Recovery Movement in Psychiatry*. Chichester: Wiley-Blackwell.

[41] Amering M, Schmolke M. (2009) *Recovery in Mental Health. Reshaping Scientific and Clinical Responsibilities*. Chichester: John Wiley & Sons, Ltd.

[42] Corrigan P, Mueser KT, Bond GR et al. (2008) *Principles and Practice of Psychiatric Rehabilitation: An Empirical Approach*. New York: Guilford Press.

[43] Roberts G, Davenport S, Holloway F et al. (2006) *Enabling Recovery. The Principles and Practice of Rehabilitation Psychiatry*. London: Gaskell.

[44] Davidson L, Tondora J, Lawless MS et al. (2009) *A Practical Guide to Recovery-Oriented Practice Tools for Transforming Mental Health Care*. Oxford: Oxford University Press.

[45] Lakeman R. (2010) Mental health recovery competencies for mental health workers: a Delphi study. *Journal of Mental Health* **19** (1): 62–74.

[46] Le Boutillier C, Leamy M, Bird VJ et al. (2011) What does recovery mean in practice? A qualitative analysis of international recovery-oriented practice guidance. *Psychiatric Services* **62**: 1470–1476.

[47] Slade M, Williams J, Bird V et al. (2012) Recovery grows up. *Journal of Mental Health* **21** (2): 99–103.

[48] Leamy M, Bird V, Le Boutillier C et al. (2011) A conceptual framework for personal recovery in mental health: systematic review and narrative synthesis. *British Journal of Psychiatry* **199**: 445–452.

[49] Slade M, Leamy M, Bacon F et al. (2012) International differences in understanding recovery: systematic review. *Epidemiology and Psychiatric Sciences* **21**: 353–364.

[50] National Collaborating Centre for Mental Health. (2009) *Core Interventions in the Treatment and Management of Schizophrenia in Primary and Secondary Care (Update)*. London: National Institute for Health and Clinical Excellence.

[51] South Australian Social Inclusion Board. (2007) *Stepping Up: A Social Inclusion Action Plan for Mental Health Reform 2007–2012*. Adelaide: Government of South Australia.

[52] Boardman J, Currie A, Killaspy H et al. (2010) *Social Inclusion and Mental Health*. London: RCPsych Publications.

[53] Tew J, Ramon S, Slade M et al. (2012) Social factors and recovery from mental health difficulties: a review of the evidence. *British Journal of Social Work* **42**: 443–460.

[54] Crowther RE, Marshall M, Bond GR et al. (2001) Vocational rehabilitation for people with severe mental illness. *Cochrane Database of Systematic Reviews* **2**: 1–55.

[55] Killackey E, Jackson H, McGorry PD. (2008) Vocational intervention in first-episode psychosis: individual placement and support v. treatment as usual. *British Journal of Psychiatry* **193**: 114–120.

[56] Repper J, Carter T. (2011) A review of the literature on peer support in mental health services. *Journal of Mental Health* **20** (4): 392–411.

[57] Clement S, Lassman F, Barley E et al. (2011) Mass media interventions for reducing mental health-health related stigma (Protocol). *Cochrane of Database of Systematic Reviews* **12**: CD009453

[58] Henderson C, Corker E, Lewis-Holmes E et al. (2012) England's time to change antistigma campaign: one-year outcomes of service user-rated experiences of discrimination. *Psychiatric Services* **63** (5): 451–457.

[59] Schrank B, Bird V, Rudnick A et al. (2012) Determinants, self-management strategies and interventions for hope in people with mental disorders: systematic search and narrative review. *Social Science & Medicine* **74**: 554–564.

[60] Copeland ME. (1999) *Wellness Recovery Action Plan*. Brattleboro: VT Peach Press.

[61] Barbic S, Krupa T, Armstrong I. (2009) A randomized controlled trial of the effectiveness of a modified recovery workbook program: preliminary findings. *Psychiatric Services* **60**: 491–497.

[62] Cook JA. (2011) Peer-delivered wellness recovery services: from evidence to widespread implementation. *Psychiatric Rehabilitation Journal* **35** (2): 87–89.

[63] Fukui S, Starnino VR, Susana M et al. (2011) Effect of wellness recovery action plan (WRAP) participation on psychiatric symptoms, sense of hope, and recovery. *Psychiatric Rehabilitation Journal* **34** (3): 214–222.

[64] Subramaniam P, Woods B. (2012) The impact of individual reminiscence therapy for people with dementia: systematic review. *Expert Review of Neurotherapeutics* **12** (5): 545–555.

[65] Bird V, Leamy M, Le Boutillier C et al. (2011) *REFOCUS: Promoting Recovery in Community Mental Health Services*. London: Rethink. Available from: researchintorecovery.com/ refocus. Accessed on 4 January 2013.

[66] Slade M, Bird V, Le Boutillier C et al. (2011) REFOCUS trial: protocol for a cluster randomised controlled trial of a pro-recovery intervention within community based mental health teams. *BMC Psychiatry* **11**: 185.

[67] Lysaker PH, Erikson M, Macapagal KR et al. (2012) Development of personal narratives as a mediator of the impact of deficits in social cognition and social withdrawal on negative symptoms in schizophrenia. *Journal of Nervous and Mental Disease* **200** (4): 290–295.

[68] Huguelet P, Mohr S, Betrisey C et al. (2011) A randomized trial of spiritual assessment of outpatients with schizophrenia: patients' and clinicians' experience. *Psychiatric Services* **62**: 79–86.

[69] Post BC, Wade NG. (2009) Religion and spirituality in psychotherapy: a practice-friendly review of research. *Journal of Clinical Psychology* **65** (2): 131–146.

[70] Hathaway W, Tan E. (2009) Religiously oriented mindfulness-based cognitive therapy. *Journal of Clinical Psychology* **65** (2): 158–171.

[71] Foresight Mental Capital Wellbeing Project. (2008) *Mental Capital and Wellbeing: Making the Most of Ourselves in the 21st Century. Final Project Report*. London: Government Office for Science.

[72] Henry J. (2007) Positive psychology and the development of well-being. In: Haworth J, Hart G (eds.), *Well-Being: Individual, Community and Societal Perspectives*. Basingstoke: Palgrave Macmillan, pp. 25–40.

[73] Slade M. (2010) Mental illness and well-being: the central importance of positive psychology and recovery approaches. *BMC Health Services Research* **10**: 26.

[74] Swanson J, Swartz M, Ferron J et al. (2006) Facilitated psychiatric advance directives: a randomized trial of an intervention to foster advance treatment planning among persons with severe mental illness. *American Journal of Psychiatry* **163**: 1943–1951.

[75] Henderson C, Flood C, Leese M et al. (2004) Effect of joint crisis plans on use of compulsory treatment in psychiatry: single blind randomised controlled trial. *BMJ* **329**: 136–140.

[76] Drake RE, Deegan PE. (2009) Shared decision making is an ethical imperative. *Psychiatric Services* **60** (8): 1007.

[77] Rapp C, Goscha RJ. (2006) *The Strengths Model: Case Management with People with Psychiatric Disabilities*, 2nd edn. New York: Oxford University Press.

[78] Seligman M, Rashid T, Parks AC. (2006) Positive psychotherapy. *American Psychologist* **61** (8): 774–788.

[79] Lopez SJ, Edwards LM. (2008) The interface of counseling psychology and positive psychology: assessing and promoting strengths. In: Brown SD, Lent RW (eds.), *Handbook of Counseling Psychology*, 4th edn. Hoboken: John Wiley & Sons, Inc., pp. 86–99.

[80] Duckworth LA, Steen TA, Seligman ME. (2005) Positive psychology in clinical practice. *Annual Review of Clinical Psychology* **1**: 629–651.

[81] Seligman MEP, Steen TA, Park N et al. (2005) Positive psychology progress: empirical validation of interventions. *Tidsskrift for Norsk Psykologforening* **42** (10): 874–884.

[82] Bird V, Le Boutillier C, Leamy M et al. (2012) Assessing the strengths of mental health service users – systematic review. *Psychological Assessment* **24**: 1024–1033.

[83] Perkins R, Slade M. (2012) Recovery in England: transforming statutory services? *International Review of Psychiatry* **24**: 29–39.

[84] Flood J. (1991) *Archaeology of the Dreamtime: The Story of Prehistoric Australia and Its People*. Sydney: Collins.

[85] Cross T, Earle K, Echo-Hawk-Solie H et al. (2000) *Cultural Strengths and Challenges in Implementing a System of Care Model in American Indian Communities*. Systems of Care: Promising Practices in Children's Mental Health, 2000 series (vol. 1). Washington, DC: Center for Effective Collaboration and Practice, American Institutes for Research, pp. 8–14.

[86] Chisholm D, Flisher AJ, Lund C et al. (2007) Scale up services for mental disorders: a call for action. *Lancet* **370** (9594): 1241–1252.

[87] Collins PY, Patel V, Joestl SS et al. (2011) Grand challenges in global mental health. *Nature* **475** (7354): 27–30.

[88] Williams J, Leamy M, Bird V et al. (2012) Measures of the recovery orientation of mental health services: systematic review. *Social Psychiatry and Psychiatric Epidemiology* **47**: 1827–1835.

[89] Slade M, Hayward M. (2007) Recovery, psychosis and psychiatry: research is better than rhetoric. *Acta Psychiatrica Scandinavica* **116** (2): 81–83.

SECTION 2
Meeting the global challenge

CHAPTER 5

Implementing evidence-based treatments in routine mental health services: Strategies, obstacles, new developments to better target care provided

Antonio Lasalvia, Sarah Tosato, Katia De Santi, Doriana Cristofalo, Chiara Bonetto and Mirella Ruggeri

Department of Public Health and Community Medicine, Section of Psychiatry, University of Verona, Verona, Italy

Introduction

Over the past two decades, the *evidence-based medicine* (EBM) paradigm – the systematic use of scientific evidence in clinical decision-making – has gained increasing attention and profoundly changed practices of health-care professionals [1]. The four fundamental principles of EBM have been outlined as (i) use the best available scientific evidence, (ii) individualise the evidence, (iii) incorporate patient preferences and (iv) expand clinical expertise. The *evidence-based practice* refers to the extent to which individual practitioners, teams and departments/hospitals follow and practise the principles of EBM. The application of the four fundamental principles is required to guide the decision-making at various levels by individual clinicians/teams and by departments/institutions as a standard practice for evidence-based practice [2].

Administrators, clinicians, user organisations and researchers generally agree that they are obliged to provide the most effective mental health treatments. Implementing evidence-based practices in routine treatment settings is a crucial part of this [3]. Once research has shown which treatments are most effective, dissemination of this information and implementation of these treatments by individual clinicians and health services as a whole becomes the goal. Over the years, in different health service settings, both public health authorities and professional organisations have developed

Improving Mental Health Care: The Global Challenge, First Edition.
Edited by Graham Thornicroft, Mirella Ruggeri and David Goldberg.
© 2013 John Wiley & Sons, Ltd. Published 2013 by John Wiley & Sons, Ltd.

various modes of implementing evidence-based practice in routine conditions, including treatment algorithms, procedures to base care on evidence-based practices and practice guidelines [4, 5].

Discrepancies between research evidence and clinical practice: The efficacy–effectiveness and the evidence–practice gaps

Despite the growing body of evidence accumulating over the years on the most effective treatments in medicine, a gap has been described between the efficacy achieved with the methodology adopted by EBM – such as randomised controlled trials (RCTs) – in experimental settings and its effectiveness when the treatment was applied in real-world clinical practice. This phenomenon, sometimes called the 'efficacy–effectiveness' gap, has been demonstrated in multiple settings within health care, including psychiatry [6], and cited as a potential barrier to achieving optimal benefit from available treatments [7]. Another problem is that extensive empirical research demonstrates that several pharmacological and psychosocial interventions are effective in improving the lives of persons with severe mental illnesses [8, 9]; but, despite this knowledge base, practices supported by research evidence are not widely offered in routine mental health services [10]. This might be called the 'evidence–practice' gap.

For instance, in the United States the Schizophrenia Patient Outcome Research Team (PORT) found that patients affected by schizophrenia were highly unlikely to receive treatment shown in research to be effective [11]; even standard medication practices supported by research were usually not followed, and as few as 10% of patients received more complex interventions, such as supported employment or family psychoeducation. The problem of poor access to evidence-based practices for persons with severe mental illness has been cited by numerous reviewers of the literature [12]. Thus, a critical challenge for the mental health field is to facilitate the widespread adoption of research-based practices in routine mental health-care settings so that persons with severe mental illness can benefit from interventions that have been shown to work [10].

More recently, discrepancies between the best available evidence, as contained in the clinical guideline recommendations, and routine practices have been reported by the SIEP-DIRECT'S (DIscrepancy between Routine practice and Evidence in psychiatric Community Treatments on Schizophrenia) Project. The SIEP-DIRECT'S Project was a multi-site research conducted in 19 community mental health services located throughout Italy, aimed at identifying discrepancies between evidence and routine practice in the treatment of patients with schizophrenia [13]. A panel of experts developed and tested a set of 103 indicators that operationalise preferred clinical practice requirements according to the National Institute for Health and Clinical Excellence (NICE) guidelines of schizophrenia (the full text of the indicators both in Italian and in English are available online at http://www.psychiatry.univr.it/page_eps/back_issues.htm [14]). The data yielded by this project demonstrate that an advanced community care model, such as the one developed in Italy over the last 30 years, has the capacity to quickly intervene, engage patients suffering from severe mental illness and interact appropriately with the agencies operating in the surrounding community and with patients' social networks. In the participating services, clinical practices concerning drug use were shown to be acceptably in line with the NICE clinical guidelines, although major discrepancies between evidence and guidelines regarding several other aspects were detected: a lack of written guidelines and protocols to use as a guide for treatment provision; an underestimation of the importance of systematically providing users with information on diagnosis, outcomes and treatments; a tendency to avoid implementing specific and structured forms of intervention and monitoring their outcomes; and difficulty in considering patients' family members as individuals directly requiring specific forms of support and who should also be regularly involved in the patient care process. The SIEP-DIRECT'S Project data indicate that too many services are still operating under the influence of these attitudes.

Although this gap between knowledge and practice is not unique to the mental health field, the challenge for public mental health systems is to ensure that evidence-based practices become more broadly available and more seamlessly integrated into existing systems of care. This effort to narrow the gap between knowledge and practice is critically predicated on a broad range of effectiveness studies that continually inform the existing knowledge base [15]. Besides political and budgetary constraints, a major obstacle to broad-based implementation is a knowledge gap related to the active ingredients of successful programmes, and to mechanisms that facilitate and catalyse the implementation of innovative programmes in mental health systems. Also, while there are emerging models related to implementation of evidence-based practices in site-specific or organisation-specific settings, models – especially evidence-based models – for broad-based, system-wide implementation are lacking [16].

It is important not only to translate the *content* of research evidence into clinical practice but also that clinicians – in clinical practice – try to adopt some of the *processes* that have been shown to be effective in RCTs, including routine outcome measurement and involvement of patients in decision-making. This implies translating the *how* from RCTs to real-world clinical care, something which has received relatively less attention [17]. This barrier thus pertains to the 'efficacy–effectiveness' gap. Progress in the domain of routine outcome assessment is the key to implementing research findings into ordinary practice and monitoring its impact. Routine and systematic measures of patients' functioning and well-being, along with disorder-specific clinical outcomes at appropriate time intervals, have been long recognised as important tools for patient management [18].

The assessment of effectiveness and efficiency should be based on the outcome of individual patients and, by aggregation, the outcomes achieved by health services. This should be performed not only through traditional or 'driven' outcome assessment (i.e. an assessment carried out by well-trained external raters using a wide variety of assessment instruments), but also on evaluation performed by clinicians in the context of their own routine practice [19]. The use of outcome instruments may actually enhance, rather than detract, the patient-centredness of the mental care experience [20]. As patient-centred approach facilitates patient participation and actively seeks the patient's perspective in the treatment interaction, this has been found to be associated with increased satisfaction [21], better treatment adherence [22] and less symptoms burden [23]. The use of patient-rated outcome measures, particularly those that capture important aspects of the patient's experience (such as quality of life, emotional distress or service satisfaction), may increase health professionals' awareness and the ability to address patients' concerns [24]. With routine collection and regular feedback to treating staff, these standardised measures, augmented in some cases by individualised patient measures, can be used to track treatment process from both staff and patient perspectives [25]. Despite the growing international consensus that outcomes should be routinely measured in clinical practice [26], routine use of this approach is unfortunately limited. A number of barriers to adoption of standardised routine outcome assessment in real-world settings have been described, including lack of familiarity with measurement instruments, lack of faith in the basic psychometric properties of available tools, lack of time and resources needed to complete and review measure, lack of concordance between measures and treatment philosophy and organisational resistance to change [27, 28]. Standardised outcome measurement will not become the routine until these barriers are addressed.

Translating research evidence into clinical practice: The case of early intervention in psychosis

The general consensus on the continuing 'evidence–practice' gap has prompted greater efforts to disseminate and implement evidence-based practices in community-based settings by highlighting the epidemiology of evidence-based health intervention data and by adapting and putting these interventions into practice over time. To accomplish this goal, researchers find themselves grappling with a number of key issues, including how to best translate intervention programmes to encourage uptake and implementation in ways that preserve the scientifically validated components of evidence-based practices and how to integrate the efforts of the various stakeholders in settings over which researchers have little control. It is therefore becoming ever more crucial to perform implementation studies and develop ways to sustain intervention programmes aimed to maintain the integrity of evidence-based treatments in real-world settings after the completion of the research phase.

The case of early intervention in psychosis seems particularly interesting in this regard and deserves specific attention. Various attempts have been made over recent years to implement specialised treatment services for young patients experiencing a first-episode of psychosis with the aim of offering evidence-based care that optimises outcomes and minimises deterioration. These services are based on mounting evidence from randomised controlled studies showing that specialised early psychosis services are more effective than treatment as usual [29, 30]. These programmes are being conducted either in stand-alone specific services or by dedicated teams working within the framework of existing community mental health services. Early intervention programmes incorporated principles of treatment shown to be effective in schizophrenia and related disorders but accurately modified to meet the specific needs of patients with first-episode psychosis (FEP) (mostly adolescents or young adults) that are largely different from those of previously treated patients with more established conditions [31]. The considerable development and interest in this area has also been reflected by government guidance on mental health policy implementation in the United Kingdom, which explicitly directs health-care providers to ensure that first-episode teams are in place and that they provide cognitive-behavioural psychological interventions for people with first-onset psychosis for the three years following presentation to services [32]. Although the enthusiasm in regard to the potential benefits of specialised early intervention services has resulted in significant shifts in policy and resource allocation in some countries (e.g. the United Kingdom), it also generated a continuing debate about the feasibility of these new shifts in service development and on their sustainability over the long run [33–37]. Although emerging evidence from recent RCTs indicates that integrated multi-element early intervention programmes have clinically important short-term benefits over standard care [38], other research reports that the interventions are effective only as long as actively implemented [39] and clinical gains made in the first one to two years of early intervention services are lost once the patient, in the subsequent phases of illness, is referred to generalist mental health teams [40]. The potential for improving outcome of FEP patients must rely not only on an earlier timing of interventions, but also on improved treatment strategies that are more suited to the earlier phase of illness and to a younger patient population. In fact, a number of clinical practice guidelines have been developed over the past few years [41], which make a number of recommendations and list several crucial service components that should be included in treatment services, such as cognitive-behavioural strategies, early family psychoeducation, assertive outreach and supported employment.

There is however emerging evidence that psychosocial interventions which have been proved to be effective are not widely provided to FEP patients in routine settings (i.e. 'evidence–practice' gap). The findings from the SIEP-DIRECT'S Project on the treatment of the first episode of schizophrenia [13] showed that Italian mental health services, while having good capacity to maintain patients 'in treatment' and a good rapidity of response to first-episode treatment demand, need improvements with regard to availability of specialised early intervention services or specific care pathways for FEP patients within generalist mental health services. The SIEP-DIRECT'S Project also found that the low frequency use of psychotherapeutic, psychosocial and rehabilitative approaches observed in the treatment of chronic patients [42] was even lower for FEP patients. This sounds somewhat paradoxical since the first episode is precisely the right time when these approaches, if applied with the required specificity, can play a key role in increasing the patient's probability of recovery. A more widespread diffusion of these practices on a nationwide scale must be considered a future priority [13].

Additional information on discrepancies between evidence and routine treatment provided to FEP patients have been given by the Psychosis Incident Cohort Outcome Study (PICOS) [43, 44]. The PICOS is a large multi-site naturalistic research which aimed to examine the relative role of clinical, social, genetic and morpho-functional brain factors in predicting symptomatic and functional outcomes in a large cohort of FEP patients receiving care from public mental health services located in a broad area (nearly 3.3 million inhabitants) of the Veneto region, north-eastern Italy. According to the data collected in the PICOS, standard care for FEP patients generally consists of personalised outpatient psychopharmacological treatment, combined with non-specific supportive clinical management at the community mental health centre level or – when required – in patients' homes. When necessary, brief hospital stays can also be arranged in small inpatient psychiatric units located in public general hospitals. Family interventions generally consist of non-specific informal support/ educational sessions [45]. However, specialised individual psychotherapeutic interventions for patients (including cognitive-behavioural therapy (CBT)) and specialised psychoeducational or cognitive-oriented family interventions are usually not provided due to the lack of trained professionals [46].

Overall, what emerges from the SIEP-DIRECT'S and the PICOS findings is a picture where service engagement for FEP patients is, on average, rather good; and as continuity of mental health care is an indicator of the quality of care, data support high quality of care provided by the Italian community-based mental health system under this respect. However, routine treatment for FEP patients seems to lack specificity: in fact, mental health care delivered by Italian mental health services does not seem to meet the most recent guidelines recommendations, and this specifically applies to the more structured psychosocial interventions and/or for those interventions with a higher 'technological content' (such as CBT or family psychoeducation).

Challenges and obstacles of implementing evidence-based treatment in early psychosis

There are a number of methodological challenges that may influence the implementation of early intervention services in routine settings [47].

One problem is that in an area such as psychological treatments, which have been proved to be the pivotal component in the early psychosis services [48], it is important to derive treatments from a sound theoretical base and build into trial design an explanatory component to test whether the hypothesised mechanism is actually that which mediates any effect. One example of an alternative explanation would be that the clinical effect of a psychological treatment is mediated inadvertently through another therapeutic mechanism, such as improved compliance with drug treatments.

The replicability of conceptual models adopted, particularly for the psychotherapeutic interventions, is a further critical issue. CBT for psychosis, for example, typically involves a range of psychological techniques focusing on different aspects of psychopathology. The emphasis, particularly in Europe, is for the approach to be individually tailored according to individual clinical priorities and case formulation [49]. In North America, the approach tends to be a more standardised, less flexible, manualised one.

The fidelity issue is also crucial when implementing evidence-based intervention in routine practice. Findings from empirical research on the psychological interventions of mental disorders suggest that therapist competence plays a key role in producing positive treatment outcomes. Yet, the extent to which these findings generalise to the complex environment of everyday clinical practice remains unclear. The relationships between therapist adherence to theoretical models (fidelity), therapist competence, training, supervision and clinical variability must be thoroughly investigated, as well as the best ways to assess these characteristics. Treatment fidelity refers to the methodological strategies used to examine and enhance the reliability and validity of interventions [50], as it is necessary to maintain validity and to ensure a fair comparison between interventions. In the absence of fidelity evaluation, ineffective techniques may be implemented and disseminated at a high cost to the community and the individual, and disentangling specific from non-specific treatment factors may prove to be difficult. Conversely, if fidelity is not considered and non-significant results are found, it is not possible to discern whether the absence of treatment effect is due to an ineffective intervention or to poor treatment fidelity. As a result, potentially beneficial treatments for specific patient populations may be prematurely disregarded. Several features of the research setting limit the generalisability of data obtained, and it currently seems much easier to manualise therapies in research settings than in the real world [51]. Although the therapy manual is considered the main vehicle for transferring empirically supported psychotherapies into clinical practice, the actual value of generalising the requirement for treatment manual adherence is debatable. In fact, some evidence suggests that best outcomes are obtained by therapists who demonstrate flexibility by adapting their interventions to their individual clients' needs [52].

Strict adherence to a highly structured manual could prove effective, on average, for clients presenting with clearly defined problems (e.g. major depression, panic disorder, social phobia) but less so for patients experiencing a more complex series of presenting problems, such as those often encountered in the framework of early psychoses. Thus, the issue of the degree to which psychotherapies must involve flexible modification and integration to be effective when applied in everyday clinical work remains an open one.

The development of model programmes integrating a range of different medical and psychological approaches should be the main focus for future development. Service configurations like those being evaluated by Early Psychosis Prevention and Intervention Center, Lambeth Early Onset and the Calgary Early Intervention programme [38], which provide comprehensive needs-led services for FEP patients throughout the onset and early critical period of the disorder, are important, though the weakness of many of these in research terms is that it remains unclear which elements of complex programmes, sometimes given to heterogeneous samples, are effective. As a result, further controlled trials designed to evaluate the effectiveness of treatments and which elements of those are effective, and for whom, are a priority.

Although there has been much attention paid to evaluating psychological interventions in recent years, less attention has been paid to the dissemination and integration of these into routine services. The skills necessary to carry out CBT and family interventions are not routinely acquired during most mental health professional basic training and require further, specialist tuition and ongoing supervision. These pose considerable challenges to trainers and service providers as current mental health services may need to be reconfigured to integrate psychological approaches into more traditional medical models of treatment. Some research has evaluated such dissemination programmes for CBT-oriented approaches with some success. Despite this promise, other studies have shown less convincing development in services [53]. However, studies evaluating the amount to which trained staff continue to implement the techniques following training have shown that there is poor adherence to the approaches, with lack of management support, not enough time due to other work demands and poor supervision as possible reasons for non-practice of the approaches [54]. These issues will need to be addressed to allow further development of evidence-based approaches in first-episode services.

Mental health services attempting to implement complex psychosocial evidence-based practices can expect to experience significant personnel change during implementation. Recent evidence suggests that staff turnover is a hindrance to implementation of evidence-based mental health service interventions.

However, putting in place a well-qualified team, examining hiring practices for the team when staff members turn over and realigning policies to create better teams as turnover occurs can benefit implementation. Finally, it appears that practitioner perspectives on the impact of turnover on implementation are in line with the quantitative outcome data suggesting that behavioural health workforce stability plays a vital role in delivery of high-quality services [55].

Implementing evidence-based early interventions in routine settings: The GET UP programme

Research on mental health interventions for FEP patients has been developed following two different strategies [48]: (a) studies evaluating specific (i.e. single-element) interventions (e.g. individual CBT) and (b) studies evaluating comprehensive (i.e. multi-element) interventions, which may include early detection strategies, individual, group and/or family therapy and case management (in addition to pharmacological treatment). The latter appear more promising [38] and have been found to be associated with symptom reduction/remission, improved quality of life, increased social and cognitive functioning, low inpatient admission rates, improved insight, high degree of satisfaction with treatment, less time spent in hospital, decreased substance abuse and fewer self-harm episodes.

Most multi-element research programmes, however, have been conducted in experimental settings and on non-epidemiologically representative samples, thereby raising the risk of underestimating the complexities of treating FEP patients in routine 'real-world' services [56]. Moreover, most early interventions have been rarely tested for their efficacy against a control group (they rather tended to adopt historical or prospective comparison design), and usually single-group studies have been carried out, which track the progress of a single group over a given period of time. With respect to practices over the last ten years, some countries have implemented specific early psychosis interventions, but even these have not yet become routinely conducted [57]. Few studies have identified barriers that may hinder the feasibility of these interventions or explore patient or family conditions that may render this type of treatment ineffective or inappropriate. Hence, efforts to implement multi-element interventions targeted to FEP patients should be accompanied by rigorous scientific methodology, with the aim of better understanding the actual effectiveness of this approach [58, 59].

The GET UP (Genetics Endophenotypes and Treatment: Understanding early Psychosis) programme, funded by the Italian Ministry of Health as part of National Health Care Research Program, was launched to fill this gap [60]. GET UP is a large research programme which consists of four partner projects (PIANO, Psychosis early Intervention and Assessment of Needs and Outcome; TRUMPET, TRaining and Understanding of service Models for Psychosis Early Treatment; GUITAR, Genetic data Utilization and Implementation of Targeted drug Administration in the clinical Routine; and CONTRABASS, COgnitive Neuroendophenotypes for Treatment and RehAbilitation of psychoses: Brain imaging, inflAmmation and StresS). The partner projects are strictly correlated, though they specifically address different areas of research. The cluster randomised controlled trial conducted in the PIANO project was the main data collection axis for the overall GET UP research programme. The PIANO trial aimed to (a) compare, at nine months, the effectiveness of a multi-component psychosocial intervention with that of treatment as usual in a large epidemiologically based cohort of FEP patients and their family members recruited from a ten-million-inhabitant catchment area; (b) identify the barriers that may hinder its feasibility in 'real-world' routine clinical settings and patient/family conditions that may render this intervention ineffective or inappropriate; and (c) identify clinical, psychological, environmental and service organisation predictors of effectiveness, compliance and service satisfaction in FEP patients treated in the Italian community mental health-care system.

Study participants were recruited from 117 community mental health centres operating for the Italian National Health Service and located in two whole regions of northern Italy (Veneto and Emilia-Romagna) and in the cities of Florence, Milan and Bolzano. The experimental treatment package consisted of standard care plus evidence-based additional psychosocial treatments: (a) cognitive-behavioural therapy for psychosis (CBTp) for patients, (b) family intervention for psychosis (FIp) and (c) case management (CM). CBTp was based on the model developed by Fowler et al. [61], Kuipers et al. [62] and Garety et al. [63]. Family intervention was based on the model proposed by Leff et al. [64] and further developed by Kuipers et al. [65]. Before beginning the trial, mental health staff applying the experimental interventions received specific training programmes in CBTp, FIp and CM. At the end of the training, an assessment of the competence achieved was performed and detailed intervention manuals based on international standards were developed and given to the professionals as a standard to be followed for their treatment. This represents the largest cluster randomised trial evaluating the effectiveness of evidence-based psychosocial intervention to FEP patients ever conducted in the international literature. Its initial findings will soon be available to the interested audience. The GET UP programme is expected to improve our knowledge base on the optimal service organisation and delivery of mental health care for patients with FEP in routine practice. Moreover, this programme will aim (a) to evaluate the feasibility of large-scale training programme on evidence-based psychosocial treatments to professionals working in routine mental health services and (b) to gain more insight on the potential barriers that may hinder implementation of effective multi-element psychosocial interventions in the routine care. In addition, the GET UP programme is expected to provide the opportunity to plug a gap in our understanding of FEP and consequently to favour (a) better knowledge of the causes of psychosis and most effective treatments, (b) development of screening and assessment programmes regarding disease susceptibility, (c) promotion of multi-dimensional standardised assessment measures for a comprehensive evaluation of new cases of psychotic patients and their family members and (d) promotion of an integrated, patient-centred care in FEP. Overall, the GET UP programme will allow us to gain more insight into both the 'efficacy–effectiveness' gap (by testing the effectiveness of multi-element psychosocial interventions in a large pragmatic trial conducted in routine service) and on the 'evidence–practice' gap (by implementing and disseminating evidence-based practices within routine mental health care) that have proved to play a crucial role in delaying knowledge transfer from clinical research to health-care interventions.

Increasing knowledge on the interplay between biological, environmental and clinical factors to better target implementation of treatments

Research on the interplay between biological, environmental and clinical factors is rich of potentiality to better target implementation of evidence-based treatments. Psychosis is a model of particular interest, for its considerable heterogeneity in outcome [66, 67]. A comprehensive review showed that the long-term favourable outcome of schizophrenia ranges between 21% and 57% depending on the outcome dimension and the diagnostic criteria used [68]. The search for consistent and reliable prognostic factors that could identify at the illness onset which patients will have a higher probability to recover completely from those with a less favourable outcome has become an important goal [43]. Finding good prognostic factors for psychosis remains a major challenge for clinical research. Some of this knowledge derives from studies that have as their main aim understanding the aetiology of psychosis, which in a near future could prove to be useful in clinical settings to improve illness treatment and prognostication. In the last years, one of the aspects that have been investigated is the mediating process involved in the complex relationships that exist between predictors and trajectories of outcome by considering the impact of biological variables, among which genetic factors and abnormalities in brain morphology and functioning play a crucial role, in predicting clinical outcome.

For example, the negative symptom cluster, once established, is more stable over time and is more likely to be associated with neurocognitive impairments [69], brain abnormalities [70] and work and social incapacity [71]. Interestingly, previous studies have reported significant relationship between genetic variations in *DTNBP1* gene and the persistence of negative symptoms over time [72–74]. It is notable that gene–symptoms relationships have emerged primarily from follow-up studies of putative schizophrenia risk genes, with only handful of replicated findings [75, 76].

Consequently, future studies should define persistent aspects of the schizophrenic profile which are more likely to represent an underlying biological pathogenesis as opposed to fluctuating, possibly environmentally mediated, symptoms. The definition of this specific clinical phenotype based on symptoms, social functioning and prognosis and its correlation with genetic risk factors will not only permit an assessment of the clinical heterogeneity of the disease but will also improve the classification of mental disorders and potentially enable the identification of useful biological markers [76]. The final aim of the identification of these genetic factors is to facilitate the search for independent risk environmental factors and enable investigation into the mechanism of interaction between genes and the environment. This approach will also be important for clinical prognostication and planning, treatment outcome and social adaptation [77, 78].

Another interesting example of the interplay between biological and clinical factors is violent behaviour that patients affected by schizophrenia display more frequently than general population [79]. Violent behaviour is a predictor of unfavourable course of schizophrenia due to the fact that it might cause hospital admission and delay discharge, increase caregiver burden, lead to arrest and incarceration and increase stigma and financial costs for schizophrenia [80]. Moreover, schizophrenia patients exhibiting this behaviour are at higher likelihood to have a substance abuse comorbidity [81] and be nonadherent to psychopharmacological treatments [82]. For all these reasons, violence in schizophrenia constitutes a major public health concern.

Although violence in schizophrenia is a complicated phenomenon that results from the interaction between many biological and social factors, it has been demonstrated that carrying the Met allele of the COMT Val[158]Met polymorphism increases the risk of violent acts [83–85]. This result is notable, because not only it adds knowledge about the molecular mechanism underlying this phenomenon but also because understanding the biological process might contribute to the future development of pharmacological agents that can influence phenotypic variables associated with schizophrenia [86].

To date, few studies have considered clinical, environmental and biological predictors in FEP. One of these is the aforementioned PICOS project [43]. It investigated the relationship between genetic patterns and clinical and social characteristics of FEP patients, both at the cross-sectional and longitudinal level, together with an extensive set of environmental, clinical, psychosocial and biological variables, and explored possible endophenotypes [87] as neurological soft signs (NSS) [88, 89], neuroimaging markers as fronto-thalamic-cerebellar grey matter deficit [90] and cognitive markers as verbal memory deficit [91].

Endophenotypes seem to be promising for understanding the molecular mechanisms underlying disease risk and manifestation because these are heritable traits that are supposed to form a causal link between genes and observable phenotypes [87]. They have the advantage of being measurable with strategies that use quantitative units of analysis and amenable to assessment in the laboratory [92]. Furthermore, the relationship between a specific endophenotype and certain genetic variants could be stronger than that with the illness itself [87].

Structural MRI studies have found that several regional cerebral changes are related with the presence of NSS in schizophrenia and a recent meta-analysis reported a strong association between NSS and cognitive impairments in psychosis, in particular between sensory and motor neurological functions and several aspects of cognitive ability including spatial, executive and language performance [93].

Consequently, the PICOS findings will help clinicians to discriminate from the beginning of the illness which patients have these neurological impairments in order to settle down specific neurocognitive and/or rehabilitative treatments.

The important results achieved through the PICOS will be further expanded in the aforementioned GET UP programme, since it focuses on genetic and neuropsychological factors that can predict the response to both psychological and psychopharmacological treatments. In fact, the clinical heterogeneity of psychosis is also associated with variability in response to antipsychotic treatment: at least 30% of the patients do not respond to antipsychotic treatment and a further proportion responds only partially or develops severe side effects. In relation to pharmacokinetics, numerous findings suggest the utility of the genotyping of metabolism enzymes (P450) linked to pharmacokinetic profiles of antipsychotic medications for the personalisation of therapeutic dosage [94]. To date, few studies have investigated the pharmacogenetics in FEP. In particular, some functional polymorphisms in genes involved in dopaminergic and serotoninergic neurotransmission pathways (DRD3, DRD2, 5-HT2C, SLC6A4) have been associated to antipsychotic drug response and/or weight gain in these patients [95]. Moreover, polymorphisms in the serotonin transporter gene were found associated with clinical response to CBT plus placebo or CBT plus bupropion [96].

The final aim of integrating biological data (from genomics, transcriptomics and proteomics) in clinical research of psychosis and genetic psychiatry research is to implement an algorithm combining clinical, cognitive and neuro-morphofunctional profiles and pharmacological and/or non-pharmacological treatment efficacy to achieve a personalisation of therapies for FEP.

Conclusion

The translation of more innovative and efficacious treatments from experimental settings to routine clinical practice occurs slowly, and when it does occur, the transformation process is influenced by complex mechanisms. Hence, it is crucial that policy makers and clinicians discuss both the delivery and the content of care on a regular basis when developing mental health-care programmes. Other factors that always need to be carefully examined are overall organisational models, specific types of intervention or intervention packages selected, quantity and quality of mental health staff training and, most of all, the methods proposed for achieving these goals and assessing their outcomes. A new generation of well-designed effectiveness trials, which carefully take into consideration this complexity, are urgently warranted [97]. Finally, subtyping psychoses by implementing research on the interplay between biological, environmental and clinical factors will increase knowledge on their aetiology and prognosis and in a near future could identify biological markers useful in clinical settings to improve illness treatment.

References

[1] Sackett DL, Rosenberg WMC, Gray JAM et al. (1996) Evidence based medicine: what it is and what it isn't. *BMJ* **312**: 71–72.

[2] Desai NG. (2006) Evidence-based practices in mental health: distant dream or emerging reality? *Indian Journal of Psychiatry* **48** (1): 1–3.

[3] Grol R, Grimshaw J. (2003) From best evidence to best practice: effective implementation of change in patients' care. *Lancet* **362**: 1225–1230.

[4] Grol R. (2001) Improving the quality of medical care: building bridges among professional pride, payer profit, and patient satisfaction. *Journal of the American Medical Association* **286** (20): 2578–2585.

[5] Gaebel W, Weinmann S, Sartorius N et al. (2005) Schizophrenia practice guidelines: international survey and comparison. *British Journal of Psychiatry* **187**: 248–255.

[6] Geddes JR, Harrison PJ. (1997) Closing the gap between research and practice. *British Journal of Psychiatry* **171**: 220–225.

[7] Tansella M, Thornicroft G. (2009) Implementation science: understanding the translation of evidence into practice. *British Journal of Psychiatry* **195** (4): 283–285.

[8] Leucht S, Tardy M, Komossa K et al. (2012) Maintenance treatment with antipsychotic drugs for schizophrenia. *Cochrane Database of Systematic Reviews* **16** (5): CD008016.

[9] Jones C, Hacker D, Cormac I et al. (2012) Cognitive behaviour therapy versus other psychosocial treatments for schizophrenia. *Cochrane Database of Systematic Reviews* **18** (4): CD008712.

[10] Torrey WC, Drake RE, Dixon L et al. (2001) Implementing evidence-based practices for persons with severe mental illnesses. *Psychiatric Services* **52**: 45–50.

[11] Lehman AF, Steinwachs DM, the co-investigators of the PORT project. (1998) Patterns of usual care for schizophrenia: initial results from the schizophrenia patient outcomes research team (PORT) client survey. *Schizophrenia Bulletin* **24**: 11–20.

[12] Drake RE, Goldman HH, Leff HS et al. (2001) Implementing evidence-based practices in routine mental health service settings. *Psychiatric Services* **52**: 179–182.

[13] Ruggeri M. (2008) Guidelines for treating mental illness: love them, hate them. Can the SIEP-DIRECT'S project serve in the search for a happy medium? *Epidemiologia e Psichiatria Sociale* **17** (4): 270–277.

[14] National Institute for Health and Clinical Excellence. (2002) Schizophrenia: full national clinical guidelines on core interventions in primary and secondary care. Available from: http://www.nice.org.uk/CG1. Accessed 5 February 2013.

[15] Barbui C, Tansella M. (2011) Cochrane reviews impact on mental health policy and practice. *Epidemiology and Psychiatric Sciences* **20**: 211–214.

[16] Ganju V. (2003) Implementation of evidence-based practices in state mental health systems: implications for research and effectiveness studies. *Schizophrenia Bulletin* **29** (1): 125–131.

[17] Weiss AP, Guidi J, Fava M. (2009) Closing the efficacy-effectiveness gap: translating both the what and the how from randomized controlled trials to clinical practice. *Journal of Clinical Psychiatry* **70** (4): 446–449.

[18] Ruggeri M. (2002) Feasibility, usefulness, limitations and perspectives of routine outcome assessment: the South Verona Outcome Project. *Epidemiologia e Psichiatria Sociale* **11** (3): 177–185.

[19] Lasalvia A, Ruggeri M. (2007) Assessing the outcome of community-based psychiatric care: building a feedback loop from 'real world' health services research into clinical practice. *Acta Psychiatrica Scandinavica Supplementum* **437**: 6–15.

[20] Lasalvia A, Ruggeri M, Mazzi MA et al. (2000) The perception of needs for care in staff and patients in community-based mental health services. The South-Verona Outcome Project 3. *Acta Psychiatrica Scandinavica* **102** (5): 366–375.

[21] Ruggeri M, Lasalvia A, Salvi G et al. (2007) Applications and usefulness of routine measurement of patients' satisfaction with community-based mental health care. *Acta Psychiatrica Scandinavica Supplementum* **437**: 53–65.

[22] McCabe R, Bullenkamp J, Hansson L et al. (2012) The therapeutic relationship and adherence to antipsychotic medication in schizophrenia. *PLoS One* **7** (4): e36080.

[23] Lasalvia A, Bonetto C, Cristofalo D et al. (2007) Predicting clinical and social outcome of patients attending 'real world' mental health services: a 6-year multi-wave follow-up study. *Acta Psychiatrica Scandinavica Supplementum* **437**: 16–30.

[24] Lasalvia A, Bonetto C, Malchiodi F et al. (2005) Listening to patients' needs to improve their subjective quality of life. *Psychological Medicine* **35** (11): 1655–1665.

[25] Lasalvia A, Bonetto C, Tansella M et al. (2008) Does staff-patient agreement on needs for care predict a better mental health outcome? A 4-year follow-up in a community service. *Psychological Medicine* **38** (1): 123–133.

[26] Slade M. (2002) Routine outcome assessment in mental health services. *Psychological Medicine* **32** (8): 1339–1343.

[27] Forsner T, Hansson J, Brommels M et al. (2010) Implementing clinical guidelines in psychiatry: a qualitative study of perceived facilitators and barriers. *BMC Psychiatry* **20**: 10–18.

[28] Hannes K, Pieters G, Goedhuys J et al. (2010) Exploring barriers to the implementation of evidence-based practice in psychiatry to inform health policy: a focus group based study. *Community Mental Health Journal* **46** (5): 423–432.

[29] McGorry PD, Krstev H, Harrigan S. (2000) Early detection and treatment delay: implications for outcome in early psychosis. *Current Opinion in Psychiatry* **13**: 37–43.

[30] Edwards J, Harris MG, Bapat S. (2005) Developing services for first-episode psychosis and the critical period. *British Journal of Psychiatry* **48** (Suppl.): 91–97.

[31] Edwards J, McGorry PD. (2002) *Implementing Early Intervention in Psychosis*. London: Martin Dunitz.

[32] Joseph R, Birchwood M. (2005) The national policy reforms for mental health services and the story of early intervention services in the United Kingdom. *Journal of Psychiatry and Neuroscience* **30** (5): 362–365.

[33] Pelosi AJ, Birchwood M. (2003) Is early intervention for psychosis a waste of valuable resources? *British Journal of Psychiatry* **182**: 196–198.

[34] Pelosi A. (2009) Is early intervention in the major psychiatric disorders justified? No. *BMJ* **337**: a710.

[35] Manchanda R, Norman RM, Malla A. (2004) Value of early intervention in psychosis. *British Journal of Psychiatry* **185**: 171.

[36] McGorry P. (2009) Is early intervention in the major psychiatric disorders justified? Yes. *BMJ* **337**: a695.

[37] Bosanac P, Patton GC, Castle DJ. (2010) Early intervention in psychotic disorders: faith before facts? *Psychological Medicine* **40**: 353–358.

[38] Bird V, Premkumar P, Kendall T et al. (2010) Early intervention services, cognitive-behavioural therapy and family intervention in early psychosis: systematic review. *British Journal of Psychiatry* **197**: 350–356.

[39] Bertelsen M, Jeppesen P, Petersen L et al. (2008) Five-year follow-up of a randomized multicenter trial of intensive early intervention vs standard treatment for patients with a first episode of psychotic illness: the OPUS trial. *Archives of General Psychiatry* **65**: 762–771.

[40] Gafoor R, Nitsch D, McCrone P et al. (2010) Effect of early intervention on 5-year outcome in non-affective psychosis. *British Journal of Psychiatry* **196**: 372.

[41] Addington D. (2009) Best practices: improving quality of care for patients with first-episode psychosis. *Psychiatric Services* **60**: 1164–1166.

[42] Semisa D, Casacchia M, Di Munzio W et al. (2008) Promoting recovery of schizophrenic patients: discrepancy between routine practice and evidence. The SIEP-DIRECT's Project. *Epidemiologia e Psichiatria Sociale* **17** (4): 331–348.

[43] Lasalvia A, Tosato S, Brambilla P et al. (2012) Psychosis Incident Cohort Outcome Study (PICOS). A multisite study of clinical, social and biological characteristics, patterns of care and predictors of outcome in first-episode psychosis. Background, methodology and overview of the patient sample. *Epidemiology Psychiatric Sciences* **21** (3): 281–303.

[44] Bertani M, Lasalvia A, Bonetto C et al. (2012) The influence of gender on clinical and social characteristics of patients at psychosis onset: a report from the Psychosis Incident Cohort Outcome Study (PICOS). *Psychological Medicine* **42**: 769–780.

[45] Lasalvia A, Gentile B, Ruggeri M et al. (2007) Heterogeneity of the Departments of Mental Health in the Veneto Region ten years after the National Plan 1994–96 for Mental Health. Which implication for clinical practice? Findings from the PICOS Project. *Epidemiologia e Psichiatria Sociale* **16**: 59–70.

[46] Bertani M, Lasalvia A, Bissoli S et al. (2008) Treatment pathways for first-episode psychotic patients within community based-mental health services in the Veneto region. Preliminary findings from the PICOS project. VIII ENMESH Conference. *Good Practice, Good Outcome*. Cracow (Poland), 23–25 May 2008.

[47] Haddock G, Lewis S. (2005) Psychological interventions in early psychosis. *Schizophrenia Bulletin* **31**: 697–704.

[48] Penn DL, Waldheter EJ, Perkins DO et al. (2005) Psychosocial treatment for first-episode psychosis: a research update. *American Journal of Psychiatry* **162**: 2220–2232.

[49] Kuipers E, Bebbington P. (2006) Cognitive behaviour therapy for psychosis. *Epidemiologia e Psichiatria Sociale* **15** (4): 267–275.

[50] Alvarez-Jimenez M, Wade D, Cotton S et al. (2008) Enhancing treatment fidelity in psychotherapy research: novel approach to measure the components of cognitive behavioural therapy for relapse prevention in first-episode psychosis. *Australian New Zealand Journal of Psychology* **42**: 1013–1020.

[51] Kidd SA, George L, O'Connell M et al. (2010) Fidelity and recovery-orientation in assertive community treatment. *Community Mental Health Journal* **46**: 342–350.

[52] Cohen DJ, Crabtree BF, Etz RS et al. (2008) Fidelity versus flexibility: translating evidence-based research into practice. *American Journal of Preventive Medicine* **35**: 381–389.

[53] Lancashire S, Haddock G, Tarrier N et al. (1997) The effects of training in psychosocial interventions for community psychiatric nurses in England. *Psychiatric Services* **48** (1): 39–41.

[54] Kavanagh D, Clark D, Piatkowska O et al. (1993) Application of cognitive-behavioural family interventions in multidisciplinary teams: what can the matter be? *Australian Psychologist* **28**: 1–8.

[55] Woltmann EM, Whitley R, McHugo GJ et al. (2008) The role of staff turnover in the implementation of evidence-based practices in mental health care. *Psychiatric Services* **59**: 732–737.

[56] Ruggeri M, Tansella M. (2008) Improving the treatment of schizophrenia in real world mental health services. *Epidemiologia e Psichiatria Sociale* **17** (4): 249–253.

[57] Cocchi A, Meneghelli A, Preti A. (2010) "Programma 2000": a multi-modal pilot programme on early intervention in psychosis underway in Italy since 1999. *Early Intervention in Psychiatry* **4** (1): 97–103.

[58] Ruggeri M, Tansella M. (2007) Achieving a better knowledge on the causes and early course of psychoses: a profitable investment for the future? *Epidemiologia e Psichiatria Sociale* **16** (2): 97–101.

[59] Ruggeri M, Lora A, Semisa D. (2008) The SIEP-DIRECT'S Project on the discrepancy between routine practice and evidence. An outline of main findings and practical implications for the future of community based mental health services. *Epidemiologia e Psichiatria Sociale* **17** (4): 358–368.

[60] Ruggeri M, Bonetto C, Lasalvia A et al. (2012) A multi-element psychosocial intervention for early psychosis (GET UP PIANO TRIAL) conducted in a catchment area of 10 million inhabitants: study protocol for a pragmatic cluster randomized controlled trial. *Trials* **13** (1): 73.

[61] Fowler D, Garety P, Kuipers E. (1995) *Cognitive Behaviour Therapy for Psychosis.* Chichester: John Wiley & Sons, Ltd.

[62] Kuipers E, Fowler D, Garety P et al. (1998) London-east Anglia randomised controlled trial of cognitive-behavioural therapy for psychosis. III: follow-up and economic evaluation at 18 months. *British Journal of Psychiatry* **173**: 61–68.

[63] Garety PA, Fowler DG, Freeman D et al. (2008) A randomised controlled trial of cognitive behavioural therapy and family intervention for the prevention of relapse and reduction of symptoms in psychosis. *British Journal of Psychiatry* **192**: 412–423.

[64] Leff J, Kuipers L, Berkowitz R et al. (1985) A controlled trial of social intervention in the families of schizophrenic patients: two year follow-up. *British Journal of Psychiatry* **146**: 594–600.

[65] Kuipers E, Leff J, Lam D. (2002) *Family Work for Schizophrenia: A Practical Guide.* London: Gaskell.

[66] Hegarty JD, Baldessarini RJ, Tohen M et al. (1994) One hundred years of schizophrenia: a meta-analysis of the outcome literature. *American Journal of Psychiatry* **151**: 1409–1416.

[67] Davidson L, McGlashan TH. (1997) The varied outcomes of schizophrenia. *Canadian Journal of Psychiatry* **42**: 34–43.

[68] Jobe TH, Harrow M. (2005) Long-term outcome of patients with schizophrenia: a review. *Canadian Journal of Psychiatry* **50** (14): 892–900.

[69] Harvey PD, Koren D, Reichenberg A et al. (2006) Negative symptoms and cognitive deficits: what is the nature of their relationship? *Schizophrenia Bulletin* **32**: 250–258.

[70] Shenton ME, Dickey CC, Frumin M et al. (2001) A review of MRI findings in schizophrenia. *Schizophrenia Research* **49**: 1–52.

[71] Bowie CR, Reichenberg A, Patterson TL et al. (2006) Determinants of real-world functional performance in schizophrenia subjects: correlations with cognition, functional capacity, and symptoms. *American Journal of Psychiatry* **163**: 418–425.

[72] Tosato S, Ruggeri M, Bonetto C et al. (2007) Association study of dysbindin gene with clinical and outcome measures in a representative cohort of Italian schizophrenic patients. *American Journal of Medical Genetics Part B: Neuropsychiatric Genetics* **144B** (5): 647–659.

[73] DeRosse P, Funke B, Burdick KE et al. (2006) Dysbindin genotype and negative symptoms in schizophrenia. *American Journal of Psychiatry* **163**: 532–534.

[74] Fanous AH, van den Oord EJ, Riley BP et al. (2004) Relationship between a high-risk haplotype in the DTNBP1 (dysbindin) gene and clinical features of schizophrenia. *American Journal of Psychiatry* **162**: 1824–1832.

[75] DeRosse P, Lencz T, Burdick KE et al. (2008) The genetics of symptom-based phenotypes: toward a molecular classification of schizophrenia. *Schizophrenia Bulletin* **34**: 1047–1053.

[76] Tosato S, Lasalvia A. (2009) The contribution of epidemiology to defining the most appropriate approach to genetic research on schizophrenia. *Epidemiologia e Psichiatria Sociale* **18** (2): 81–90.

[77] Rosenman S, Korten A, Medway J et al. (2003) Dimensional vs. categorical diagnosis in psychosis. *Acta Psychiatrica Scandinavica* **107**: 378–384.

[78] Allardyce J, Gaebel W, Zielasek J. (2007) Deconstructing psychosis conference February 2006: the validity of schizophrenia and alternative approaches to the classification of psychosis. *Schizophrenia Bulletin* **33**: 863–867.

[79] Wessely S. (1997) The epidemiology of crime, violence and schizophrenia. *British Journal of Psychiatry Supplement* **32**: 8–11.

[80] Volavka J. (2002) *Neurobiology of Violence*. Washington, DC: American Psychiatric Publishing.

[81] Fazel S, Gulati G, Linsell L et al. (2009) Schizophrenia and violence: systematic review and meta-analysis. *PLoS Medicine* **6**: e1000120.

[82] Velligan DI, Weiden PJ, Sajatovic M et al. (2009) The expert consensus guideline series: adherence problems in patients with serious and persistent mental illness. *Journal of Clinical Psychiatry* **70**: 1–46.

[83] Singh JP, Volavka J, Czobor P et al. (2012) A meta-analysis of the Val158Met COMT polymorphism and violent behavior in schizophrenia. *PLoS One* **7** (8): e43423.

[84] Bhakta SG, Zhang JP, Malhotra AK. (2012) The COMT Met158 allele and violence in schizophrenia: a meta-analysis. *Schizophrenia Research* **140**: 192–197.

[85] Tosato S, Bonetto C, Di Forti M et al. (2011) Effect of COMT genotype on aggressive behaviour in a community cohort of schizophrenic patients. *Neuroscience Letters* **495**: 17–21.

[86] Jones G, Zammit S, Norton N et al. (2001) Aggressive behaviour in patients with schizophrenia is associated with catechol-O-methyltransferase genotype. *British Journal of Psychiatry* **179**: 351–355.

[87] Gottesman II, Gould TD. (2003) The endophenotype concept in psychiatry: etymology and strategic intentions. *American Journal of Psychiatry* **160**: 636–645.

[88] Dazzan P, Murray RM. (2002) Neurological soft signs in first-episode psychosis: a systematic review. *British Journal of Psychiatry Supplement* **43**: s50–s57.

[89] Tosato S, Dazzan P. (2005) The psychopathology of schizophrenia and the presence of neurological soft signs: a review. *Current Opinion in Psychiatry* **18** (3): 285–288.

[90] Marcelis M, Suckling J, Woodruff P et al. (2003) Searching for a structural endophenotype in psychosis using computational morphometry. *Psychiatry Research* **122**: 153–167.

[91] Paulsen JS, Heaton RK, Sadek JR et al. (1995) The nature of learning and memory impairments in schizophrenia. *Journal of the International Neuropsychological Society* **1**: 88–99.

[92] Mazzoncini R, Zoli M, Tosato S et al. (2009) Can the role of genetic factors in schizophrenia be enlightened by studies of candidate gene mutant mice behaviour? *World Journal of Biological Psychiatry* **10**: 778–797.

[93] Chan RC, Xu T, Heinrichs RW et al. (2010) Neurological soft signs in non-psychotic first-degree relatives of patients with schizophrenia: a systematic review and meta-analysis. *Neuroscience and Biobehavioral Review* **34** (6): 889–896.

[94] Kirchheiner J, Nickchen K, Bauer M et al. (2004) Pharmacogenetics of antidepressants and antipsychotics: the contribution of allelic variations to the phenotype of drug response. *Molecular Psychiatry* **9** (5): 442–473.

[95] Lencz T, Robinson DG, Napolitano B et al. (2010) DRD2 promoter region variation predicts antipsychotic-induced weight gain in first episode schizophrenia. *Pharmacogenetics and Genomics* **20**: 569–572.

[96] Bloch B, Reshef A, Cohen T et al. (2010) Preliminary effects of bupropion and the promoter region (HTTLPR) serotonin transporter (SLC6A4) polymorphism on smoking behavior in schizophrenia. *Psychiatry Research* **175** (1–2): 38–42.

[97] Ruggeri M, Lasalvia A, Bonetto C (2013) A new generation of pragmatic trials of psychosocial interventions is needed. *Epidemiology and Psychiatric Sciences* **22** (2).

CHAPTER 6

The need for new models of care for people with severe mental illness in low- and middle-income countries

Ruben Alvarado[1], Alberto Minoletti[1], Elie Valencia[1], Graciela Rojas[2] and Ezra Susser[3,4,5]

[1] Faculty of Medicine, Salvador Allende School of Public Health, University of Chile, Santiago, Chile
[2] Department of Psychiatry, Clinical Hospital, University of Chile, Santiago, Chile
[3] Department of Epidemiology, Mailman School of Public Health, Columbia University, New York, NY, USA
[4] Department of Psychiatry, College of Physicians and Surgeons, Columbia University and New York State Psychiatric Institute, New York, NY, USA
[5] Department of Psychiatry, University of Göttingen, Göttingen, Germany

Introduction

The previous chapters in this book provide an important context for this one. They show that mental disorders contribute significantly to the burden of disease throughout the world; call for giving higher priority to health care for people with mental disorders in all countries, especially low- and middle-income countries (LAMICs); and describe key initiatives to help achieve this end. They also emphasise that while mental health care still receives fewer resources and lower priority than other sectors of health care, progress is palpable. Indeed, in some LAMICs, we may be approaching a historic turning point for the scaling up of mental health services.

This chapter focuses on the need for new models of community-based care for people with severe mental disorders in LAMICs. We propose that, in LAMICs, community-based care for severe mental illness is required to meet the needs of those who are most disadvantaged and disabled, and that such care is feasible and sustainable. However, many of the models for community care of those with severe mental illness used in high-income countries (HICs) are neither feasible nor sustainable in LAMICs. First, we offer a broad perspective on what is needed to further develop and scale up community-based care in LAMICs. Second, we introduce the distinctive context of Latin America and describe a new

Improving Mental Health Care: The Global Challenge, First Edition.
Edited by Graham Thornicroft, Mirella Ruggeri and David Goldberg.

initiative to promote community-based care in the region. Third, we examine the remarkable progress that has been made in Chile towards implementing community-based care for severe mental illness. The Chilean experience offers an important model, not previously described in English language publications. The fourth and final part draws out the global implications of these findings. As noted earlier, many important topics in global mental health are beyond the scope of this chapter but covered elsewhere in the book. One example directly relevant to community mental health services in LAMICs is the importance of following WHO's recommendations on the use of antipsychotic medications in primary health services and increasing the availability of these medications.

Development of community-based care in LAMICs

Population studies

Population studies of severe mental illness are essential for planning services, but are still very limited in LAMICs. For many common mental disorders such as depression and anxiety, we now have substantial information from population studies in LAMICs, at least for prevalence. This information has been largely derived from community surveys conducted across the globe. The methods used in these surveys [1] are not suitable, however, for severe mental disorders such as schizophrenia. A concerted global effort is needed to conduct population studies of severe mental illness. To illustrate, we consider the available information on incidence rates, burden of disease and treatment gap for schizophrenia.

Epidemiologic investigations of the occurrence and causes of schizophrenia in HICs have advanced rapidly in recent years [2, 3]. But comparable progress has not been made in LAMICs. With respect to incidence, the landmark Ten Country Study begun in the late 1970s set a standard for estimating a 'treated incidence rate' that is still followed today [4]. The standard included the ascertainment of new onset cases at the time of first treatment contact with any health service within a clearly defined population. In the 'developing country' sites of the Ten Country Study, incidence rates were derived for rural and urban Chandigarh, India. Subsequently, numerous studies have used a similar approach to obtain incidence rates in HICs, but very few have done so in LAMICs. Examples include studies of incidence rates in some Caribbean countries [5] and in Sao Paulo, Brazil [6]. But in many large and important regions, there are still no published incidence studies that meet this standard. Furthermore, in some regions, the ordinary standards may not suffice.

In parts of Africa, for example, a reliable estimate of 'treated incidence' requires comprehensive ascertainment of new onset cases treated outside the health-care system, for example, by traditional healers. To do so, one may need to access a very large number of traditional healer practices and screen for psychoses in collaboration with them. (Ezra Susser is currently piloting this approach together with a South African colleague [7, 8]) in a semirural area of KwaZulu-Natal, South Africa.) Thus, we still know very little about the treated incidence of schizophrenia in LAMICs. We know still less about 'true' incidence, which includes untreated cases, a significant proportion in many LAMICs [9, 10].

A WHO report estimated that schizophrenia was the cause of 2.8% of the years lost to disability, ranking seventh among all diseases [11]. Among adolescents and young adults (15–44 years), schizophrenia was ranked third. Due to sparse data, these estimates are uncertain for LAMICs. Based on evidence from a variety of sources, however, it is safe to assume that schizophrenia and other severe mental disorders make a substantial contribution to burden of disease. It is also important to note that people with schizophrenia have higher mortality rates and shorter longevity than the general population. The difference appears to be roughly comparable to the difference between cigarette smokers and non-smokers. The causes include increased mortality from cardiovascular disease and suicide, poorer living conditions and inadequate access to general health care.

Although there is a significant lack of good-quality treatment in all countries, the vast majority of people with schizophrenia in HICs receive at least some kind of treatment. This is not always the case in LAMICs, and, furthermore, the variation among LAMICs is substantial. In a study that estimated the treatment gap for individuals with schizophrenia in 50 LAMICs [12], a larger gap was correlated with fewer resources (especially psychiatrists and mental health nurses) and fewer community-based facilities. These estimates do not include the provision of mental health care by traditional healers. In some locales, traditional healers are pervasive and locally accessible. Since few countries have integrated traditional healers with other forms of mental health care, however, their contributions (positive and negative) are largely unknown and unquantifiable at the present time. With further progress towards building community-based services, traditional healers might become measurable components of the network of services in such locales.

Community-based care in LAMICs

Given what we already know from other sources, improvements in community mental health care for people with severe mental illness in LAMICs should not await the accumulation of population studies. These processes should occur in parallel and will benefit one another. To characterise community-based care, the principles articulated by Thornicroft and Tansella [13] offer a useful starting point. Though based primarily on research in HICs, the following principles, drawn from their work, are also relevant to LAMICs:

- Reduce as much as possible the number of patients that live in psychiatric hospitals for large periods of their lives, moving those who are able to community-based residence and avoiding admitting new patients for prolonged periods of time.
- Develop a network of mental health services within the community, with good accessibility for the population and high ability to resolve the acute and crisis phases of the disorder, allowing the person to maintain their family and

community ties, not lose their various roles and minimise the social stigma associated with these diseases.

- Build a legal system that protects human and civil rights of these individuals, especially in the acute phase of the illness.
- Provide medical and psychosocial interventions, on an ongoing basis, which meet the needs of each patient and are quality-assured.
- Integrate work with the family and/or informal caregivers of these individuals who need information, specific skills development and support for their unique needs.
- Coordinate work with community organisations (education, police and justice, athletic, civic participation, etc.) to achieve the greatest social integration possible for every person.

For LAMICs, we suggest a special emphasis on five points consistent with these principles. Community-based mental health-care services should be (a) close to the communities that use them; (b) accessible to all affected individuals and their families/caregivers; (c) based in, but not limited to, primary care; (d) provided not only in clinics but also in homes and other social environments where affected individuals conduct their daily lives; and (e) shaped with the active involvement of affected individuals, their families and communities.

Demonstration projects in many regions of the globe support the use of community-based mental health care along these lines for people with severe mental illness in LAMICs. In Africa, the foundational study was the Aro Village experiment in Nigeria led by Lambo and colleagues [14–18]. This and subsequent demonstration projects in Africa suggest that community-based care is both feasible and useful for people with severe mental illness [19–23]. Similar inferences can be drawn from demonstration projects elsewhere in the globe; in a later section, we discuss examples from Latin America.

Indeed, we propose that the need for community-based care is, if anything, greater in LAMICs than in HICs. Hospitals are not readily accessible to patients and their families, especially for rural populations. The high cost of long-term hospital care pre-empts the development of the wider range of services required to promote social integration and improve quality of life. Mental health clinics improve upon hospital care in many ways, but often include only a few of the elements of community-based care described earlier.

The need to develop and test new models in LAMICs

The strong evidence base from HICs and the promising results from demonstration projects in LAMICs offer useful guidance for improving care for people with severe mental illness in the present time. But the full development and scale-up of community-based care in LAMICs is likely to be much more effective if we specify what we still do not know about community-based services in LAMICs and directly address these gaps in knowledge. We pose three questions here and return to answer them later in the chapter, for the context of Latin America.

First, how can community-based programmes be sustained over the long run? Very few of the demonstration projects, from Aro Village onwards, were able to continue as governments and societies changed. Again, Thornicroft and Tansella offer a useful starting point. They propose a stepped-care model, which considers the incorporation of components of greater complexity and specialisation, to the extent that countries have more resources to do so. This general guidance is not sufficient, however, to sustain actual applications in particular contexts.

Second, how can we extract features of community-based care in HICs to develop models that are likely to be feasible, effective and sustainable in LAMICs? Some of the models that have produced strong results in HICs are, in our view, not sustainable on any wide scale in LAMICs. Assertive Community Treatment (ACT), for example, is a team-based approach which involves intensive care over a long period, and the creation of a virtually distinct and self-contained system of care. We think that the transplantation of a costly system that does not fit well with or make optimal use of existing local resources is not a sustainable approach. Other models are more adaptable to LAMICs, but still cannot be transplanted without adaptation. Generally, LAMICs have less-developed policies and programmes, fewer services based in the community and fewer resources of all kinds (especially specialised). Strategies that consider these contextual differences must be designed.

Third, how can we strengthen the evidence base for the use of community-based care for severe mental illness? As explained elsewhere in this book, the results of randomised controlled trials (RCTs) are not the only kind of evidence that should be considered. Nonetheless, we think that RCTs are an essential component for building strong evidence-based approaches. As yet, only two RCTs have been published that tested a model of community-based mental health care for schizophrenia in the context of a LAMIC (see papers by Ran et al. and Chaterjee et al. cited in Chapter 7).

The context of Latin America

Although Latin America includes a plethora of countries and cultures, there are enough commonalities to make it meaningful to consider community mental health care across the region. The commonalities are most apparent in the southern part of the continent, where the official language is usually Spanish or Portuguese, the economic status is usually middle-income and the political history often includes a period of oppressive dictatorship followed by democratic government. Across a broader swath of Latin America, a common factor is the accelerating growth of large urban areas, where there are stark inequalities and sizable marginalised communities that lack basic infrastructure. Last but not least, somewhat parallel developments have occurred in mental health services. Regional policies for mental health services have been developed, though their implementation varies across countries, as described later. In the next section, we illustrate how a single country diverged from the regional pattern and yet maintained an adherence to regionally developed principles, underscoring that there is indeed a common thread to be found within the various experiences of Latin American countries.

As early as the 1950s, Latin American researchers began epidemiological studies that used case ascertainment and random sampling methods to assess the prevalence of mental disorders among residents of different countries [24–26]. These studies prompted new public health approaches to addressing the high burden of mental disorders and first attempts to build mental health services in the community. The hegemonic role of mental hospitals as the main form of treatment began to be questioned, and debates arose about alternative models based on general hospitals and primary care centres, as well as the need to implement day hospitals, group homes and sheltered workshops to facilitate the social integration of people with severe mental disorders. A few pilot experiences were carried out in some Latin American countries, where psychiatrists, general practitioners and other health professionals put some of these ideas into practice [27–29]. Although the community model was never implemented in full due to lack of political support and resources, these early experiences helped to raise awareness and generate learning about alternatives to mental hospitals.

Most of these innovative programmes were downsized or shut down by the dictatorships that plagued several countries of the region during the 1970s. Instead, more mental hospitals were built, until their number exceeded 250, with about 150 000 long-stay beds. In most of the region, these hospitals were virtually the only public service for care of severe mental illness that was accessible to the whole population, and they generally lacked the staff and resources to provide meaningful care. Thus, patients were cut off from their social and family environment, with no rehabilitation programmes, intensive use of physical restraints and other human rights violations [30, 31].

A new cultural and political atmosphere emerged as Latin American countries began the return to democracy. The social movements that led this change were also eager to finally begin to address long-ignored social problems. The community orientation for delivering mental health services found a receptive audience. Particularly influential were the work of Franco Basaglia in Brazil [32] and then Benedetto Saraceno in Nicaragua [33–35]. The central ideas that took root were that it was possible to transform the asylums into a network of community centres, and that patients could become citizens with the same rights as other people.

The Caracas Declaration

The Regional Conference for the Restructuring of Psychiatric Care in Latin America, convened by the Pan American Health Organization (PAHO/WHO) with the support of multiple global institutions and held in Caracas in 1990, played a major role in the eventual development of mental health services in the community [36–38]. The conference brought together key stakeholders and generated an influential position statement, the Caracas Declaration, which set forth the conceptual framework for the reform movement that unfolded in Latin America in the ensuing years. In the Declaration, conference attendees endorsed their commitment to transforming antiquated hospital-based mental health delivery systems into comprehensive community-based delivery systems. They regarded primary care as the main vehicle for delivering mental health services, also calling for the adoption of the Local Health Systems Model and the integration of social and health-care networks. In addition, the Declaration called for legislative action aimed at anchoring the reform process in a legal framework and protecting the human rights of people with mental health problems.

The momentum generated in Caracas was furthered through the PAHO/WHO Initiative for the Restructuring of Psychiatric Services whose goal was to promote and support mental health reform initiatives in Latin America, in collaboration with a large number of countries, international organisations and experts. The principles of the Caracas Declaration have been ratified, and expanded, in an ongoing process that continues up to the present time.

The new mental health-care model supported by PAHO/WHO and regional leaders has been increasingly incorporated in national policies, plans and legislation. Among the cornerstones of the new model are promotion of self-care and informal care, inclusion of mental health into primary care (especially for common mental disorders), decentralisation of specialised outpatient care for severe mental illness, development of day care programmes and psychosocial rehabilitation, and integration of mental health services in general hospitals. Most countries have ratified the global and Pan American treaties regarding human rights of people with mental disorders and disabilities, and PAHO/WHO has undertaken numerous awareness-raising and training activities in almost all Latin American countries. The actual implementation of the model has been highly variable across countries, as we discuss later. Nonetheless, since the Caracas Declaration, almost all Latin American countries have at least established some community mental health centres and tried to downsize and improve the psychiatric hospitals [38].

Local initiatives

In parallel with these regional efforts, many local initiatives emerged, some of which were highly innovative as well as influential. Here we have space only to mention two of them. Both included the full array of services described earlier as community-based mental health care for people with severe mental illness. These two programmes were established in adjacent provinces in the Patagonia region of Argentina, and yet were quite distinctive and were developed independently of one another. In fact, it seems somewhat remarkable that these two innovative programmes were initiated separately within the same remote region, and that both developed into influential models cited by international organisations such as WHO and the World Mental Health Federation.

In the province of Rio Negro, Hugo Cohen led a bold initiative to replace institutional care in mental hospitals with community-based mental health services [39]. This was one of the earliest attempts to radically transform public mental health services in Latin America, and helped to galvanise the process across the region. Despite early success, however, it proved difficult to sustain progress. This can be attributed in large part to the insufficient support provided by successive governments in the province for community services. Consequently, the Rio Negro programme has suffered some setbacks in recent years. Backed by community participation and legislation, the mental health programme has developed a comprehensive network of community services in the public sector, through 27 years of experience. The main components of this network are primary care teams, general hospitals with specialised interdisciplinary mental health teams, psychosocial rehabilitation with strong intersectoral links, group homes and social firms to offer employment to people with mental disability.

In the province of Neuquén, José Lumerman established in the 1990s a non-government organisation (NGO) to provide community mental health services [40]. There were few inpatient beds in Neuquén (most patients with severe and chronic mental illness were sent to La Borda hospital in Buenos Aires) but also virtually no community mental health services. Initially, Lumerman attempted to create such services within the public system, but his efforts were blocked by government agencies. He then went outside the public sector to set up a community-based programme that was supported primarily by reimbursements for care from the Seguridad Social (a form of health insurance accessible to most but not all people). Since there were very few psychiatrists or other specialised resources, the programme was built with the local resources that were available, using an approach that would now be called 'task shifting'. For example, the province did have an excellent public health system and a large number of general doctors; hence, general doctors were recruited and trained to lead mental health teams.

The programme also recruited people from outside the health professions, such as artists and actors, to participate in the rehabilitation process. This programme has sustained its progress, with continual expansion and improvement over a period of more than 15 years. It now offers high-quality care to virtually all people in the city of Neuquén, and to many elsewhere in the province, and is affiliated in various ways with the public health system.

It is useful to consider the reasons why these two excellent programmes have proved sustainable, one in the public sector and the other as an NGO. We propose that it is related to the enormous and ongoing efforts made by both programmes to sustain relationships with all key stakeholders. These include not only the government health sector but also education, justice and other sectors, the families and patients themselves, the general doctors of the province, the local media, the governing party of the province and the administrators of the local Seguridad Social. For example, the governing party and the chief of the local Seguridad

Social changed often, and each time, new relationships had to be developed and sustained. It was only possible to do so because the programmes had become embedded in the community by the involvement and support of such a wide range of stakeholders.

The current state

The many promising signs of progress are real, but one should not be deceived by them. The principles endorsed at Caracas and afterwards are still not matched by the political will to transform mental health care in most countries of the region. Based on the knowledge already generated by local experiences across the region, three Latin American countries, Brazil, Chile and Panama, are actually implementing radical transformations of the mental-hospital-based model. On average, the number of beds in mental hospitals in these three countries was reduced by approximately 62% in the last ten years. Along with this reduction in hospital beds, these three countries have significantly increased overall expenditures on mental health care, as well as the percentage of mental health expenditures allocated to general hospitals, outpatient facilities and community services. There are also user and family organisations that frequently participate in the elaboration of policies, plans and legislation. Thus, three countries have now demonstrated that it is feasible to develop community mental health services for people with severe mental illness as an alternative to hospital care. They have done so at a rapid rate, and evaluations suggest that the transformation has been beneficial to patients and their families.

These achievements are not matched, however, by most other countries in the region. In other Latin American countries, overall, the average reduction in mental hospital beds was approximately 24% in the last ten years. Most countries have also lagged in providing increased funding for mental health care, and in redistributing funding from mental hospitals to community services. The median of health budget allocated to mental health in Latin America is still lower than the median of countries worldwide with similar income levels. Thus, 22 years after Caracas Declaration, most countries of the region continue to maintain a model of services for severe mental disorders based primarily on psychiatric hospitals that consume on average over 75% of the national mental health budgets.

Some other countries, such as Argentina, are currently making plans to follow the example set by Brazil, Chile and Panama. These plans provide hope (though still no hard evidence) that progress will accelerate in the near future. If it does not, and the pace of downsizing of mental hospitals and increase of community services remains the same as in the last ten years, Latin America will take over 50 years to implement the Caracas Declaration (and subsequent commitments that built upon it) across the region.

Latin American countries have also lagged in implementing the human rights legislation that was integral to the Caracas Declaration. The region is below the world average for countries with similar income levels in the percentage of countries that have specific and enforceable mental health legislation. This leaves people with severe mental disorders vulnerable to human rights violations in two out of three countries in the region.

On the other hand, we should not disregard the significant progress that has been made in the development of community mental health services in Latin America. Although Brazil is a single country, it represents a large part of the continent, in terms of both geography and population. Community mental health care in Chile offers a highly advanced exemplar for other countries, as we shall describe later. Local initiatives continue to develop across the region. Virtually all countries now have a significant number of mental health centres located in the community, especially in urban areas, albeit not enough.

Furthermore, these varied developments provide an opportunity to develop multi-country studies to help identify factors hindering and favouring the implementation of community services and the downsizing of mental hospitals, and to compare the effectiveness of alternative strategies for doing so. At the same time, countries with major advances in community services have created appropriate conditions to study the incorporation of new strategies and interventions that could further improve access, quality and equity. This will foster progress towards community-based care in its full sense (as described earlier in the chapter and articulated similarly in the PAHO/WHO model).

The RedeAmericas

All the authors of this chapter are involved in a new regional initiative termed RedeAmericas (RA) [41]. The primary but not exclusive focus of the RA is on community-based care for severe mental disorders in urban areas of Latin America. Participating sites are in Argentina (Buenos Aires, Cordoba, Neuquén), Brazil (Rio de Janeiro), Chile (Santiago), Colombia (Medellín) and the United States (New York). The relevance to this chapter is that the RA seeks to address the three questions posed in the first section. As we have already commented on the first question (How can community-based programmes be sustained over the long run?), we discuss the other two here.

The second question was: how can we extract features of community-based care in HICs such that the models applied in particular LAMIC contexts are likely to be feasible, effective and sustainable? As one example of how this might be done, we describe how we selected an intervention for use in the RA over the course of a prolonged dialogue. We chose to adapt the model of Critical Time Intervention (CTI) [42–45], previously tested in HICs but not LAMICs, for the following reasons. First, CTI is a time-limited nine-month intervention targeted at critical points of transition and explicitly designed so as to have an enduring effect (demonstrated in RCTs in HICs). This makes it attractive for Latin America, because to reach the entire population with limited resources, there must be turnover in the persons receiving the intervention. Second, CTI is designed to be an adjunctive component that complements but does not substitute for existing health and mental health care. This makes it adaptable to the varying service systems encountered across Latin America. Third, CTI relies upon *in vivo* services delivered in the community by mental health workers who meet with patients wherever they spend their time. This crucial feature of community-based care is still absent in most community mental health centres in Latin America; services tend to be provided at the clinic rather than within the social environment of the community. Five years of pilot testing in Rio de Janeiro convinced us that CTI was indeed adaptable.

For the RA, CTI was adapted to CTI-Task Shifting (CTI-TS). CTI-TS has three features relevant to this context that were not included in previous RCTs of CTI (though included in some other applications). First, the targeted critical period of transition is the nine months after first contact with mental health services for a psychotic disorder. We reasoned that the long-term pattern of patients' and families' relationships with mental health services would be partly shaped by their early encounters. Second, the intervention is delivered by pairs comprising a Peer Support Worker and a Community Mental Health Worker. The use of Peer Support Workers, with equivalent pay and status to other workers, is somewhat novel in Latin America, but we thought it was important to introduce and evaluate this component. Among other reasons, the inclusion of Peer Support Workers in mental health services could help to promote and model social integration. Third, CTI-TS emphasises the connection of the patient to both primary care and mental health services. The connections of patients with severe mental illnesses to primary care services tend to be weak in Latin America, and are an essential component of community-based care. We also thought that the process of connecting patients to both these services would contribute to strengthening communication and ongoing ties between primary care and mental health services.

The third question was: how can we strengthen the evidence base for the use of community-based care for severe mental illness? We have noted earlier that we consider RCTs to be an essential component of the evidence base, currently missing for LAMICs. In the RA, however, we chose to test the feasibility of a *regional* RCT of CTI-TS done in three countries. This would not be feasible in all regions, but we thought it would be feasible in Latin America, because of the commonalities among countries and the history of mental health policies that were regionally developed and promoted. A regional RCT could have a major impact on scaling up effective services across the region. By contrast, results from a series of trials using different interventions in various countries could not be readily translated into a regional policy. A regional RCT is challenging because essentially the same intervention has to be applied to settings that differ in their service systems as well as in other ways. Thus, the intervention has to specify what components can be adapted to a specific context and what components must remain the same across contexts. Nonetheless, given the potential benefits, we thought it well worth testing whether a regional RCT could be done.

The experience of Chile

Chile is an example of a country that, in the past 50 years, has undergone a transition from being within the low-income group to being a higher-middle-income country and, throughout its recent history, has gone through different stages in the development of mental health services. These transformations were strongly influenced by Chile's political and social context. The country's experience can serve as a model for LAMICs.

The history of mental health services in Chile can be divided into four stages. The first three will be described briefly, and we will expand on what has happened in the last two decades.

As in other countries, the first stage was characterised by care centred in large psychiatric hospitals. The first of these hospitals, the Insane Asylum of Our Lady of Angeles, was founded in 1852 in Santiago. It was later renamed National Insane Asylum, and then Psychiatric Hospital, in 1952. In the first half of the twentieth century, other psychiatric institutions – generally smaller and shorter-lived – were constructed outside of the capital [46].

The second phase was marked by the development of various psychiatric and community mental health initiatives, in a period spanning from the late 1960s to 1973. The most noteworthy programme, of greatest impact, was led by Dr. Juan Marconi [24, 47] in the south of Santiago. He is credited with generating a school of thought, integrating the health and university systems and training many generations of professionals that influenced mental health policies that are still relevant today. Marconi's model consisted of a system of delegation of functions, or task shifting, from the specialist to the community, passing through professionals, primary care specialists and community leaders. Through a structured educational system, well adapted to the local culture, with training programmes and support manuals, the new model reached the whole community. It is important to note that these initiatives occurred within a historical and political context which made them possible – both within the country and in a large part of Latin America – where there was a deepening of democratic structures, increased social participation and governments that developed strong social transformations through social policies inspired by principles of solidarity and social justice.

The third stage was characterised by the termination of these community-based initiatives and the concentration of services within psychiatric hospitals once again. This occurred between 1973 and 1990, during the dictatorship of General Pinochet. There was significant health reform in this period, with the decentralisation of government-administered health services, separating primary care from the rest of the system (assigning its administration to municipal governments) and introducing initiatives for the development of a private system (both for insurance companies and health providers). However, these changes hardly affected mental health care, since it remained centred inside psychiatric hospitals.

The last stage began with the return of democracy in 1990, and has continued until today, marked by the progressive and sustained implementation of the National Mental Health and Psychiatry Plan, which was instated in 1993, with a second version in 2000 [48, 49]. This plan includes various aspects of mental health policy, but we will focus on the care of people with severe mental disorders, which was defined as a priority issue.

The first aspect was the deinstitutionalisation of people who lived in chronic wards of large psychiatric hospitals. Between 1990 and 2010, the total number of long-stay beds in mental hospitals decreased from 3160 to 1086 (a reduction of 65.6%) [49]. At the same time, 172 community group homes (for 1412 people) and 44 rehabilitation units for 848 people were created, neither of which existed in 1990 [49].

A second aspect was the creation of alternatives to hospitalisation. By 2010, there were 45 day hospitals (for 752 people), 58 ambulatory care units and 75 community mental health centres [49]. Meanwhile, the number of short-term beds in general hospitals increased from 239 to 517. All of this was accompanied by an increase in specialised human resources (psychiatrists, psychologists, nurses, social workers, etc.).

A third aspect was the establishment of user and/or family groups throughout the country, which work cooperatively with mental health services. These groups were involved, for example, in the development of innovative projects for protected employment (as well as many other programmes). This progressive empowerment of users and families has brought about discussions in recent years of various legal initiatives that aim to ensure that these individuals' human and civil rights are respected.

What factors made these achievements possible? The story is still in development, and our responses are necessarily partial, but we think it is appropriate to highlight the following points:

- The articulation of National Mental Health and Psychiatry Plans, both versions of which were products of a participative process and the consensus of different stakeholders. These have been used as a guide for policy decisions and the use of resources.
- The presence of leaders of this policy, at national and regional levels, who are able to influence health authorities. These leaders have consistently implemented the National Plans over time and have ensured coordination within the country.
- The creation of strong ties between mental health policy and general health policy in the country. This has facilitated the linking and coordination of priorities for mental health and general health, the assimilation of the new systems of financial allocation and many other developments.

- The recognition that support is needed for an ongoing process of development, with the coordination of different components and the introduction of new components.
- Collaborative work with other institutions that are politically relevant. As an example, work with academia enables the continual training of mental health teams, the development of investigations to evaluate programmes and build an evidence base and the effective use of information systems such as registers.

Since 2004, Chile has introduced a 'system of explicit guarantees' for access, opportunity, quality and financing for receiving care for priority health issues, including the first episode of schizophrenia. Through this system, all people that require care can demand medical attention for their health problems, in the public or private system, under certain explicit standards. An evaluation that was carried out in the first years of the programme showed that the system met the majority of the standards, but the main weaknesses were in the use of psychosocial interventions and in those designed to meet the day-to-day needs of these individuals [50].

Though there are still inequalities within the country in regard to access to specialised, professional tools and resources (particularly in rural zones), in the past two decades, there has been a fundamental change in the model of care. Key challenges for the future are increasing the coverage (especially through better detection of cases in primary care), improving the quality of care that aims to meet everyday needs, fighting against stigma and for greater social integration, caring for informal caregivers and expanding the development of employment programmes. Active efforts to help address these challenges are ongoing; the system is not considered complete or static. The CTI-TS intervention of the RA is one example of new initiatives that, if proven effective, could help address some of these challenges.

Implications for global mental health

We offer five general proposals that follow from or extend the discussion in this chapter. First, we suggest that it is important to give special attention to the most disabled and disadvantaged persons with mental illness in LAMICs. Thus, we have chosen to focus on community-based care for people with severe mental illness. This does not imply that other mental disorders, or other forms of care, do not merit similar attention. In fact, these are discussed elsewhere in this book. Rather, it reflects our view that we should not overlook the most vulnerable groups as we extend mental health care more broadly to the general population.

Second, the engagement and support for families and other informal caregivers, similarly, needs to be kept at the forefront in global mental health. The impact of severe mental disorder on the health and quality of life of caregivers has been well recognised since the nineteenth century [51], became prominent in research in the decades after World War II [51–53] and is further elaborated in recent research. In LAMICs, the vast majority of people with severe mental illness live with their families, and this might actually promote recovery in some contexts [54]. Given scarce resources, however, the burden on families can be inordinate. Thus, we need to respond to the larger role assumed by caregivers in these contexts, not only to reduce their burden but also to help them derive psychological and social benefits from their long-term caregiving roles.

Third, we think it is necessary to consider such questions within the context of particular regions. Latin America is distinctive from other LAMICs in its history, social and economic development, and current state of mental health services. It also has the potential for launching regional initiatives, demonstrated already by past efforts. The consideration of these distinctive features is needed as a complement to global perspectives on mental health care in order to translate these perspectives into regional and local changes.

Fourth, we propose that mental health initiatives in LAMICs are more likely to be meaningful and sustainable when they build on local resources, are adapted to local context and devote ongoing attention to garnering the support of all key stakeholders. This point would probably be endorsed by everyone in the global mental health field and may appear to be familiar rhetoric. But it is more often found in theory than in practice. We have provided examples of both local and country level initiatives that did put this principle into practice and, perhaps as a result, proved to be sustainable and to continue to develop over time.

Finally, though not discussed in this chapter, we believe that one of the key challenges for global mental health will be the provision of services that are accessible and useful to all people, at least within a given area. Taking the example of Latin America, the large urban areas comprise significant numbers of people at economic levels ranging from extreme wealth to extreme poverty. These urban areas also bring together people of many cultural backgrounds. It will not be easy to develop mental health services that can be used by all or even most of these groups, and we do not claim to know how to do so. But if we cannot do so, we are likely to find that a tiered and fragmented system of care emerges.

Acknowledgement

Ezra Susser gratefully acknowledges the Dr. Lisa Oehler Foundation, University of Göttingen, Germany.

References

[1] Kessler RC, Ustun TB. (2004) The World Mental Health (WMH) Survey Initiative Version of the World Health Organization (WHO) Composite International Diagnostic Interview (CIDI). *International Journal of Methods in Psychiatric Research* **13** (2): 93–121.

[2] McGrath JJ, Susser ES. (2009) New directions in the epidemiology of schizophrenia. *Medical Journal of Australia* **190** (4 Suppl.): S7–S9.

[3] Kirkbride JB, Susser E, Kundakovic M et al. (2012) Prenatal nutrition, epigenetics and schizophrenia risk: can we test causal effects? *Epigenomics* **4** (3): 303–315.

[4] Jablensky A, Sartorius N, Ernberg G et al. (1992) Schizophrenia: manifestations, incidence and course in different cultures. A World Health Organization ten-country study. *Psychological Medicine Monograph Supplement* **20**: 1–97.

[5] Bhugra D, Hilwig M, Hossein B et al. (1996) First-contact incidence rates of schizophrenia in Trinidad and one-year follow-up. *British Journal of Psychiatry* **169** (5): 587–592.

[6] Menezes PR, Scazufca M, Busatto G et al. (2007) Incidence of first-contact psychosis in Sao Paulo, Brazil. *British Journal of Psychiatry Supplement* **51**: s102–s106.

[7] Burns JK. (2010) Mental health services funding and development in KwaZulu-Natal: a tale of inequity and neglect. *South African Medical Journal* **100** (10): 662–666.

[8] Burns JK, Jhazbhay K, Kidd M et al. (2011) Causal attributions, pathway to care and clinical features of first-episode psychosis: a South African perspective. *International Journal of Social Psychiatry* **57** (5): 538–545.

[9] Phillips MR, Zhang J, Shi Q et al. (2009) Prevalence, treatment, and associated disability of mental disorders in four provinces in China during 2001–05: an epidemiological survey. *Lancet* **373** (9680): 2041–2053.

[10] Alem A, Kebede D, Fekadu A et al. (2009) Clinical course and outcome of schizophrenia in a predominantly treatment-naive cohort in rural Ethiopia. *Schizophrenia Bulletin* **35** (3): 646–654.

[11] World Health Organization. (2001) *The World Health Report 2001: Mental Health: New Understanding, New Hope*. Geneva: World Health Organization.

[12] Lora A, Kohn R, Levav I et al. (2012) Service availability and utilization and treatment gap for schizophrenic disorders: a survey in 50 low- and middle-income countries. *Bulletin of the World Health Organization* **90** (1): 47–54B.

[13] Thornicroft G, Tansella M. (2009) *Better Mental Health Care*. Cambridge: Cambridge University Press.

[14] Lambo TA. (1956) Neuropsychiatric observations in the western region of Nigeria. *British Medical Journal* **2** (5006): 1388–1394.

[15] Lambo T. (1961) A plan for the treatment of the mentally ill in Nigeria: the village system at Aro. In: Linn L (ed.), *Frontiers in General Hospital Psychiatry*. New York: International Universities Press, pp. 215–231.

[16] Lambo T. (1966) Patterns of psychiatric care in developing African countries: the Nigerian Village program. In: David HP (ed.), *International Trends in Mental Health*. New York: McGraw Hill, pp. 147–153.

[17] Lambo T. (1968) Experience with a program in Nigeria. In: Williams R, Ozarin L (eds.), *Community Mental Health: An International Perspective*. San Francisco: Jossey-Bass, pp. 97–110.

[18] Asuni T. (1967) Aro hospital in perspective. *American Journal of Psychiatry* **124** (6): 763–770.

[19] Schulsinger F, Jablensky A. (1991) The national mental health programme in the United Republic of Tanzania. A report from WHO and DANIDA. *Acta Psychiatrica Scandinavica Supplementum* **364**: 1–132.

[20] Kilonzo GP, Simmons N. (1998) Development of mental health services in Tanzania: a reappraisal for the future. *Social Science & Medicine* **147** (4): 419–428.

[21] Lund C, Oosthuizen P, Flisher AJ et al. (2010) Pathways to inpatient mental health care among people with schizophrenia spectrum disorders in South Africa. *Psychiatric Services* **61** (3): 235–240.

[22] Baumgartner J. (2004) Measuring disability and social integration among adults with psychotic disorders in Dar es Salaam, Tanzania. PhD thesis. University of North Carolina at Chapel Hill.

[23] Ngoma MC, Prince M, Mann A. (2003) Common mental disorders among those attending primary health clinics and traditional healers in urban Tanzania. *British Journal of Psychiatry* **183**: 349–355.

[24] Marconi J, Varela A, Rosenblat E et al. (1955) A survey on the prevalence of alcoholism among the adult population of a suburb of Santiago. *Quarterly Journal of Studies on Alcohol* **16** (3): 438–446.

[25] Rodriguez J, Kohn R, Aguilar-Gaxiola S (eds.). (2009) *Epidemiología de los Trastornos Mentales en América Latina y el Caribe* [Epidemiology of Mental Disorders in Latin America and the Caribbean]. Washington, DC: Organización Panamericana de la Salud.

[26] Rodríguez J, Kohn R, Levav I. (2009) Epidemiología de los Trastornos Mentales en América Latina y el Caribe [Epidemiology of Mental Disorders in Latin America and the Caribbean]. In: Rodriguez J (ed.), *Salud Mental en la Comunidad* [Community Mental Health]. Washington, DC: Organización Panamericana de la Salud.

[27] Mariategui J, Adis Castro G (eds.). (1970) *Estudios sobre Epidemiología Psiquiátrica en América Latina* [Studies on Psychiatric Epidemiology]. Buenos Aires: ACTA.

[28] Minoletti A, Pemjean A. (1973) Salud Mental en el Norte de Chile: Un Desafío Teórico y Operacional [Mental health in the north of Chile: a theoretical and operational challenge]. *Acta Psiquiátrica y Psicológica de América Latina* **19**: 434–444.

[29] Mari JJ, Garcia de Oliveira Soares B, Silva de Lima M et al. (2009) Breve historia de la epidemiología psiquiátrica en América Latina y el Caribe [Brief history of psychiatric epidemiology in Latin America and the Caribbean]. In: Rodriguez J, Kohn R, Aguilar-Gaxiola S (eds.), *Epidemiología de los Trastornos Mentales en América Latina y el Caribe* [Epidemiology of Mental Disorders in Latin America and the Caribbean]. Washington, DC: Organización Panamericana de la Salud, pp. 3–19.

[30] Marconi J. (1976) Política de salud mental en América Latina [Policy of mental health in Latin America]. *Acta Psiquiatrica y Psicologica de America Latina* **22** (2): 112–120.

[31] León CA. (1976) Perspectiva de la salud mental de la comunidad en América Latina [Outlook of community mental health in Latin America]. *Boletín de la Oficina Sanitaria Panamericana* **81** (2): 122–138.

[32] Fusar-Poli P, Bruno D, Machado-De-Sousa JP et al. (2011) Franco Basaglia (1924–1980): three decades (1979–2009) as a bridge between the Italian and Brazilian mental health reform. *International Journal of Social Psychiatry* **57** (1): 100–103.

[33] Saraceno B, van OM, Batniji R et al. (2007) Barriers to improvement of mental health services in low-income and middle-income countries. *Lancet* **370** (9593): 1164–1174.

[34] Saraceno B. (2007) Mental health systems research is urgently needed. *International Journal of Mental Health Systems* **1** (1): 2.

[35] Saraceno B, Dua T. (2009) Global mental health: the role of psychiatry. *European Archives of Psychiatry and Clinical Neuroscience* **259** (Suppl. 2): S109–S117.

[36] Gonzalez R, Levav I. (1991) *Reestructuracion de la Atencion Psiquiatrica. Bases Conceptuales y Guias para su Implementacion* [Restructuring of Psychiatric Care. Conceptual Bases and Guidelines for Its Implementation]. HPA/MND I.9I. Washington, DC: Organización Panamericana de la Salud.

[37] Levav I, Restrepo H, Guerra de MC. (1994) The restructuring of psychiatric care in Latin America: a new policy for mental health services. *Journal of Public Health Policy* **15** (1): 71–85.

[38] Caldas de Almeida JM, Horvitz-Lennon M. (2010) Mental health care reforms in Latin America: an overview of mental health care reforms in Latin America and the Caribbean. *Psychiatric Services* **61** (3): 218–221.

[39] Cohen H, Natella G. (2009) Argentina: El programa de salud mental en la provincia de Río Negro. In: Rodríguez J (ed.), *Salud Mental en la Comunidad*. Washington, DC: Organización Panamericana de la Salud serie PALTEX.

[40] Collins PY, Adler F, Boero M et al. (1999) Using local resources in Patagonia: primary care and mental health in Neuquen, Argentina. *International Journal of Mental Health* **28** (3): 3–16.

[41] RedeAmericas. (2012). Available from: http://cugmhp.org/redeamericas. Accessed on 4 January 2013.

[42] Susser E, Valencia E, Conover S et al. (1997) Preventing recurrent homelessness among mentally ill men: a "critical time" intervention after discharge from a shelter. *American Journal of Public Health* **87** (2): 256–262.

[43] Herman DB, Conover S, Gorroochurn P et al. (2011) Randomized trial of critical time intervention to prevent homelessness after hospital discharge. *Psychiatric Services* **62** (7): 713–719.

[44] Cavalcanti MT, Carvalho MC, Valencia E et al. (2011) Adaptation of critical time intervention for use in Brazil and its implementation among users of psychosocial service centers (CAPS) in the municipality of Rio de Janeiro. *Ciencia e Saude Coletiva* **16** (12): 4635–4642.

[45] Critical Time Intervention. (2012). Available from: http://www.criticaltime.org/. New York: Critical Time Intervention. Accessed on 4 January 2013.

[46] Escobar E. (1990) Historia del Hospital Psiquiátrico (1852–1952) [History of psychiatric hospital (1852–1952)]. *Revista de Psiquiatría* **7**: 361–368.

[47] Marconi J. (1973) La revolución cultural chilena en programas de salud mental [Chilean cultural revolution in the programs of mental health]. *Acta Psiquiátrica y Psicológica de América Latina* **19** (1): 17–33.

[48] Ministerio de Salud. (2000) *Plan Nacional de Salud Mental y Psiquiatría* [National Plan of Mental Health and Psychiatry]. Santiago: Ministerio de Salud.

[49] Minoletti A, Sepulveda R, Horvitz-Lennon M. (2012) Twenty years of mental health policies in Chile: lessons and challenges. *International Journal of Mental Health* **41** (1): 21–37.

[50] Markkula N, Alvarado R, Minoletti A. (2011) Adherence to guidelines for treatment compliance in the Chilean National Program for first-episode schizophrenia. *Psychiatric Services* **62**: 1463–1469.

[51] Susser E, Baumgartner JN, Stein Z. (2010) Commentary: Sir Arthur Mitchell – pioneer of psychiatric epidemiology and of community care. *International Journal of Epidemiology* **39** (6): 1417–1425.

[52] Clausen J, Yarrow M. (1955) Mental illness and the family. *Journal of Social Issues* **11**: 3–5.

[53] Grad J, Sainsbury P. (1963) Mental illness and the family. *Lancet* **1** (7280): 544–547.

[54] Susser E, Collins P, Schanzer B et al. (1996) Topics for our times: can we learn from the care of persons with mental illness in developing countries? *American Journal of Public Health* **86** (7): 926–928.

CHAPTER 7

The role of primary care in low- and middle-income countries

David Goldberg[1], Graham Thornicroft[1] and Nadja van Ginneken[2,3]

[1] Health Service and Population Research Department, Institute of Psychiatry, King's College London, London, UK
[2] Nutrition and Public Health Intervention Research Department, London School of Hygiene and Tropical Medicine, London, UK
[3] Sangath, Goa, India

Introduction

The World Bank divides LAMICs into three broad groups, mainly on the basis of their gross national income (GNI) [1]. Countries in the low-income group account for 798 million people living in predominantly rural areas. Those in the low- to middle-income groups comprise 2.52 billion people with 39% living in urban areas, and those in the upper-middle-income group include 2.45 billion people, with 57% living in urban areas.

These three groups are compared with high-income countries in Table 7.1, which shows not only the mean GNI of each group but the effect that this has on the proportion of the total health spend that is devoted to mental illness, as well as the median mental health spend per 100 000 population at risk. All the LAMICs spend about 75% of their mental health spend on hospital services, in contrast to the high-income countries that only spend 54% of their much larger income in this way. The much larger sums devoted to mental disorders in high-income countries means that much larger sums can be spent on drug treatments for mental disorders.

These gross inequalities inevitably have consequences for the manpower that can be employed in the mental health services. It can be seen from Table 7.2 that low-income countries will only have on average 5 psychiatrists for each ten million population, in contrast to the high-income countries with 859 psychiatrists. Even more disturbing is the fact that when these data are compared with those published seven years earlier, the low-income countries have lost one psychiatrist for each ten million people, while the high-income countries have gained

Improving Mental Health Care: The Global Challenge, First Edition.
Edited by Graham Thornicroft, Mirella Ruggeri and David Goldberg.
© 2013 John Wiley & Sons, Ltd. Published 2013 by John Wiley & Sons, Ltd.

Table 7.1 Relative financial indicators for countries in income bands relevant to mental illness from *WHO Mental Health Atlas* [2].

Country income group	Mean GNI per capita[a] ($)	% of health spend on mental illness	Median mental health spend/100 K ($)	Mean annual spend on psychiatric drugs/100 K ($)
Low income	530	0.55	20 000	1 700
Lower-middle income	1 623	1.9	50 000	17 200
Upper-middle income	5 886	2.38	376 000	82 700
High income	40 197[b]	5.1	4.48 M	2.63 M

[a] From World Bank.
[b] OECD countries.

Table 7.2 Manpower in mental health by income level of country, rates per 100 000 population from *World Mental Health Atlas* [2].

Country income	Psychiatrists/100 K	Other MDs/100 K	Nurses/100 K	Clinical psychologists/100 K	Social worker/100 K	Other health worker/100 K
Low income	0.05 (−0.01)*	0.06	0.42	0.02	0.01	0.12
Lower-middle income	0.54 (+0.03)	0.21	2.93	0.14	0.13	1.34
Upper-middle income	2.03 (+0.31)	0.87	9.72	1.49	0.76	13.3
High income	8.59 (+0.65)	1.49	29.13	3.79	2.16	17.09
World median	1.27	0.33	4.95	0.33	0.24	2.09

Numbers in parenthesis indicate change since 2005, as % change.
* Significant at 5%.

65 extra psychiatrists. It can be seen that all classes of mental health workers are in very short supply in low-income countries. In many low-income countries, the only medical services available to dispersed populations are provided by nurses, and unless they are allowed to prescribe drugs or learn simple psychological interventions, the situation cannot possibly improve. Thus, while only a minority (27%) of such nurses in low-income countries are not allowed to prescribe even a limited range of drugs, similar figures for lower-middle- and upper-middle-income countries are 70% and 87%, respectively [2].

When one recalls that many of the psychiatrists in lower-income countries are practising in major cities, it is clear that in most rural areas it is impossible for mental illness services to be efficiently provided as an entirely specialist service. In 1973, the World Health Organization (WHO) formulated its policy to provide mental health services in the health services of the developing countries by incorporating them into primary care services [3]. This important policy document has influenced all the developments in services in primary care that have developed since, but clearly much had to be done before the policy could be developed into services in primary care. One early study showed that psychological disorders were common in four quite different developing countries, with an overall mean of nearly 14% of consecutive attenders who met current standards for mental disorders, and noted that patients with mental disorders presented for treatment with mainly somatic complaints, so that symptoms of depression and anxiety were most common, and psychotic symptoms occurred in only 3% of mentally disordered patients [4].

It became clear that the first requirement for the implementation of this policy was a huge expansion of mental health manpower, and an early paper on training showed how health ancillaries could be trained to first suspect and then confirm the diagnoses of psychosis, depression and epilepsy [5]. This paper stressed the need to discover what the trainees knew before the training course and provided them with simple algorithms for making the various diagnoses as well as providing them with a few basic psychotropic drugs. The role of mental health professionals in providing this training was described, as well as the role of supervisors of this work.

Setting up mental illness services in primary care

During the next 20 years, training manuals for primary health-care (PHC) staff were prepared in many LAMICs, and demonstration projects were set up in many countries. Successful initiatives have been implemented in the Indian subcontinent and several African countries, demonstrating how integrating mental health into general health care results in more accessible, affordable and acceptable services and care. A modest investment of resources into primary care has the potential to reduce the burden of mental disorders considerably [6, 7]. Uganda is one successful example. Having identified mental health as a priority,

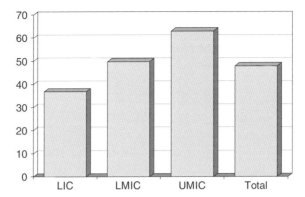

Figure 7.1 Percentage of primary health-care clinics in which psychotropic medicines are available, by country income group. LIC, low-income countries; LMIC and UMIC, lower- and upper-middle-income countries. Data derived from WHO AIMS study [9].

small mental health units (offering inpatient and outpatient care) are being constructed at regional hospitals; other reforms include curriculum changes and substantial training and re-training of health-care providers; new guidelines, training manuals, monitoring tools and support supervision teams; increased supply of psychotropic medications; and mass public education. Uganda's integration of mental health into primary care and investment of resources has improved access to affordable, and less stigmatising, mental health care [8].

However, with severe shortages of funds for mental disorders in many countries to support newly trained staff and psychotropic drugs, progress was still at best poor across the developing world, and most mentally disordered patients are still not being either diagnosed or treated (see Figure 7.1) [9]. At the national level, the proportion of people with diagnosable mental disorders who receive health-care interventions ('coverage') is at best between 27% and 30.5% across Europe [10, 11] and the United States [12], respectively, and at worst this has been documented as a treated annual prevalence rate of 2% in Nigeria [13]. Especially since the 2007 Lancet series of mental health papers [6], the significance of this 'treatment gap' is increasingly appreciated worldwide [14–16].

Evidence-based interventions in low- and middle-income countries: The Mental Health GAP

The Department of Mental Health and Substance Abuse at the WHO has recognised the importance of this challenge by launching as its centrepiece the Mental Health Global Action Programme (mhGAP) in 2008 [17]. The first major product of this programme is the mhGAP Implementation Guide (MIG) [18]. This is a landmark mental health publication by the WHO as it is a document designed for direct use by first- and second-level practitioners (district medical officer and primary care staff), and until this point, WHO has more often focused upon providing governmental level technical assistance and advice [19].

The mhGAP Intervention Guide contains case findings and treatment guidelines for nine categories of mental and neurological disorders which are common in low-income settings and which have a major public health impact:

1 Depression
2 Psychoses
3 Epilepsy/seizures
4 Developmental disorders
5 Behaviour disorders
6 Dementia
7 Alcohol use disorders
8 Drug use disorders
9 Self-harm/suicide

The MIG is based upon very thorough use of existing literature reviews, and upon 93 newly commissioned systematic reviews addressing important clinical questions where there was uncertainty. The procedures used were those recommended by the WHO for creating transparent, evidence-based guidelines using the *Grading of Recommendations Assessment, Development and Evaluation* (GRADE) methodology [19]. The draft MIG proposals were then modified in light of a detailed feasibility exercise and subject to scrutiny in relation to their acceptability to service users and carers, and their human rights implications [20]. It is therefore reasonable to consider the MIG as being simplified treatment guidelines specifically designed for primary care/district-level non-specialist staff, which are based upon the strongest possible current evidence of effective mental health interventions in low- and middle-income settings.

Yet, the fundamental public health questions go beyond the formulation of guidelines and include: (a) Can such guidelines be put into practice in routine clinical settings? (b) If so, do they confer patient benefit? (c) Does their use contribute to an increase in the treated prevalence (coverage) rates for specified conditions? In short, it is clear from over two decades of research that the creation of guidelines is necessary but not sufficient for evidence-based practice. As a consequence, there has been the recent rapid development of 'implementation science' [21] with some applications in the field of mental health [22]. A recent review has summarised the factors which have been identified as facilitators or barriers to the implementation of mental-illness-related clinical guidelines [23] and distinguished between: (a) the adoption in principle of guidelines, (b) early implementation and (c) their sustained use over time.

The work leading up to the preparation of the mhGAP appears to have caused a new wave of projects to train PHC staff for the assessment and treatment of mental illness. In recent years, there has been progress in many LAMICs. In low-income countries, courses have been set up in Burundi [24], Equatorial Guinea [25], Guinea-Brissau [26], Kenya [27, 28], Tanzania [29], Uganda [8, 30–32] and Haiti [33]. In lower-middle-income countries, they have been set up in India [5, 34], Pakistan [35, 36], Iraq [37], Nigeria [38], Sudan [39], Sri Lanka [36] and Syria [40], while in upper-middle-income countries, they have been set up in Colombia [41], Jordan [36], Lebanon [42], Peru [43], Russia [44, 45] and South Africa [46]. These various courses vary a great deal in intensity and duration, but they appear to represent an emergence of a determination to introduce these services across a wide front.

There are two essential conditions that must be met before a new training course can be set up: first, the course should have managerial support with the agreement of either the local or the national government, and, second, there must be a local trainer available who can give time not just to the course itself but to providing support after the new service is set up. While these reports are encouraging, most LAMICs have either not carried out or not published details of such courses by mid-2012.

Different forms of collaboration between psychiatric and primary care services

'Stepped care' refers to offering an inexpensive treatment to mildly ill patients, a more elaborate and more expensive treatment to moderately or severely ill patients, and referral to a mental health professional in a separate service only for those who have not responded to a treatment in primary care or those who are actively suicidal. At each level, there are usually specific indications for a movement to the next stage. In the context of depression, it may refer to health information, CCBT or physical exercise for the mildly ill; an active psychological or pharmacological treatment for the moderately or severely ill; and specialist referral only for those few patients who have not responded. It can be seen that stepped care is particularly suited for government- or insurance-funded services, where cost reduction is important – therefore, it is routinely used by the National Institute for Health and Clinical Excellence (NICE) in the United Kingdom, for example.

'Shared care' refers to efforts to involve primary care in the routine management of people with *severe mental disorders* (schizophrenia or bipolar illness) who are maintained on stable medication. The mental health service offers support from a specialised nurse to the GP and undertakes to re-admit the patient should a severe relapse occur. Care from primary care is much less stigmatising for the patient, and the mental health service is able to continue to accept new referrals from primary care, since it is not faced with an ever-increasing load of psychotic patients.

'Collaborative care' is a somewhat more elaborate version of shared care and typically has three components:
- A dedicated coordinator of the intervention supported by a multi-professional team.
- Joint determination of the plan of care.
- Long-term coordination and follow-up coordination of both mental and physical health care.

The dedicated coordinator is typically located within the primary care team, rather than being an emissary of the mental health team. Indeed, help is often provided by a behavioural scientist, typically a clinical psychologist in high-income countries, but often a lay health worker in low-income countries. Nor need the collaboration refer necessarily to the mental health service at all – in collaborative care of diabetes, for example, it may refer to the specialist service for diabetes.

Evidence of effectiveness and cost-effectiveness of collaboration between the two services

Any novel treatment typically costs more money, at least in the short term. Where health costs are free at the point of delivery, or are largely reimbursed by medical insurance companies, it makes sense to offset any advantages gained by the new treatment against the cost of it. Before one can transfer the cost of a quality-adjusted life year (QALY) from one country to another, one must establish that health costs for items of service are comparable, and that the amount of money devoted to health care is also equivalent.

The amount a rich country is prepared to pay for a QALY is by no means the same as a poor one. But in a poor country, individual items of care may be much less, and this will affect the amount they are prepared to pay for each QALY. Whereas a high-income country like the United Kingdom spends 10% of its health budget on mental health, lower-income countries spend less than 1% (Table 7.1). A high-income country will be able to spend much greater sums on a QALY than a low-income country, but this will be counterbalanced by the fact that the cost of care is very much less in the latter.

Fortunately, there are now a number of well-conducted effectiveness and cost-effectiveness studies in LAMICs. An early study by Chisholm and colleagues [47] compared two localities each in India and Pakistan. For three of these localities, providing a mental health service in primary care, there were improvements over time in symptoms, disability and quality of life, while total economic costs were reduced. A more recent paper [48] estimates the additional cost per capita of scaling up mental health expenditure to provide pharmacological and/ or psychosocial treatment of schizophrenia, bipolar disorder, depression and hazardous alcohol use in LAMICs. This was found to be between $1.85 and $2.60 per year in low-income countries and $3.20 and $6.25 per year in lower-middle-income countries, which represents an additional annual investment of $0.18–0.55 per capita.

Many effective treatments for depression are inexpensive, and these include antidepressants, problem solving and behavioural activation. A specially trained lay health worker is capable of delivering effective mental health interventions. Araya and others [49] allocated 240 low-income female patients with severe depression in Santiago, Chile, to usual care or care administered by a three-month, multi-component intervention led by a non-medical health worker, which included a psychoeducational group intervention, structured and systematic follow-up and drug treatment. At six months' follow-up, 70% of the intervention group compared with 30% of the usual-care group had recovered. A later paper [50] considered outcome at six months and found that after adjusting for initial severity, women receiving the stepped-care programme had a mean of 50 additional depression-free days over six months relative to patients allocated to usual care. The stepped-care programme was marginally more expensive than usual care (an extra 216 Chilean pesos per depression-free day). The authors concluded that small investments to improve depression appear to yield larger gains in poorer environments. These data have been re-examined to evaluate the cost-effectiveness of usual care versus 'improved stepped care' [51], where it was shown that the latter treatment was likely to lead to a greater reduction in lifetime episodes of depression and a greater number of quality-adjusted days. However, there is an increased cost/QALY gained, of I$468 against I$113 for usual care. Since this is within the amount that Chile is prepared to pay, the stepped-care model should be preferred to usual care.

A study by Patel and others [52] assigned patients with common mental disorders to either collaborative stepped care (CSC) by lay health counsellors or to enhanced usual care. The CSC condition meant that all patients with high scores on a screening questionnaire were given psychoeducation by the lay counsellors, but patients with higher scores were offered an antidepressant by the primary care physician. Psychoeducation taught patients strategies to alleviate symptoms, such as breathing exercises for anxiety symptoms and scheduling activities for symptoms of depression. Moderately or severely ill patients who were offered drug treatment could also have group interpersonal psychotherapy from the lay health worker.

Those who failed to respond to the more active treatments, or who were actively suicidal, were referred on to a mental health specialist. For the control intervention, physicians and patients in usual care practices received screening results and were given the treatment manual prepared for primary care physicians. The CSC intervention turned out to be effective in the public clinics, but not in private clinics. The authors observe that in the public clinics, larger numbers of patients tend to be seen for shorter periods by a doctor, and the privacy needed to discuss interpersonal difficulties is not always possible.

A later paper [53] followed these patients up for 12 months and found a 30% decrease in the prevalence of common mental disorders among those with baseline ICD-10 diagnoses (risk ratio (RR)=0.70, 95% CI 0.53–0.92) and a similar effect among the subgroup of participants with depression (RR=0.76, 95% CI 0.59–0.98). Suicide attempts/plans showed a 36% reduction over 12 months (RR=0.64, 95% CI 0.42–0.98) among baseline ICD-10 cases. Strong effects were observed on days out of work and psychological morbidity, and modest effects on overall disability. In contrast, there was little evidence of impact of the intervention on any outcome among participants attending private facilities. A detailed qualitative study [54] investigated the factors producing the effectiveness of the lay health counsellors. They were female college graduates, recruited from the local community, who were trained to lead the intervention in a structured two-month course to deliver a range of psychosocial treatments (psychoeducation, interpersonal therapy, referral to appropriate agencies, adherence support) for common mental disorders. They acted as a case manager for all patients who screened positive and took overall responsibility for the intervention delivery, working in close collaboration with the primary care physician and the psychiatrist for all non-drug treatments and supporting adherence with antidepressants for those who were prescribed the drug by the primary care physician. The key factors which enhance the acceptability and integration of the counsellors in primary care are training, systematic steps to build trust, the passage of time, the observable impacts on patient outcomes and supervision by a visiting psychiatrist. However, a paper by the same group [55] indicated that if three treatments were compared – antidepressant, psychotherapy and placebo with usual care – then only the antidepressant was superior to the placebo.

Chisholm and Saxena [56] compared strategies for intervening in five different neuropsychiatric disorders in LAMICs. They assessed them in terms of percentage of remissions achieved and reduction in disability. Best results were found for older anticonvulsants and antidepressants versus newer drugs, and for population-based measures for the control of alcohol problems.

Although Puerto Rico is officially a high-income country, the GNI of its inhabitants is low compared with the rest of the United States ($15 500 against $47 340), nearer the top end of upper-middle-income countries. We therefore include a study by Vera and others [57] in which 179 PHC patients were randomly assigned to collaborative care or usual care. The collaborative care intervention involved enhanced collaboration among physicians, mental health specialists and care managers paired with depression-specific treatment guidelines, patient education and follow-up. It was found to significantly improve clinical symptoms and functional status of depressed patients with coexisting chronic general medical conditions.

Other studies of interventions in primary care in LAMICs for common mental disorders

Although they do not meet the aforementioned requirements for evaluations of collaborative, stepped or shared care models, a wealth of other types of programmes integrating mental health into PHC have shown the effectiveness of various health professionals in providing care.

For example, medical officers have been successfully used to deliver interventions for common mental disorders in Uganda [58] and Iran [59], and nurses for delivering care for alcohol problems in Thailand [60] and child mental health services in South Africa [61].

Lay health workers have provided care for maternal depression in Jamaica [62] and shown that such care produced benefits in both child development and maternal depression, provided that there had been at least 45 visits.

Other studies have been less encouraging: primary care doctors in Africa have been shown to have low recognition rates of anxiety and depression [63] and much inappropriate prescribing has been reported in LAMICs [64, 65].

Things that can, and do, go wrong

There is a long list of reasons why mental illness services do not achieve nationwide acceptance, even in countries that have examples of excellent services in demonstration sites. However, none of them apply universally.

A centrally mandated and funded national plan, but poor local acceptance

India is a good example of this, with a series of national plans that are not, or only imperfectly, taken up locally. Goel [66] himself a retired central planner, suggests that 'a top–down approach to planning, and unrealistic expectations from low-paid or poorly motivated primary healthcare personnel play an important role and may result in the failure of even adequately funded programmes'. There is good evidence for this: an independent assessment of 20 widely dispersed districts reported that only 10% of the districts fully used the funds allocated for setting up these services. Twenty percent of the districts did not use the funds at all, and the remaining 70% of districts had only partially used them. Even with adequate funds, 75% of the districts were unable to maintain a regular supply of drugs. When planning is divorced from the ground realities, poor governance, managerial incompetence and unrealistic expectations from low-paid/poorly motivated PHC personnel play an important role and may result in the failure of even adequately funded programmes.

Failures at local level

Wig and Murthy [67] write that the most important failure in India is the low involvement of the health workers and doctors in care. Instead, in almost all of the centres, the district mental health programme (DMHP) has become 'extension clinics' where psychiatric teams visit once a month or so and conduct clinics. They also point to the lack of coordination between the DMHP team and the medical college where the team is located. Isaac [68] points out that there is almost no involvement of the private and non-governmental sectors in the national mental health programme, and recommends that such partnerships need to be developed.

In Sri Lanka [69] and South Africa [70, 71], the lack of community awareness and stigma towards mental disorders lead to poor attendance within Western medical settings and non-cooperation. These as well as other studies have shown that involving the community and the family and having outreach community health workers to provide follow-up support but also psychoeducation improves understanding, attendance at clinics and acceptance of treatment.

Poor supervision of the trained staff

Many authors underscore the importance of providing ongoing supervision to staff newly undertaking this work. It is not sufficient to provide a training course unless such supervision is available. Many studies have highlighted that primary care workers and those at community level may have poor attitudes towards mental health and also feel disempowered to treat these conditions [36, 72]. In addition, in many LAMICs, there is a problem of attrition of health workers at PHC level [73]. Several studies have suggested that increased supervision/mentorship, motivation and ongoing adequate training help improve retention and motivation to treat [36, 72, 73]. In areas with few trained mental health professionals, there are logistical problems in providing such support – the good results reported in the cost-effectiveness studies above all had such support. In low-income countries, such staff are already overstretched, and other solutions need to be found. Quosh [40] describes how new trainers were trained to meet the needs of refugees flowing into Syria from Iraq by using mental health professionals as 'master trainers' who trained a second rank of primary care staff, school staff and community workers to provide training to staff who will actually carry out the mental health work. These 'second rank' staff may also provide supervision to the staff after basic training has been provided. Alternatively, a telephone hotline supervision service may be provided, as described in Uganda [58].

Local managers assign low priority to mental health work

Ssebunnya and others [32] describe a health district in Uganda where a single nurse is the sole mental health worker but is often diverted to general nursing duties. Her hospital manager asserted, 'we don't have mental health staff in the hospital. Mental health has not been one of the immediate priority areas....

I can't bring in a psychiatric nurse if I don't have the general nurses to take care of general patients'. In similar fashion, Omigbodun [74] describes primary care mental health services in two districts in Nigeria and found virtually no mental health services were being provided in either district. She concludes that 'current training is not effective and virtually none of what was learnt appears to be used by PHC workers in the field'.

The availability and quality of psychotropic drugs

In many low-income countries, psychotropics must compete with other needs for drugs and are either unavailable or very scarce. It is difficult to provide help to many epileptics or those with severe psychoses without them, and psycho-therapeutic help for depression is time-consuming if antidepressants are not available. As might be expected, the situation is not quite so bad in upper-middle-income countries (see Tables 7.1 and 7.2). The quality of drugs is also a major issue as in LAMIC drug suppliers, even those who provide government-run clinics, do not always provide reliable drugs [75].

Community services for severe mental disorders in low-income countries

Various surveys report problems with inappropriate psychotropics, or needless polypharmacy in PHC [75, 76]. Two studies have addressed the treatment of severe mental disorders in low-income countries by arguing for an alternative to the mental hospital. A study by Ran and others [77] in Chengdu, China, assigned families with a member suffering from schizophrenia to three groups: drug management plus family intervention, drug management only and a control condition where medication was neither encouraged nor discouraged. This showed that the combined intervention was effective in that relatives' attitude to the patient and the patient's cooperation with medication was improved, and most importantly, the relapse rate over nine months in this group (16.3%) was much less than either the drug-only group (37.8%) or the control group (61.5%). Chatterjee and others [78] showed that patients with chronic schizophrenia in rural India had a superior response to the combination of community-based rehabilitation and outpatient care than they did to outpatient care alone.

Using traditional healers to supplement PHC services

Working closely with traditional healers has a number of potential advantages to the primary care mental health system. These healers typically have the confidence of the local population but use a completely different frame of reference for understanding mental health problems. Such healers typically make use of suggestion and altered states of consciousness to aid the healing process, and the healer usually inspires confidence in his clients and may make use of involvement of the family and other community members to assist the healing process. In contrast, medical officers in LAMICs may not be accustomed to family interventions and often rely on pharmacological agents to assist them.

It is clearly advantageous for each set of healers to have greater understanding of what the other healers are good at, as this may lead to patients being referred to the most effective set of healers. Thus, a faith healer may do a more effective job with a case of hysterical aphonia or paralysis, while a Western medical officer will typically be more effective with epileptic seizures, acute psychoses and severely depressed patients. This may be the theory, but it does not seem to be the practice.

Lam and others [79] subjected a set of practitioners of Chinese traditional medicine to the standard ten-week training course made available to medical officers in mental health skills. The traditional practitioners indeed rated themselves as more confident in both the diagnosis and management of mental health problems and declared that they were more confident at referring appropriate patients to Western physicians – but at follow-up there was no evidence that an increased number had been so referred. Saeed and others [80] compared the diagnoses made by faith healers in Pakistan for 139 of their patients who consented to be seen by a psychiatrist using standard research instruments. Not surprisingly, there was no relationship between these two assessments. Patients considered to have either depression or anxiety by the psychiatrist were most often considered to be cases of 'saya' (a belief that an evil spirit had cast his or her shadow on the patient) but were also likely to receive six other different diagnostic assessments. While Western psychiatry is based on the pattern of symptoms that a patient has, the faith healers are concerned to identify the cause of the problem and direct their energies to that. The patient and his or her family are typically told that *they are not to blame* but have been possessed by a jinn, *churail* or spirit.

Others have also been positive about the contribution that might potentially be made by traditional healers, although they have not carried out the sort of formal studies described earlier. Razali [81] considered that the Malay traditional healers or *bomohs* might make a positive contribution by the exercise of their psychotherapeutic skills, while Robertson [82] reviews three studies of the work of traditional healers in South Africa and finds that their patients were generally appreciative of the treatment they had received, although it was not possible to reconcile the theoretical approach with that used by medical officers. He concludes that 'collaboration with traditional healers should urgently be promoted, as they are clearly providing a significant mental health service to certain sectors of the population. However, much more knowledge needs to be gained about what form of collaboration would be most appropriate'.

What are the positive arguments for mental health services based in primary care?

The majority of patients seeking help in primary care are consulting because of somatic symptoms. If these are caused by a physical disease, they hope to have this detected, and appropriate treatment given for it. Treatment at this venue is both less stigmatising and more accessible. However, a substantial proportion of these patients appear to have no obvious physical cause for their somatic symptoms, but on enquiry will be found to have a combination of anxious, depressive and somatic symptoms, most often in association with life problems. Just as the traditional healer seeks a cause for the presenting symptoms, this careful description of current symptoms, combined with symptomatic treatment and advice about how to deal with distressing thoughts or current life problems, is our nearest equivalent to this. Without the necessary mental health awareness, doctors run the risk of reinforcing the patients' physical symptoms, while neglecting the cause of their distress. In addition to this, the major disorders such as acute psychosis, severe depression and epilepsy are more effectively detected and treated by Western medical concepts.

References

[1] World Bank. (2012) *List of Economies*. Washington, DC: World Bank. Available from: http://data.worldbank.org/country. Accessed on 5 February 2013.

[2] World Health Organization. (2011) *World Mental Health Atlas*. Geneva: World Health Organization.

[3] World Health Organization. (1975) *Organisation of Mental Health Services in the Health Services of the Developing Countries*. Technical Support Services #564. Geneva: World Health Organization.

[4] Harding TW, de Arango MV, Baltazar J et al. (1980) Mental disorders in primary health care, a study of their frequency and diagnosis in four developing countries. *Psychological Medicine* **10**: 231–241.

[5] Murthy RS, Wig NN. (1983) The WHO collaborative study for extending mental health care: a training approach to enhancing the availability of mental health manpower in a developing country. *American Journal of Psychiatry* **140**: 1486–1490.

[6] Saxena S, Thornicroft G, Knapp M et al. (2007) Resources for mental health: scarcity, inequity, and inefficiency. *Lancet* **370**: 878–889.

[7] World Health Organization. (2008) *Closing the Gap in a Generation. Health Equity Through Action on the Social Determinants of Health*. Geneva: World Health Organization.

[8] Kigozi F. (2007) Integrating mental health into primary health care – Uganda's experience. *South African Psychiatry Review* **10**: 17–19.

[9] World Health Organization. (2009) *Mental Health Systems in Selected Low- and Middle-Income Countries: A WHO-AIMS Cross-National Analysis*. Geneva: WHO.

[10] Alonso J, Lepine JP. (2007) Overview of key data from the European Study of the Epidemiology of Mental Disorders (ESEMeD). *Journal of Clinical Psychiatry* **68** (Suppl. 2): 3–9.

[11] Wittchen HU, Jacobi F. (2005) Size and burden of mental disorders in Europe – a critical review and appraisal of 27 studies. *European Neuropsychopharmacology* **15**: 357–376.

[12] Kessler RC, Demler O, Frank RG et al. (2005) Prevalence and treatment of mental disorders, 1990 to 2003. *New England Journal of Medicine* **352** (24): 2515–2523.

[13] Wang PS, Aguilar-Gaxiola S, Alonso J et al. (2007) Use of mental health services for anxiety, mood, and substance disorders in 17 countries in the WHO world mental health surveys. *Lancet* **370** (9590): 841–850.

[14] Dua T, Barbui C, Clark N et al. (2011) Evidence based guidelines for mental, neurological and substance use disorders in low- and middle-income countries: summary of WHO recommendations. *PLoS Medicine* **8**: 1–11.

[15] Thornicroft G. (2007) Most people with mental illness are not treated. *Lancet* **370** (9590): 807–808.

[16] Eaton J, McCay L, Semrau M et al. (2011) Scale up of services for mental health in low-income and middle-income countries. *Lancet* **378** (9802): 1592–1603.

[17] World Health Organization. (2008) *Mental Health Gap Action Programme. Scaling Up Care for Mental, Neurological, and Substance Use Disorders*. Geneva: World Health Organization.

[18] World Health Organization. (2010) *mhGAP Intervention Guide for Mental, Neurological and Substance Use Disorders in No-Specialized Health Settings*. Geneva: World Health Organization.

[19] Barbui C, Dua T, van Ommeren M et al. (2010) Challenges in developing evidence-based recommendations using the GRADE approach: the case of mental, neurological, and substance use disorders. *PLoS Medicine* **7** (8): e1000322.

[20] Hill S, Pang T. (2007) Leading by example: a culture change at WHO. *Lancet* **369** (9576): 1842–1844.

[21] Madon T, Hofman KJ, Kupfer L et al. (2007) Public health. Implementation science. *Science* **318** (5857): 1728–1729.

[22] Thornicroft G, Lempp H, Tansella M. (2011) The place of implementation science in the translational medicine continuum. *Psychological Medicine* **41** (10): 2015–2021.

[23] Tansella M, Thornicroft G. (2009) Implementation science: understanding the translation of evidence into practice. *British Journal of Psychiatry* **195**: 283–285.

[24] Ventevogel P, Ndayisaba H, van de Put W. (2011) Psychosocial assistance and decentralised mental health care in post conflict Burundi 2000–2008. *Intervention* **9** (3): 315–331.

[25] Morón-Nozaleda MG, Gómez de Tojeiro J, Cobos-Muñoz D et al. (2011) Integrating mental health into primary care in Africa: the case of Equatorial Guinea. *Intervention* **9** (3): 304–314.

[26] de Jong TVM. (1996) A comprehensive public mental health programme in Guinea-Bissau: a useful model for African, Asian and Latin-American countries. *Psychological Medicine* **26**: 97–108.

[27] Jenkins R, Kiima D, Okonji M et al. (2010) Integration of mental health into primary care and community health working in Kenya: context, rationale, coverage and sustainability. *Mental Health in Family Medicine* **7** (1): 37–47.

[28] Jenkins R, Kiima D, Njenga F et al. (2010) Integration of mental health into primary care in Kenya. *World Psychiatry* **9** (2): 118–120.

[29] Mbatia J, Jenkins R. (2010) Development of a mental health policy and system in Tanzania: an integrated approach to achieve equity. *Psychiatric Services* **61** (10): 1028–1031.

[30] Baingana F, Onyango Mangen P. (2011) Scaling up of mental health and trauma support among war affected communities in northern Uganda: lessons learned. *Intervention* **9** (3): 291–303.

[31] Bhana A, Petersen I, Baillie KL et al. (2010) The MHapp Research Programme Consortium. Implementing the World Health Report 2001 recommendations for integrating mental health into primary health care: a situation analysis of three African countries: Ghana, South Africa and Uganda. *International Review of Psychiatry* **22** (6): 599–610.

[32] Ssebunnya J, Kigozi F, Kizza D et al. (2010) MHaPP Research Programme Consortium. Integration of mental health into primary health care in a rural district in Uganda. *African Journal of Psychiatry* **13**: 128–131.

[33] Budosan B, Frederique Bruno R. (2011) Strategy for providing integrated mental health/psychosocial support in post earthquake Haiti. *Intervention* **9** (3): 225–236.

[34] Chowdhury AN, Brahma A, Banerjee S et al. (2006) Community mental health service by IRMC model involving multi-purpose health workers in Sundarban, India. *International Medical Journal* **13** (3): 185–190.

[35] Naqvi HA. (2010) Primary care psychiatry in Pakistan: issues and challenges. *Journal of Pakistan Medical Association* **60** (10): 794–795.

[36] Budosan B. (2011) Mental health training of primary health care workers: case reports from Sri Lanka, Pakistan and Jordan. *Intervention* **9** (2): 125–136.

[37] Sadik S, Abdulrahman S, Bradley M et al. (2011) Integrating mental health into primary health care in Iraq. *Mental Health in Family Medicine* **8** (1): 39–49.

[38] Makanjuola V. (2010) Impact of a one week intensive training of the trainers of community health workers in South-West of Nigeria. *Asia-Pacific Psychiatry* **2010** (2): A6, Conference proceedings of the 14th Pacific Rim College of Psychiatrists Scientific Meeting, Brisbane.

[39] El Gaili DE, Magzoub MM, Schmidt HG. (2002) The impact of a community-oriented medical school on mental health services. *Education for Health* **15** (2): 149–157.

[40] Quosh C. (2011) Takamol: multi-professional capacity building in order to strengthen the psychosocial and mental health sector in response to refugee crises. *Intervention* **9** (3): 249–264.

[41] Climent CE, de Arango MV, Plutchick R. (1983) Development of an alternative, efficient, low-cost mental health delivery system in Cali, Colombia. Part II: the urban health centre. *Social Psychiatry* **18**: 95–102.

[42] Hijazi Z, Weissbecker I, Chammay R. (2011) The integration of mental health into primary health care in Lebanon. *Intervention* **9** (3): 265–278.

[43] Kohan I, Pérez-Sales P, Huamaní Cisneros M et al. (2011) Emergencies and disasters as opportunities to improve mental health systems: Peruvian experience in Huancavelica. *Intervention* **9** (3): 237–248.

[44] Jenkins J, Bobyleva Z, Goldberg D et al. (2009) Integrating mental health into primary care in Sverdlovsk. *Mental Health in Family Medicine* **6**: 29–36.

[45] Zakroyeva A, Goldberg D, Gask L et al. (2008) Training Russian family physicians in mental health skills. *European Journal of General Practice* **14** (1): 19–22.

[46] van Deventer C, Couper I, Wright A et al. (2008) Evaluation of primary mental health care in North West province – a qualitative view. *South African Journal of Psychiatry* **14** (4): 136–140.

[47] Chisholm D, James S, Sekar K et al. (2000) Integration of mental health care into primary care. Demonstration cost-outcome study in India and Pakistan. *British Journal of Psychiatry* **176**: 581–588.

[48] Chisholm D, Lund C, Saxena S. (2007) Cost of scaling up mental healthcare in low- and middle-income countries. *British Journal of Psychiatry* **191**: 528–535.

[49] Araya R, Rojas G, Fritsch R et al. (2003) Treating depression in primary care in low-income women in Santiago, Chile: a randomised controlled trial. *Lancet* **361**: 995–1000.

[50] Araya R, Flynn T, Rojas G et al. (2006) Cost-effectiveness of a primary care treatment program for depression in low-income women in Santiago, Chile. *American Journal of Psychiatry* **163** (8): 1379–1387.

[51] Siskind D, Araya R, Kim J. (2010) Cost-effectiveness of improved primary care treatment of depression in women in Chile. *British Journal of Psychiatry* **197**: 291–296.

[52] Patel V, Weiss H, Chowdhary N et al. (2010) Effectiveness of an intervention led by lay health counsellors for depressive and anxiety disorders in primary care in Goa, India (MANAS): a cluster randomised controlled trial. *Lancet* **376**: 2086–2095.

[53] Patel V, Weiss HA, Chowdhary N et al. (2011) Lay health worker led intervention for depressive and anxiety disorders in India: impact on clinical and disability outcomes over 12 months. *British Journal of Psychiatry* **199**: 459–466.

[54] Pereira B, Andrew G, Pednekar S et al. (2011) The integration of the treatment for common mental disorders in primary care: experiences of health care providers in the MANAS trial in Goa, India. *International Journal of Mental Health Systems* **5**: 26.

[55] Patel V, Chisholm D, Rabe-Hesketh S et al. (2003) Efficacy and cost-effectiveness of drug and psychological treatments for common mental disorders in general health care in Goa, India: a randomised, controlled trial. *Lancet* **361** (9351): 33–39.

[56] Chisholm D, Saxena S. (2012) Cost-effectiveness of strategies to combat neuropsychiatric conditions in Sub-Saharan Africa and South East Asia: mathematical modelling study. *BMJ* **344**: e609.

[57] Vera M, Perez-Pedrogo C, Huertas SE et al. (2010) Collaborative care for depressed patients with chronic medical conditions: a randomized trial in Puerto Rico. *Psychiatric Services* **61** (2): 144–150.

[58] Ovuga E, Boardman J, Wasserman D. (2007) Integrating mental health in to primary health care: local initiatives from Uganda. *World Psychiatry* **6**: 60–61.

[59] Sharifi V. (2009) Urban mental health in Iran: challenges and future directions. *Iranian Journal of Psychiatry and Behavioural Sciences* **3** (1): 9–14.

[60] Noknoy S, Rangsin R, Saengcharnchai P et al. (2010) RCT of effectiveness of motivational enhancement therapy delivered by nurses for hazardous drinkers in primary care units in Thailand. *Alcohol & Alcoholism* **45** (3): 263–270.

[61] Pillay AL, Lockhat MR. (1997) Developing community mental health services for children in South Africa. *Social Science & Medicine* **45** (10): 1493–1501.

[62] Baker-Henningham H, Powell C, Walker S et al. (2005) The effect of early stimulation on maternal depression: a cluster randomised controlled trial. *Archives of Disease in Childhood* **90**: 1230–1234.

[63] Patel V. (1996) Recognition of common mental disorders in primary care in African countries: should 'mental' be dropped? *Lancet* **347** (9003): 742–744.

[64] Patel V, Andrade C. (2003) Pharmacological treatment of severe psychiatric disorders in developing world: lessons from India. *CNS Drugs* **17** (15): 1071–1080.

[65] Linden M, Lecrubier Y, Bellantuono C et al. (1999) The prescribing of psychotropic drugs by primary care physicians: an international collaborative study. *Journal of Clinical Psychopharmacology* **19** (2): 132–140.

[66] Goel DS. (2011) Why mental health services in low- and middle-income countries are under-resourced, under-performing: an Indian perspective. *National Medical Journal of India* **24**: 94–97.

[67] Wig NN, Murthy RS. (2009) Mental health care in India – past, present and future. *The Tribune*, October 10.

[68] Isaac M. (2011) National mental health programme: time for reappraisal. In: Kulhara P, Avasthi A, Thirunavukarasu M (eds.), *Themes and Issues in Contemporary Indian Psychiatry.* New Delhi: Indian Psychiatric Society.

[69] Ganesan M. (2011) Building up mental health services from scratch: experiences from East Sri Lanka. *Intervention* **9** (3): 359–363.

[70] Peterson I, Ssebunnya J, Bhana A et al. (2011) Research Programme Consortium. Lessons from case studies of integrating mental health into primary health care in South Africa and Uganda. *International Journal of Mental Health Systems* **5**: 8.

[71] Peterson I, Lund C. (2011) Mental health service delivery in South Africa from 2000 to 2010: one step forward, one step back. *South African Medical Journal* **101**: 751–757.

[72] Sharma S, Piachaud J. (2011) Iraq and mental health policy: a post invasion analysis. *Intervention* **9** (3): 332–344.

[73] Kakuma R, Minas H, van Ginneken N et al. (2011) Human resources for mental health care: current situation and strategies for action. *Lancet* **378** (9803): 1654–1663.

[74] Omigbodun OO. (2001) A cost-effective model for increasing access to mental health care at the primary care level in Nigeria. *Journal of Mental Health Policy and Economics* **4**: 133–139.

[75] Cohen, A. (2001) *The Effectiveness of Mental Health Service in Primary Care: The View from the Developing World.* Geneva: World Health Organization.

[76] Hanlon C, Wondimagegn D, Alem A. (2010) Lessons learned in developing community mental health care in Africa. *World Psychiatry* **9** (3): 185–189.

[77] Ran MS, Xiang MZ, Chan CLW et al. (2003) Effectiveness of psychoeducational intervention for rural Chinese families experiencing schizophrenia. A randomised controlled trial. *Social Psychiatry and Psychiatric Epidemiology* **38**: 69–75.

[78] Chatterjee S, Patel V, Chatterjee A et al. (2003) Evaluation of a community-based rehabilitation model for chronic schizophrenia in rural India. *British Journal of Psychiatry* **182**: 57–82.

[79] Lam TP, Mak KY, Goldberg D et al. (2012) Western mental health training for traditional Chinese medicine practitioners. *Acta Psychiatrica Scandinavica* **126** (6): 440–447.

[80] Saeed K, Gater R, Husain A et al. (2000) The prevalence, classification of mental disorders among attenders of native faith healers in rural Pakistan. *Social Psychiatry and Psychiatric Epidemiology* **35** (10): 480–485.

[81] Razali SM. (2009) Integrating Malay traditional healers into primary health care services in Malaysia: is it feasible? *International Medical Journal* **16**: 13–17.

[82] Robertson BA. (2006) Does the evidence support collaboration between psychiatry and traditional healers? Findings from three South African studies. *South African Psychiatry Review* **9**: 87–90.

CHAPTER 8

Meeting the challenge of physical comorbidity and unhealthy lifestyles

Lorenzo Burti, Loretta Berti, Elena Bonfioli and Irene Fiorini

Department of Public Health and Community Medicine, Section of Psychiatry, University of Verona, Verona, Italy

Introduction

There is an increasing evidence for a substantially increased *mortality* and *physical comorbidity* among people with severe mental illness (SMI) as compared to the general population [1–3]. Several *risk factors* have been consistently found, including medication side effects, patient's scarce concern with health and consequential *unhealthy lifestyle* and discrimination by health professionals, with resulting inadequate medical care [4–10]. Risk factors related to lifestyle are modifiable through interventions leading to health promotion, but these have to be adapted to fit the characteristics and special needs of patients with severe mental disorders [11–13]. These patients appreciate the increased attention provided by the staff to their physical health and are likely to try to change their lifestyle.

An exploratory intervention project

An exploratory project was accomplished in the South-Verona Community Psychiatric Service (CPS) in 2006. The nurses of the Community Mental Health Centre routinely monitor patients' vital parameters and weight, assist those in treatment with insulin, collect orders and serve lunch. They reported patients' physical ailments and unhealthy lifestyle to the mental health teams and suggested to intervene in collaboration with the Department of Prevention of the local health authority – a real bottom-up initiative. A health promotion programme including diet education and a group-walking activity was conjointly designed and implemented and involved most of the staff and the patients

Improving Mental Health Care: The Global Challenge, First Edition.
Edited by Graham Thornicroft, Mirella Ruggeri and David Goldberg.
© 2013 John Wiley & Sons, Ltd. Published 2013 by John Wiley & Sons, Ltd.

attending the Centre. The initiative was very successful in terms of participation, satisfaction and continuation: patients changed their orders for lunch and started to assume a healthier diet and enjoyed group walking, which they still maintain twice a week. This experience encouraged the authors to design and implement a comprehensive survey and an intervention study. In preparation for the study, the authors also conducted a systematic review and meta-analysis on weight management interventions in psychotic patients [14].

The mentally ill are a high-risk group and tend to be neglected. While campaigns of health promotion are becoming a growing concern for international organisations, they may incur the risk that disadvantaged groups like the mental health patients remain somehow excluded from these actions. The European Union (EU) documents like the White Paper 'A Strategy for Europe on Nutrition, Overweight and Obesity related health issues' [15] or the Green Paper 'Promoting healthy diets and physical activity: a European dimension for the prevention of overweight, obesity and chronic diseases' [16] deal with the general population and vulnerable groups like the children and the poor. Unfortunately, the mentally ill tend to remain neglected, in that they are not mentioned among the vulnerable groups even though they represent a particularly vulnerable, disadvantaged socio-economic group. This happens at the same time when mental health attracts wide European attention as reflected in seminal EU documents like the Mental Health Action Plan for Europe and the Mental Health Declaration for Europe adopted in Helsinki in 2005 [17]. Thus, a paradox arises: the mental health and the physical health of mental patients are individually, and separately, stressed, with the risk of uncoordinated interventions. This goes against the principle of *equity*, a founding principle of modern health services.

The socially disadvantaged population groups, which include the greatest part of mental health patients, use the complete range of preventive health services to the lowest degree. In a public-health-oriented system, a desirable goal is that all intervention policies that may have either a direct or indirect impact on health be designed to favour the less affluent individuals and to reduce social inequalities as far as possible. Instead, studies exploring the possible relationship between the provision of health promotion interventions and indicators of health need suggest that health promotion interventions have often tended to benefit populations at lower risk of ill health [18]. This 'inverse care law' also applies to clinical check-ups: patients at greater risk of ill health, for example those in social classes 4 and 5, are less easily persuaded to attend health checks. These findings are parallel to those of the Acheson Report, which describes the 'inverse prevention law', in which 'communities most at risk of ill health tend to experience the least satisfactory access to the full range of preventive services such as cancer screening, immunisation programmes and health promotion' [19].

Finally, these problems and possible solutions must be framed in a global context, taking into account countries with different levels of income. In Europe, there is a broad variety of mental health systems, varying from those still based on mental hospitals to those essentially based on community mental health, with a number of nations falling in between with various mixes of services. Case reports indicate that in many low- and middle-income countries, people in psychiatric hospitals lack access to basic health care including general health examinations, dental care, vaccines, medications and treatments for cuts and bed sores [20]. In low-income countries, even simple forms of intervention may be far beyond the resources available. Across the low- and middle-income group countries, more than three-quarters of people needing mental health care do not even receive the most basic mental health services [21]; thus, screening, diagnosis and treatment of potential comorbid physical illness remain a mere wish. Therefore, a matrix taking into account both income of the country and the appropriate level and type of intervention has to be designed after the model suggested by WHO [22].

In low-income countries, both physical and mental disorders must be treated in primary care. In affluent countries, instead, where health-care systems are complex and the risk of poor cooperation between general health and mental health systems is strong, the physical health care of mental patients may fall through the gaps of health systems and be severely neglected. Therefore, health promotion programmes targeted to the psychiatric population have to be considered a key feature of modern mental health systems of care. In fact, poor mental health often goes hand in hand with chronic disease [23]. Mental health and long-term illness have major impact on each other and should be viewed holistically. For instance, even a mild to moderate depression affects an individual's ability to undertake health-promoting behaviours. Demonstrations that the simultaneous attention to and treatment of mental and physical illness improve the prognosis of both and lower the cost of treatment might help change this situation [7].

Background: From the early studies to a widespread interest in physical comorbidity of mental patients

The seminal reviews and meta-analyses of Brown [24] on the excess mortality of people with schizophrenia, and of Harris and Barraclough [1] on the excess mortality of people with mental disorder, provided stringent empirical evidence of a phenomenon that had been known for more than a century: premature death in these populations. There are many hypotheses about why people with psychiatric disorders are more likely to die than the rest of the population, and they are sometimes supported by inconsistent data. Psychiatric patients are at higher risk of suicide, accidental or violent death in general. The association that links psychiatric morbidity to a higher mortality from natural causes is less clear and has to be investigated using a multi-causal model. This excessive comorbidity has become more debated now because it is partly iatrogenic, in that it results from the side effects of antipsychotic drugs [25]. In the last few years, there has been a growing concern that the well-known side effects of antipsychotics may have further contributed to the shortened lifespan of people with schizophrenia.

Many first-generation and second-generation antipsychotics can cause significant weight gain, metabolic syndrome (MS), diabetes mellitus and cardiovascular disorders [26]. Antipsychotic medication may also cause the prolongation of QT-time, with serious ventricular arrhythmias, and predisposition to sudden cardiac death [27, 28]. There is a high frequency of concurrent pathological conditions in the psychiatric population [29–31] as well as smoking and other unhealthy lifestyle habits, tendency to self-neglect and poor quality of living conditions and care [32–34]. Other data suggest that medical assistance is often less adequate for psychiatric patients than for people without psychiatric disorders [35–37]. Furthermore, the limited ability of people with mental disorders to recognise and communicate their symptoms of organic diseases might be another possible explanation. An interesting finding is that the differential mortality gap for somatic reasons of people with schizophrenia and the general population has worsened in recent decades possibly as a result of deinstitutionalisation: since hospitalised patients are protected against alcohol abuse, while psychiatric patients followed by a community-based service are not [38]. This relative protection of long-stay inpatients is responsible for the strong reduction of mortality for liver cirrhosis, which is one of the main health policy indicators, according to the European Community list of avoidable causes of death.

The 15-year follow-up study by Brown and colleagues [39] examined the reasons for any excess mortality in a community cohort with schizophrenia in the United Kingdom. People with schizophrenia die for the same natural causes as the rest of the general population, for example, poverty, cigarettes and alcohol, unhealthy diet and lack of exercise. According to Goff and colleagues [38], the factor most strongly contributing to excess mortality is cardiovascular disease (CVD): cardiac deaths are elevated more than sixfold. Koponen and colleagues [27] report that in schizophrenic patients, the CVDs nowadays consist of 40–45% of all natural deaths, and patients with schizophrenia have been reported to be three times as likely to experience sudden unexpected death. Deaths related to respiratory illness (chronic obstructive pulmonary disease and pneumonias) are elevated approximately fivefold, but, in absolute terms, are much less frequent than cardiac deaths. Rates of human immunodeficiency virus and infectious hepatitis are also higher among patients with schizophrenia, and substance abuse may also contribute to elevated mortality rates in schizophrenia.

Physical diseases in comorbidity

A recent comprehensive review of the comorbidity of schizophrenia with physical illness has been published by Leucht and colleagues [2, 40], listing a wide range of conditions including infectious diseases, neoplasms, musculoskeletal diseases, digestive system disorders, diseases of the mouth and jaw, respiratory tract diseases, nervous system diseases, urological and genital diseases, CVDs, skin and connective tissue diseases and nutritional and metabolic diseases.

An elevated prevalence of bacterial infections, especially tuberculosis, is reported among mental patients. People with SMI appear to have increased rates of sexually transmitted diseases [41]. Patients with HIV infection face a range of problems: complex medical treatments, stigmatisation, neuropsychiatric complications of the infection and premature death [42]. An increased prevalence of hepatitis in people with schizophrenia compared to the general population has been reported in various countries [43, 44]. Both hepatitis B virus and hepatitis C virus infections are major causes of liver disease, including cirrhosis and hepatocellular carcinoma [41].

Results from studies of cancer rates in patients with schizophrenia are highly heterogeneous [45]. It is long known that people with schizophrenia have a reduced prevalence of cancer. There are several possible explanations: genetic factors that lead to schizophrenia on the one hand may protect from cancer on the other, certain antipsychotic drugs may protect against tumours and frequent hospitalisations include better access to medical care [2]. On the other hand, a higher risk for lung cancer is reported and is consistent with the high rate of smokers among persons with schizophrenia. The increased risk for breast cancer and tumours of the corpus uteri may result from hormonal factors, such as higher prolactinaemia following the long-term intake of neuroleptics [46].

Studies on musculoskeletal diseases consistently found osteoporosis in people with schizophrenia compared to normal controls. Preventive measures should be part of any treatment of patients with schizophrenia. These include information about a balanced diet with sufficient amounts of calcium and vitamin D; motivation to regular weight-bearing exercise; avoidance of tobacco, caffeine and alcohol and sufficient exposure to sunlight.

The dental status of people with schizophrenia is usually poor. The reasons leading to dental conditions are various. McCreadie and colleagues [47] listed the following: first, the majority of patients only go to the dentist when they have trouble with their teeth or gums; few go for a regular check-up. It is, therefore, not surprising that more patients have fillings and extractions. Also, fewer of the patients clean their teeth daily [48].

Respiratory tract diseases are more prevalent in people with SMI; they are thought to be the result of the high rates of smoking or passive smoking [49]. Diseases of the respiratory system (and cardiovascular system) account for much of the excess morbidity and mortality [50]. As to the nervous system diseases, the reduced causation of extrapyramidal side effects is considered among the main reasons for the success of second-generation antipsychotics. However, they account for other detrimental side effects like the metabolic ones. Schizophrenia-like psychoses are said to have a strong association with epilepsy, which may be congenital or acquired, particularly when there is a temporal lobe focus [51]. An association between schizophrenia and Alzheimer's disease has not been clearly demonstrated so far. A reduced pain sensitivity is reported in people with schizophrenia, and it may contribute to the decreased seeking of medical help.

Systematic studies on urological and genital diseases have revealed that sexual dysfunction is highly prevalent in both untreated and treated schizophrenia patients, affecting 30–80% of women and 45–80% of men.

Sexual dysfunction is considered by many schizophrenic patients to be more troublesome than most other symptoms and adverse drug effects and is a major cause of poor quality of life, negative attitude to therapy and treatment non-compliance [52]. Antipsychotic drugs are implicated in sexual dysfunction: many new and old antipsychotic drugs increase prolactin levels with short-term side effects (galactorrhea, gynaecomastia, menstrual irregularities, incontinence, sexual and reproductive dysfunction including diminished libido and impaired orgasm in both sexes and erectile or ejaculatory dysfunction in males) and long-term side effects (risk of pituitary tumours, breast cancer and osteoporosis) [53]. Although many of these are definitively connected to elevated prolactin levels, some, such as breast cancer and pituitary tumours, require further study [54]. As to prostate cancer, studies consistently found reduced incidences may be due to the anti-proliferative activity of some antipsychotics. Obstetric complications are instead increased in mothers with schizophrenia.

Prevalence of heart failure, arrhythmia and stroke is higher in people with schizophrenia than in control populations [55]. The high prevalence of smoking, obesity, poor diet and sedentary lifestyle may contribute to their higher CVD mortality. Another risk factor is represented by the cardiac side effects of antipsychotic drugs which can prolong the QT interval with the risk of arrhythmias and sudden cardiac death. Another component has to do also with the lesser care that people with schizophrenia receive when physically ill: they are less likely to receive diagnostic attention and medically necessary procedures compared to the non-mentally-ill population.

The MS and related issues will be treated in the section on risk factors. Here we limit to mention polydipsia which may occur in schizophrenia with the risk of water intoxication with hyponatraemia that can cause neurological symptoms such as nausea, vomiting, delirium, ataxia, seizures, coma and even death. In the long run, polydipsia may cause osteoporosis, dilatation of urinary tracts, cardiac failure, hypertension and malnutrition.

Risk factors

Risk factors such as weight, medication side effects, MS and institutionalisation have a critical role in the increased rates of physical illnesses in schizophrenia [56]. Among medication side effects, weight gain is common: it plays a role in MS and is a risk factor for CVD. Hyperlipidemia and diabetes have been reported with disturbing frequency. The National Cholesterol Education Program's Adult Treatment Panel III report (ATP III) [57] identified MS as a multiplex risk factor for CVD and insulin resistance, besides other conditions, notably polycystic ovary syndrome, fatty liver, cholesterol gallstones, asthma, sleep disturbances and some forms of cancer [58]. ATP III identified six components in MS: abdominal obesity, atherogenic dyslipidemia, raised blood pressure, insulin resistance (and glucose intolerance), pro-inflammatory state and prothrombotic state. Clinical criteria to diagnose MS include waist circumference, elevated levels of triglycerides and fasting glucose, low levels of high-density lipoprotein and high blood pressure; when three out of five of these characteristics are present, a diagnosis of MS can be made [58]. The prevalence of MS in people with SMI has been estimated to be in the range of 30–60% [59].

Heiskanen et al. [60] found that the frequency of MS was two to four times higher in a group of people with schizophrenia, treated with both atypical and typical neuroleptics, than in an appropriate reference population. The measurement of waist circumference can be used, along with fasting blood glucose or blood pressure, as a screening tool for MS [61]. Prevention is the optimal management strategy, and this can be best achieved through lifestyle interventions such as regular physical exercise and a healthy diet [59]. Established risk factors should also be considered when selecting the most appropriate antipsychotic medication for an individual patient, based on differences in the potential effect of individual medications in inducing weight gain, in increasing risk of diabetes or in worsening lipid profile [61].

The American Psychiatric Association's guidelines for the treatment of schizophrenia suggest that, where patients require treatment in a residential facility, this should be in the least restrictive setting that will ensure patient safety and allow for effective treatment [62]. Overall, community residential facilities have been found to be less regimented than hospital wards and more facilitative of patient autonomy [63]. A number of studies have found that the majority of patients with longer-term mental health problems prefer living in the community, rather than in a hospital [64], and report a higher quality of life than those in traditional hospital settings [65]. Sheltered care has also been related to better health status than hospital settings [66]. Indeed, gains in quality of life and autonomy are important benefits that may be associated with the move to a variety of smaller residences [65].

However, even in a country like Italy where the closure of all mental hospitals (MHs) has been accomplished and patients deemed to require long-term residential care are admitted to residential facilities (RFs), the risks of institutionalisation remain. In a study by de Girolamo and collaborators [65], they found that patients who had been admitted at least once in an MH are more likely to be illiterate, to cooperate poorly, to be inactive in the RF, to be physically impaired and to have lower Global Assessment of Functioning scores [67]; death rates are more than threefold those of general population [29]. They are also judged less likely to be discharged within the following six months; few patients, anyhow, did show any progress towards recovery during the study. Thus, institutionalisation may represent a risk factor for physical illnesses among psychiatric patients.

The reasons for this may involve poor nutritional habits, physical inactivity, heavy smoking and long-term exposure to psychoactive drugs [65] or poor living and care conditions in psychiatric facilities [32].

Lifestyles

The risk factors listed earlier have a critical role in the increased rates of physical illnesses in schizophrenia [56]. Since there are a number of well-established modifiable risk factors that can be addressed to help reduce overall risk in patients with schizophrenia, attention to factors that precipitate these risks is particularly crucial if the long-term health of patients is to be increased [61]. There is a growing consensus that a crucial aspect of intervention may be helping patients to improve their lifestyle especially regarding exercise, diet, smoking, alcohol and substance abuse. Levels of physical activity in patients with schizophrenia tend to be poor: they are substantially less active than the general population and worsen dramatically after the first psychotic episode [68].

Patients with schizophrenia consume a poor diet, which is high in fat and low in fibre [39, 69, 70], having less than 50% of the recommended intake of fruits and vegetables on average [64]. In a study, Brown et al. [39] found that no subject in the sample ate as many as five portions of fruits or vegetables a day, as recommended by WHO [15]. McCreadie [70] examined in detail the dietary intake of 102 people with schizophrenia in Dumfries and Glasgow. Their fruit and vegetable consumption averaged 16 portions per week (less than half the recommended intake), and very few patients made acceptable dietary choices across a range of foodstuffs. Poor diet can have a detrimental effect on physical health by increasing weight, leading to obesity and potentially inducing MS and cardiovascular effects [71].

In a review by Kelly and McCreadie [72], the prevalence of smoking in schizophrenia was estimated to be among 75–92%, much higher than that of the general population (30–40%). The 'self-therapy' smoking hypothesis is supported by a New Zealand study on women, where the improvement in a variety of psychiatric symptoms was greater than in women patients who did not smoke. In this study, it was also observed that smoking had the effect of a 'mood elevator' and was a supportive factor for the patient in resolving daily tasks [73]. The high incidence of smoking means that people with schizophrenia are at greater risk of experiencing the associated detrimental effects such as coronary disease, weight increase, MS and respiratory morbidity and mortality [38]. Smoking, in fact, is a plausible explanation for the excess respiratory disease mortality, also in consideration of excess lung cancer mortality [31, 32].

The abuse of drug and alcohol is a considerable problem in patients with severe mental health illness: nearly 35% of people with schizophrenia will abuse alcohol at some point during their lives [74]. In addition, the presence of a substance use disorder contributes to the prevalence of particular types of medical conditions over and above the effect of SMI alone as stated by Dickey et al. [75]. Drug and alcohol abuse may also increase the risk of suicide [76].

Interventions

Overall, it is clear that patients with schizophrenia require integrated care that addresses both mental and physical health needs. Simple and practical guidelines should be available for use by health-care services to reinforce, monitor and encourage the maintenance of physical health. For this reason, in 2002, the Mount Sinai Conference [4] developed recommendations for monitoring the physical health of patients who take antipsychotic medication. The National Institute for Health and Clinical Excellence guidelines for schizophrenia [77] recommend reducing smoking, doing appropriate physical exercise and having a healthy diet as important aspects of physical health care in schizophrenia. Regular physical health check-ups that include the monitoring of blood pressure, cardiovascular condition, weight, blood glucose or diabetes, lipid profiles and drug-related adverse events are also important.

Aside from the specific content of national and general guidelines, various local centres have taken action to promote physical health in mental illness, with promising results. These initiatives focus on simple interventions such as regular walking groups [71]: walking, either in the form of supervised group walks or unsupervised home-based walking, is one of the easiest, safest and most inexpensive types of exercise to promote, and it is also one of the most popular forms of exercise among those with and without chronic illness [13]. Even after years of inactivity, increasing physical activity reduces the risk of mortality [78]. Physiological benefits of regular exercise can include reductions in the relative risks of atherosclerosis, obesity and hypertension and improvements in lipid profiles and glucose tolerance. In addition, by providing distraction and social interaction, exercise has the potential to help reducing participants' perceptions of auditory hallucinations, raising self-esteem and improving sleep patterns and general behaviour [79]. Exercise may also help improve mood, decrease common symptoms such as lack of energy and psychosocial withdrawal and relieve comorbid depression and anxiety [80].

In the systematic review of randomised controlled trials by Bonfioli and associates [14], psychoeducational and/or cognitive-behavioural interventions aimed at weight loss (or prevention of weight gain) in patients with psychosis were compared with treatment as usual. An average of $-0.98 \, kg/m^2$ reduction in the mean body mass index of psychotic subjects resulted at the end of the intervention phase. A reduction of 0.98 points in the body mass index corresponds to a loss of 3.12% of the initial weight. This percentage is below the 5–10% weight loss deemed sufficient to improve weight-related complications such as hypertension, type II diabetes and dyslipidemia. However, outcomes associated with metabolic risk factors may have greater health implications than weight changes alone.

The efficacy of several strategies in changing unhealthy behaviours, such as cigarette smoking, excessive alcohol intake and poor diet, have been tested [81, 82]. Bradshaw and colleagues [11] showed that properly controlled smoking cessation is a safe intervention for people with schizophrenia and does not lead to deterioration in positive symptoms or increase in medication side effects. Brief advice from a physician to quit smoking has been found to improve cessation rates dramatically, and cognitive-behavioural programmes focused on practical problem-solving, skills training and the provision of support are an integral part of the current guidelines for smoking cessation interventions for the general population [38]. The evidence of efficacy for interventions on alcohol and substance abuse is still weak. Cleary et al. [83] reviewed randomised controlled trials on the topic of substance use in the severely mentally ill and found no compelling evidence to support any one psychosocial treatment over another to reduce substance use by people with serious mental illnesses.

Motivational interviewing seems more promising in relation to alcohol abuse and smoking, while its efficacy in changing habits such as poor physical exercise, diet and HIV risk behaviours is still controversial [84, 85]. However, other methods of promoting lifestyle changes have shown various degrees of efficacy: for example, it seems that giving advice only is less efficacious than involving the patients in promoting their health [81]. However, health promotion campaigns targeted at a population level, such as for cigarette smoking, appear to have a small but significant impact in reducing prevalence rates [86], as even a low percentage of success of a campaign represents large absolute numbers of people who change their health behaviour such as quitting smoking.

Empowerment also seems beneficial: the setting approach to health promotion should focus on strengthening individual abilities and resources of people with mental illness to empower them to achieve their fullest health potential by making healthy choices. There is evidence based on multi-level research designs that empowering initiatives can improve health outcomes [87].

The health promotion study in South Verona (PHYSICO I)

This study investigated the prevalence of physical comorbidity, risk factors and poor health behaviour (especially related to diet and physical exercise) in people with an ICD-10 diagnosis of affective and non-affective functional psychotic disorder in contact with the South-Verona CPS [88]. The assessment procedure consisted of a physical health examination, laboratory tests and an interview on socio-demographic data, physical health status, risk factors, lifestyles and quality of life. Two current methods were used to assess the cardiovascular risk in the sample: the Italian 'Cuore risk index' [89] and the diagnosis of the MS according to the ATP III definition [58]. This index was the result of a project to develop a ten-year coronary risk predictive equation specific to the Italian population.

One hundred and ninety-three subjects were included (i.e. provided written informed consent) and completed the assessment. Results showed that the diseases of the circulatory system, including hypertension and coronary heart disease, were the most represented. Nervous system diseases including severe diseases like stroke or Alzheimer's disease and less severe ailments like migraine were in second place. Metabolic diseases including diabetes and thyroid dysfunctions came third, together with diseases of the musculoskeletal system/connective tissue. Almost half of the subjects for whom the Cuore index was calculated were at risk for CVDs, especially the majority of males of the age group 50–69 years, among whom seven subjects were at high risk and were referred to the cardiologist. The MS occurred in slightly less than one-third of the subjects in the sample, mainly males aged 50–69 years.

Lifestyles (dietary habits, physical activity, smoking habits and alcohol consumption) were recorded and analysed according to the methodology proposed by the Progressi delle Aziende Sanitarie per la Salute in Italia (PASSI) study report [90]. The PHYSICO sample presented a higher percentage of overweight/ obesity and of smoking habits and a lower percentage of adherence to WHO recommendations for diet and physical activity than the general population sample. While a lower percentage of PHYSICO patients declared that they consumed alcohol, a higher percentage more of those who did consume it admitted risky drinking habits, such as drinking between meals. PHYSICO has proceeded to phase II, a 24-month intervention study on health education interventions of diet and physical activity in the whole area of the Mental Health Authority of Greater Verona, including four psychiatric services serving a population of 400000. The total sample size amounts to 400 subjects (100 per centre). Experimental and control subjects are tested at baseline, at monthly intervals and after the end of the intervention period with the same instruments of PHYSICO I. Primary outcome criteria are based on WHO recommendations on diet and exercise. In particular, (a) eating at least five servings of fruits or vegetables a day (400–500 g daily) and (b) engaging in moderate physical activity (like brisk walking) for at least 30 minutes on at least five days a week [91]. The design of the intervention programme has been improved in 2010 by participating in the National Project for Physical Activity (PNPAM) which resulted in the publication of the guidelines for the promotion of healthy lifestyles in psychiatric patients [92]. This manual has been included among the 'best practices of healthy physical-sports programmes' recommended in the Euro Sport Health project (www.eurosporthealth.eu). The intervention proper lasts six months and includes educational sessions on the importance of diet and fitness, motivational interviews, monitoring the participation in the programme and health behaviour for diet and fitness and regular physical exercise under the guidance and the supervision of an expert trainer. Control subjects receive treatment as usual.

Conclusions

People with SMI are affected by higher and premature mortality than the general population. Physical comorbidity is also increased with notable excess cardiovascular, respiratory, nutritional and metabolic diseases. Medication side effects, increased weight, diabetes, hypertension and patient's unhealthy lifestyle are the most common risk factors, together with stigma, leading to discrimination by health professionals and patient's neglect. In addition, physical comorbidity is the area less enhanced by the progress in the treatment of SMI: some evidence is robust, but several points are still obscure or controversial. The same hypotheses on the reasons why people with psychiatric disorders are more likely to die than the rest of the population are manifold and sometimes based on inconsistent data. Therefore, this is an area requiring systematic and well-designed research. Since some risk factors depend upon patients' lifestyle, preventive interventions in diet education, physical activity, smoke and substance abuse are possible. It is fundamental that the professionals of mental health have the necessary competence and a solid commitment to care for the physical besides the mental health of their patients.

Sartorius has observed that 'in many countries psychiatrists have taken off their white coats, shed the symbols of being physicians, forgetting that they are medical doctors … [Therefore] a revision of the curricula for training health professionals, at undergraduate and postgraduate level [should take place]' [7]. Psychiatrists should lead a change towards a comprehensive model of care in all the different professionals working with them in a mental health facility. This is professionally and ethically due, and it is likely to elicit an interested and satisfied participation in the patients involved, with positive effects in diminishing risk factors, reducing the gap between psychiatry and medicine at large, lowering stigma, improving the prognosis and decreasing costs. Finally, it must be stressed that the first step is acknowledging that the problem exists. While scholars are well aware of it, first-line clinical personnel may ignore, overlook or even not consider it to be a problem, especially in institutional care, in degraded environments and in low-income countries.

References

[1] Harris EC, Barraclough B. (1998) Excess mortality of mental disorder. *British Journal of Psychiatry* **173**: 11–53.
[2] Leucht S, Burkard T, Henderson JH et al. (2007) Physical illness and schizophrenia: a review of the literature. *Acta Psychiatrica Scandinavica* **116**: 317–333.
[3] Fleischacker WW, Cetkovich-Bakmas M, De Hert M et al. (2008) Comorbid somatic illnesses in patients with severe mental disorders: clinical, policy and research challenges. *Journal of Clinical Psychiatry* **64** (4): 514–519.

[4] Marder SR, Essock SM, Miller AL et al. (2004) Physical health monitoring of patients with schizophrenia. *American Journal of Psychiatry* **161**: 1349.

[5] Chafetz L, White MC, Collins-Bride G et al. (2005) The poor general health of severely mentally ill: impact of schizophrenic diagnosis. *Community Mental Health Journal* **41** (2): 169–184.

[6] Nasrallash HA, Meyer JM, Goff DC et al. (2006) Low rates of treatment for hypertension, dyslipidemia and diabetes in schizophrenia: data from a CATIE schizophrenia trial sample at baseline. *Schizophrenia Research* **86**: 15–22.

[7] Sartorius N. (2007) Physical illness in people with mental disorders. *World Psychiatry* **6** (1): 3–4.

[8] Vreeland B. (2007) Bridging the gap between mental and physical health: a multidisciplinary approach. *Journal of Clinical Psychiatry* **68** (4): 26–33.

[9] Likouras L, Douzenis A. (2008) Do psychiatric departments in general hospitals have an impact on the physical health of mental patients? *Current Opinion in Psychiatry* **21**: 398–402.

[10] De Hert M, Correll CU, Bobes J et al. (2011) Physical illness in patients with severe mental disorders. I. Prevalence, impact of medications and disparities in health care. *World Psychiatry* **10**: 52–77.

[11] Bradshaw T, Lovell K, Harris N. (2005) Healthy living interventions and schizophrenia: a systematic review. *Journal of Advanced Nursing* **49** (6): 634–654.

[12] McCreadie R, Kelly C, Connolly M et al. (2005) Dietary improvement in people with schizophrenia. *British Journal of Psychiatry* **187**: 346–351.

[13] Richardson C, Faulkner G, McDevitt J et al. (2005) Integrating physical activity into mental health services for persons with serious mental illness. *Psychiatric Services* **56** (3): 325–331.

[14] Bonfioli B, Berti L, Goss C et al. (2012) Health promotion lifestyle interventions for weight management in psychosis: a systematic review and meta-analysis of randomised controlled trials. *BMC Psychiatry* **12**: 78.

[15] Commission of the European Communities. (2007) White Paper "A strategy for Europe on nutrition, overweight and obesity related health issues". Brussels: European Union. Available from: http://europa.eu/legislation_summaries/public_health/health_determinants_lifestyle/c11542c_en.htm. Accessed on 2 January 2013.

[16] Commission of the European Communities. (2005) Green Paper "Promoting healthy diets and physical activity: a European dimension for the prevention of overweight, obesity and chronic diseases". Brussels: European Union. Available from: http://ec.europa.eu/health/ph_determinants/life_style/nutrition/documents/nutrition_gp_en.pdf. Accessed on 2 January 2013.

[17] World Health Organisation (WHO). (2005) *Mental Health Declaration for Europe*. Helsinki, 12–15 January 2005 EUR/04/5047810/6. Available from: http://www.euro.who.int/__data/assets/pdf_file/0008/88595/E85445.pdf. Accessed on 5 February 2013.

[18] Gillam SJ. (1992) Provision of health promotion clinics in relation to population need: another example of the inverse care law? *British Journal of General Practice* **42**: 54–56.

[19] Acheson D. (1998) *Independent Inquiry into Inequalities in Health*. The Acheson Report. November 26 . Available from: http://www.dh.gov.uk/en/Publicationsandstatistics/Publications/PublicationsPolicyAndGuidance/DH_4097582. Accessed on 2 January 2013.

[20] World Health Organisation (WHO). (2010) *Mental Health and Development: Targeting People with Mental Health Conditions as a Vulnerable Group*. Geneva: World Health Organisation, pp. 15–17. Available from: http://www.who.int/mental_health/policy/mhtargeting/en/index.html. Accessed on 2 January 2013.

[21] World Health Organisation (WHO). (2011) *Who Highlights Global Underinvestment in Mental Health Care*. Geneva: World Health Organisation. Available from: http://www.who.int/mediacentre/news/notes/2011/mental_health_20111007/en/. Accessed on 2 January 2013.

[22] World Health Organization (WHO). (2001) *The World Health Report 2001. Mental Health: New Understanding, New Hope*. Geneva: World Health Organization. Available from: http://www.who.int/whr/2001/en/. Accessed on 2 January 2013.

[23] World Health Organisation (WHO). (2010) *Empowering People with Chronic Physical Illness for Better Mental Health*. Geneva: World Health Organisation. Available from: http://www.euro.who.int/en/what-we-do/health-topics/noncommunicable-diseases/mental-health/news/news/2010/14/chronic-physical-illness-and-mental-health. Accessed on 2 January 2013.

[24] Brown S. (1997) Excess mortality of schizophrenia. *British Journal of Psychiatry* **171**: 502–508.

[25] Leucht S, Fountoulakis K. (2006) Improvement of the physical health of people with mental illness. *Current Opinion in Psychiatry* **19** (4): 411–412.

[26] Weinmann S, Read J, Aderhold V. (2009) Influence of antipsychotics on mortality in schizophrenia: systematic review. *Schizophrenia Research* **113**: 1–11.

[27] Koponen H, Alaräisänen A, Saari K et al. (2008) Schizophrenia and sudden cardiac death – a review. *Nordic Journal of Psychiatry* **62** (5): 342–345.

[28] Appleby L, Shaw J, Amos T. (2000) Sudden unexplained death in psychiatric inpatients. *British Journal of Psychiatry* **174**: 405–406.

[29] Baxter DN. (1996) The mortality experience of individuals on the Salford psychiatric case register. I. All cause mortality. *British Journal of Psychiatry* **168**: 772–779.

[30] Hansen Hoyer E, Mortensen PB, Olesen AV. (2000) Mortality and causes of death in a total sample of patients with affective disorders admitted for the first time between 1973 and 1993. *British Journal of Psychiatry* **176**: 76–82.

[31] Lichtermann D, Ekelund J, Pukkala E. (2001) Incidence of cancer among persons with schizophrenia and their relatives. *Archives of General Psychiatry* **58** (6): 573–578.

[32] D'Avanzo B, La Vecchia C, Negri E. (2003) Mortality in long-stay patients from psychiatric hospitals in Italy-results from the Qualyop Project. *Social Psychiatry and Psychiatric Epidemiology* **38**: 385–389.

[33] Green A, Patel J, Goisman R. (2000) Weight gain from novel antipsychotic drugs: need for action. *General Hospital Psychiatry* **22**: 224–235.

[34] Homel P, Casey D, Allison DS. (2002) Changes in body mass index for individuals with and without schizophrenia, 1987–1996. *Schizophrenia Research* **55**: 277–284.

[35] Munk-Jørgensen P, Mors O, Mortensen PB et al. (2000) The schizophrenic patient in the somatic hospital. *Acta Psychiatrica Scandinavica* **102**: 99.

[36] Folsom DP, McCahill M, Bartels SJ. (2002) Medical comorbidity and receipt of medical care by older homeless people with schizophrenia or depression. *Psychiatric Services* **53** (11): 1456–1460.

[37] Druss BG, Bradford DW, Rosenheck RA. (2000) Mental disorders and use of cardiovascular procedures after myocardial infarction. *Journal of American Medical Association* **283** (4): 506–511.

[38] Goff DC, Cather C, Evins AE et al. (2005) Medical morbidity and mortality in schizophrenia: guidelines for psychiatrists. *Journal of Clinical Psychiatry* **66** (2): 183–194.

[39] Brown S, Birtwistle J, Roe L et al. (1999) The unhealthy lifestyle of people with schizophrenia. *Psychological Medicine* **29**: 697–701.

[40] Leucht S, Burkhard T, Henderson JH et al. (2007) *Physical Illness and Schizophrenia: A Review of the Evidence*. Cambridge: Cambridge University Press.

[41] Rosenberg SD, Goodman LA, Osher FC et al. (2001) Prevalence of HIV, hepatitis B, and hepatitis C in people with severe mental illness. *American Journal of Public Health* **91** (1): 31–37.

[42] De Hert M, Wampers M, Van Eyck D et al. (2009) Prevalence of HIV and hepatitis C infection among patients with schizophrenia. *Schizophrenia Research* **108** (1–3): 307–308.

[43] Lawrence D, Holman CDJ, Jablensky AV. (2001) *Preventable Physical Illness in People with Mental Illness*. Perth: University of Western Australia.

[44] Nakamura Y, Koh M, Miyoshi E et al. (2004) High prevalence of the hepatitis C virus infection among the inpatients of schizophrenia and psychoactive substance abuse in Japan. *Progress in Neuropsychopharmacology and Biological Psychiatry* **28**: 591–597.

[45] Catts VS, Catts SV, O'Toole BI et al. (2008) Cancer incidence in patients with schizophrenia and their first-degree relatives – a meta-analysis. *Acta Psychiatrica Scandinavica* **117** (5): 323–336.

[46] Grinshpoon A, Barchana M, Ponizovsky A et al. (2005) Cancer in schizophrenia: is the risk higher or lower? *Schizophrenia Research* **73**: 333–341.

[47] McCreadie RG, Stevens H, Henderson J et al. (2004) The dental health of people with schizophrenia. *Acta Psychiatrica Scandinavica* **110** (4): 306–310.

[48] Friedlander AH, Marder SR. (2002) The psychopathology, medical management and dental implications of schizophrenia. *Journal of the American Dental Association* **133**: 603–610.

[49] Robson D, Gray R. (2007) Serious mental illness and physical health problems: a discussion paper. *International Journal of Nursing Studies* **44**: 457–466.

[50] Filik R, Sipos A, Kehoe PG et al. (2006) The cardiovascular and respiratory health of people with schizophrenia. *Acta Psychiatrica Scandinavica* **113** (4): 298–305.

[51] David A, Malmberg A, Lewis G et al. (1995) Are there neurological and sensory risk factors for schizophrenia? *Schizophrenia Research* **14** (3): 247–251.

[52] Baggaley M. (2008) Sexual dysfunction in schizophrenia: focus on recent evidence. *Human Psychopharmacology Clinical & Experimental* **23**: 201–209.

[53] Byerly M, Suppes T, Tran QV. (2007) Clinical implications of antipsychotic-induced hyperprolactinemia in patients with schizophrenia spectrum or bipolar spectrum disorders: recent developments and current perspectives. *Journal of Clinical Psychopharmacology* **27** (6): 639–661.

[54] Bostwick JR, Guthrie SK, Ellingrod VL. (2009) Antipsychotic-induced hyperprolactinemia. *Pharmacotherapy* **29** (1): 64–73.

[55] Bresee LC, Majumdar SR, Patten SB. (2010) Prevalence of cardiovascular risk factors and disease in people with schizophrenia: a population-based study. *Schizophrenia Research* **117**: 75–82.

[56] Mitchell AJ, Malone D. (2006) Physical health and schizophrenia. *Current Opinion in Psychiatry* **19**: 432–437.

[57] National Institutes of Health. (2002) *Third Report of the National Cholesterol Education Program (NCEP) Expert Panel on Detection, Evaluation, and Treatment of High Blood Cholesterol in Adults (Adult Treatment Panel III)*. NIH Publication No. 02-5215. Bethesda: National Institutes of Health. Available from: http://www.nhlbi.nih.gov/guidelines/cholesterol/atp3full.pdf. Accessed on 2 January 2013.

[58] Grundy SM, Brewer HB, Cleeman JI et al. (2004) Definition of metabolic syndrome: report of the National Hearth, Lung and Blood Institute/American hearth Association Conference on scientific issues related to definition. *Circulation* **109**: 433–438.

[59] Expert Consensus Meeting, Dublin, 14–15 April 2005, consensus summary British Association for Psychopharmacology. (2005) Metabolic and lifestyle issues and severe mental illness – new connections to well-being? *Journal of Psychopharmacology* **19** (6): 118–122.

[60] HeiskanenT, Niskanen L, Lyytikainen R. (2003) Metabolic syndrome in patients with schizophrenia. *Journal of Clinical Psychiatry* **64**: 575–579.

[61] Van Gaal LF. (2006) Long-term health considerations in schizophrenia: metabolic effects and the role of abdominal adiposity. *European Neuropsychopharmacology* **16**: S142–S148.

[62] Lehman AF, Kreyenbuhl J, Buchanan RW et al. (2004) The schizophrenia patient outcomes research team (PORT): updated treatment recommendations 2003. *Schizophrenia Bulletin* **30**: 193–217.

[63] Cullen D, Carson J, Holloway F et al. (1997) Community and hospital residential care: a comparative evaluation. *Irish Journal of Psychological Medicine* **14**: 92–98.

[64] Taylor TL, Killaspy H, Wright C et al. (2009) A systematic review of the international published literature relating to quality of institutional care for people with longer term mental health problems. *BMC Psychiatry* **9**: 55.

[65] de Girolamo G, Picardi A, Santone G et al. (2005) The severely mentally ill in residential facilities: a national survey in Italy. *Psychological Medicine* **35**: 421–431.

[66] Cournos F. (1987) The impact of environmental factors on outcome in residential programs. *Hospital and Community Psychiatry* **38**: 848–852.

[67] Endicott J, Spitzer RL, Fleiss JL et al. (1976) The global assessment scale. A procedure for measuring overall severity of psychiatric disturbance. *Archives of General Psychiatry* **33**: 766–771.

[68] Janney CA, Richardson CR, Holleman RG et al. (2008) Gender, mental health service use and objectively measured physical activity: data from the National Health and Nutrition Examination Survey (NHANES 2003–2004). *Mental Health and Physical Activity* **1**: 9–16.

[69] McCreadie R, MacDonald E, Blacklock C et al. (1998) Dietary intake of schizophrenic patients in Nithsdale, Scotland: case control study. *BMJ* **317**: 784–785.

[70] McCreadie RG, on behalf of the Scottish Schizophrenia Lifestyle Group. (2003) Diet, smoking and cardiovascular risk in people with schizophrenia: descriptive study. *British Journal of Psychiatry* **183**: 534–539.

[71] von Hausswolff-Juhlin Y, Bjartveit M, Lindström E et al. (2009) Schizophrenia and physical health problems. *Acta Psichiatrica Scandinavica* **119** (Suppl. 438): 15–21.

[72] Kelly C, McCreadie R. (2000) Cigarette smoking and schizophrenia. *Advances in Psychiatric Treatment* **6**: 327–332.

[73] Haustein KO, Haffner S, Woodcock BG. (2002) A review of the pharmacological and psychopharmacological aspects of smoking and smoking cessation in psychiatric patients. *International Journal of Clinical Pharmacology and Therapeutics* **40** (9): 404–418.

[74] Llorca PM. (2008) Monitoring patients to improve physical health and treatment outcome. *European Neuropsychopharmacology* **18**: S140–S145.

[75] Dickey B, Normand S, Weiss R et al. (2002) Medical morbidity, mental illness, and substance use disorders. *Psychiatric Services* **53** (7): 861–867.

[76] Schneider B. (2009) Substance use disorders and risk for completed suicide. *Archives of Suicide Research* **13** (4): 303–316.

[77] National Institute for Clinical Excellence (NICE). (2002) Schizophrenia: core interventions in the treatment and management of schizophrenia in primary and secondary care. Clinical Guideline 1. London: National Institute for Clinical Excellence. Available from: http://www.nice.org.uk. Accessed on 2 January 2013.

[78] Blair S, Kohl H, Barlow C et al. (1995) Changes in physical fitness and all-cause mortality. A prospective study of healthy and unhealthy men. *Journal of the American Medical Association* **273** (14): 1093–1098.

[79] Faulkner G, Sparkes A. (1999) Exercise as therapy for schizophrenia: an ethnographic study. *Journal of Sport and Exercise Psychology* **21**: 52–96.

[80] McDevitt J, Wilbur J. (2006) Exercise and people with serious, persistent mental illness. *American Journal of Nursing* **106** (4): 50–54.

[81] Ashenden R, Silagy C, Weller D. (1997) A systematic review of the effectiveness of promoting lifestyle change in general practice. *Family Practice* **14** (2): 160–176.

[82] Kok G, van den Borne B, Mullen PD. (1997) Effectiveness of health education and health promotion: meta-analyses of effects studies and determinants of effectiveness. *Patient Education and Counselling* **30**: 19–27.

[83] Cleary M, Hunt GE, Matheson SL et al. (2008) Psychosocial interventions for people with both severe mental illness and substance misuse. *Cochrane Database of Systematic Reviews* **1**: CD001088.

[84] Burke BL, Arkowitz H, Menchola M. (2003) The efficacy of motivational interviewing: a meta-analysis of controlled clinical trials. *Journal of Consulting and Clinical Psychology* **71**: 843–861.

[85] Dunn C, Deroo L, Rivara F. (2001) The use of brief interventions adapted from motivational interviewing across behavioral domains: a systematic review. *Addiction* **96**: 1725–1742.

[86] Smith TW, Orleans CT, Jenkins CD. (2004) Prevention and health promotion: decades of progress, new challenges, and an emerging agenda. *Health Psychology* **23**: 126–131.

[87] Weiser P, Becker T, Losert C et al. (2009) European network for promoting the physical health of residents in psychiatric and social care facilities (HELPS): background, aims and methods. *BMC Public Health* **9**: 315.

[88] Berti L. (2010) The physical co-morbidity and poor health behaviour of South Verona patients with functional psychoses. A prevalence study and the design of a protocol of a health promotion randomised controlled study – PHYSICO. PhD dissertation in Psychological and Psychiatric Sciences. University of Verona.

[89] Ferrario M, Chiodini P, Chambless LE et al. (2005) Prediction of coronary events in a low incidence population. Assessing accuracy of the CUORE Cohort Study prediction equation. *International Journal of Epidemiology* **34**: 413–421.

[90] Bertoncello L., Michieletto F., Milani S.; Gruppo PROFEA. (2005) Progressi delle Aziende Sanitarie per la Salute in Italia (PASSI). Available from: http://www.epicentro.iss.it/passi/pdf/Passi_Veneto.pdf. Accessed on 5 February 2013.

[91] World Health Organisation (WHO). (2005) *Avoiding Heart Attacks and Strokes: Don't Be a Victim – Protect Yourself.* Geneva: World Health Organization. Available from: http://www.who.int/cardiovascular_diseases/resources/avoid_heart_attack_report/en/. Accessed on 2 January 2013.

[92] Bellotti C, Berti L, Bonfioli E et al. (2011) Più salute nel disagio – indirizzi operativi per la promozione degli stili di vita sani nelle persone con patologia psichiatrica: attività fisica e alimentazione, Verona: Ulss 20.

CHAPTER 9

Complex interventions in mental health services research: Potential, limitations and challenges

Thomas Becker and Bernd Puschner
Department of Psychiatry II, Ulm University, Bezirkskrankenhaus Günzburg, Germany

Introduction

This text discusses some trials testing the efficacy and effectiveness of complex interventions for people with severe mental illness in Europe which the authors were involved in or are aware of. It focuses on the issue of treatment process and on which factors determine whether interventions work. This is an important topic which has obvious implications for mental health-care planning and evaluation research. The availability of evidence on the efficacy of complex interventions in controlled trials does not guarantee success when the intervention is rolled out in routine practice at a regional or national level. Discrepancies between internal and external validity are important, and the question of implementation of innovative interventions and service models is not trivial. Relationships between interventions and outcome can be complex. There is a definition by Andrews et al. [1] of outcome as 'the effect on a patient's health status that is attributable to an intervention'. Eagar [2] distinguished between two distinct models of the relationship between intervention and outcome: 'before and after' and 'with or without', with the latter approach being particularly relevant in chronic disease states where the goal of the intervention might be to maintain current health status which would be rated as a good outcome if the alternative were potential decline [3]. In view of the complex relationship between intervention and outcome, this chapter discusses some of the issues that are relevant in understanding randomised controlled trials (RCT) in the field of complex interventions in mental health care.

Improving Mental Health Care: The Global Challenge, First Edition.
Edited by Graham Thornicroft, Mirella Ruggeri and David Goldberg.
© 2013 John Wiley & Sons, Ltd. Published 2013 by John Wiley & Sons, Ltd.

Process evaluation: What is its importance?

Complex interventions are the rule rather than the exception in mental health services research, and process evaluation is considered crucial in understanding controlled trials performed in this field [4, 5]. It is important to understand the results of controlled trials irrespective of whether the intervention has shown an effect [4, 5]. Negative study results can be due to a true lack of efficacy or to a failure to adequately implement the intervention tested. The treatment system context in which trials are performed and any incentive systems influencing patient and clinician behaviour can impinge on trial results. The description of mechanisms and trajectories leading from intervention to outcome and a road map guiding process evaluation are important, and this will be complemented by new evidence as the trial progresses. Process evaluation should be planned prior to the analysis of study outcomes, and it should not be performed post hoc in the face of negative study results.

There are examples of integral process evaluation, for example, in

- a trial of peer education for gay men that had no apparent impact on HIV risk behaviour (the intervention being largely unacceptable to peer educators recruited to deliver it);
- trials of day care for preschool children and of supportive health visiting for new mothers (with unpredicted economic effects of day care and reasons for low uptake of health visiting in a culturally diverse population);
- a trial of a secondary prevention programme for cardiovascular disease (with patients viewing heart attacks as self-limited episodes and being therefore less willing to adopt long-term lifestyle changes [5]); and
- a UK multisite mixed-method cluster RCT of an intervention introducing general practitioners to a mental health problem severity rating to improve appropriateness of referral to community mental health teams which resulted in no difference in appropriateness of referral (with low implementation of the intervention indicating that uncertainty remained about whether a severity-focused measure can help in the referral process, and with the authors concluding that more attention needs to be paid to human and organisational factors in managing the interface between services [6]).

There are suggestions for methodological approaches to evaluation such as the 'evolving RCT' in mental health [4], patient preference RCTs [7, 8] or the 'realistic evaluation approach' [9], which all aim at elucidating how interventions work, what service factors influence outcome and how mechanisms acting in a given context produce outcomes.

Five examples of complex intervention trials and understanding processes

DIALOG: 'A complex intervention that worked'

Regular meetings of patient and clinician are the basis of community mental health care. There have been attempts to improve patient–clinician communication using communication checklists or new communication technologies [10, 11]. Building on these attempts at structuring patient–clinician communication, the DIALOG (structuring patient–clinician dialogue) trial was a cluster RCT in six European centres [12]. A total group of 134 key workers were allocated to DIALOG or treatment as usual. The study included 507 people with schizophrenia or related disorders. Every other month for one year, key workers asked patients to assess satisfaction with quality of life and treatment, and to request additional or different types of support. Responses were fed back immediately in screen displays, compared with previous ratings and discussed. Subjective quality of life was defined as primary outcome in this trial, and unmet needs and treatment satisfaction were used as secondary outcomes. After 12 months, patients receiving the DIALOG intervention had better subjective quality of life, fewer unmet needs and higher treatment satisfaction. The authors concluded that an intervention structuring patient–clinician dialogue with the aim of focusing on patients' views positively influenced quality of life, needs for care and treatment satisfaction [12]. There were variations in the number of structured communications for individual patients (of approximately five per patient). The intervention did not significantly increase the time spent by key workers and patients in meetings with each other, and patient and key worker views were positive [12].

Van den Brink et al. [13] tested whether the effectiveness of structured patient–clinician communication varied between different countries and explored setting characteristics associated with outcome. Positive effects were found on quality of life and treatment satisfaction in all centres, but reductions in unmet needs were only seen in two centres, and in positive, negative and general symptoms in one centre. The intervention was most effective in settings where patients had high levels of unmet needs and suffered from high symptom levels. The authors argued that differences in patient populations served and mental health care provided should be studied with respect to their influence on intervention effectiveness [13].

Hansson et al. [14], in another DIALOG publication, addressed the issue of 'what works for whom in a computer-mediated communication intervention in community psychiatry?' by looking at factors that moderate outcome. The intervention effect, in terms of quality of life, was stronger in patients with a better relationship with their key worker and shorter duration of illness at baseline. Patients receiving the DIALOG intervention who were in competitive employment or had a shorter duration of illness showed greater reduction of unmet needs. The authors concluded that there is a lack of research on moderators of psychosocial interventions in community-based mental health. They emphasised that, in the given study design, it was not possible to test whether specific elements of the intervention were related to the moderator effects.

EMM: 'A feedback of outcome intervention not sufficiently strong'

There has been a continuous move, in mental health-care modernisation, towards quality assurance and treatment monitoring in routine care. Continuous monitoring of patient outcome has been recommended as a means to improve quality of health services several decades ago. The approach has been refined since, for example, in quality management of psychotherapy interventions [15, 16]. Knaup et al. [17] conducted a meta-analysis on the effectiveness of feedback of treatment outcome during the course of therapy, that is, outcome management (OM) for improving the quality of mental health care. A systematic literature search of controlled trials using OM in mental health services published in the English or German language identified 12 studies that met inclusion criteria. Feeding back outcome showed a small but significant positive short-term effect on mental health which did not prevail in the long run. Subgroup analyses revealed no significant differences regarding feedback modalities. OM did not contribute to a reduction of treatment duration. The authors argued that more targeted research is needed and stated that more specific questions such as differential effectiveness in subgroups (e.g. by diagnosis), cost-effectiveness issues and active ingredients of OM should be addressed.

Puschner et al. [18], in a German cluster RCT (the EMM, i.e. Ergebnismonitoring und –management/outcome monitoring and management study), recruited 294 adult patients with mental illness who received care in a general psychiatry and psychotherapy inpatient service in a South German rural setting. Participants with a wide range of diagnoses were asked to provide information on treatment outcome via weekly computerised standardised assessments using the German version of the Outcome Questionnaire 45.2 (Ergebnisfragebogen 45, EB-45), a standardised measure of mental well-being. Patients and clinicians in the intervention group received continuous (weekly) feedback of outcome. Clinicians in the intervention group were invited to participate in monthly quality circles with EMM research workers to ensure intervention quality. Patients were found to be willing and able to regularly provide outcome data, and patients valued feedback. However, use of feedback in conversations between patient and clinician was reported to be rare. OM failed to impact on patient-rated outcome during inpatient treatment. The authors concluded that OM was feasible in a routine inpatient psychiatric care setting but failed to show an overall short-term effect. In the practice of the EMM study, active use of OM was apparently limited. OM, in this trial, was broad and patient-oriented, that is, based on patient-rated outcome using a generic instrument, and some clinicians expressed doubts whether EB-45 was an adequate measure, especially due to its lack of items specifically addressing psychotic symptoms.

Many clinicians, in this study, disliked treatment recommendations, especially in case of marked discrepancy between EB-45 outcome data and clinical judgement. This could have added to the scepticism regarding OM among clinicians. Also, even though OM was intense (weekly assessments and feedback), implementation might have been too weak. The approach taken is likely to have confided too much in OM becoming an integral part of routine practice. The study should have been complemented by strategies to encourage active use of the intervention tool among clinical staff. Such measures could have included
- a focus on specific clinical syndromes,
- an elaboration of behavioural or interaction elements of the feedback algorithm and
- clinical support tools.

Also, outcome monitoring (using EB-45) was provided in both the OM and the control group, and this addition to ward routine, by itself, could have been an effective add-on with additional outcome feedback not producing an incremental effect in the intervention group. Thus, one conclusion regarding the EMM trial is that a lack of determination in implementing the intervention could have accounted for the non-superiority of OM. On the whole, the EMM intervention turned out to pass largely unnoticed. The authors concluded that effective interventions require a higher degree of commitment. Services and professionals involved in a trial need to sustain and support the new intervention and prepare the ground for effectiveness; otherwise, research will either be experienced as 'difficult' or 'a nuisance' or an 'end in itself'. Even worse, once such trials have been completed, it is impossible to state whether an intervention is truly ineffective or whether setting, context or implementation has prevented it from reaching effectiveness.

EQOLISE: 'Intervention worked but failed to do so in one site'

Supported employment (SE) is an intervention that has shown superiority over traditional forms of vocational rehabilitation (VR) in integrating people with severe mental illness in competitive employment [19]. The majority of trials of SE, however, were conducted in the United States (nine US vs six non-US studies) [19]. Therefore, considering the importance of the issue, there were strong reasons to conduct a randomised trial of SE in European centres. Burns et al. [20], in an RCT of SE (specifically, of Individual Placement and Support, IPS), included 312 patients with severe mental illness in six European centres to receive IPS ($n=156$) or vocational services (VR; $n=156$). Patients were followed up for 18 months. The difference between the proportions of people entering competitive employment in the two groups was chosen as primary outcome.

The heterogeneity of IPS effectiveness was explored with prospective meta-analyses to establish the effect of local welfare systems and labour markets. IPS was found to be more effective than vocational services for all vocational outcomes (55% of patients assigned to IPS working for at least one day vs 28% of patients assigned to vocational services). Patients assigned to the control group were significantly more likely to drop out of the service and to be readmitted to hospital than were those assigned to IPS. Local unemployment rates accounted for a substantial amount of the heterogeneity in IPS effectiveness. The authors concluded that the trial demonstrated the effectiveness of IPS in widely differing labour market and welfare contexts across Europe confirming the SE service to be an effective approach for job integration among people with severe mental illness in a European context [20].

Also, there were no differences in clinical and social functioning between IPS and control patients at the 18-month follow-up with those working having better clinical and social outcomes. There were indications that IPS was better than the control service at helping more unwell patients into work [21]. In an EQOLISE (Enhancing the Quality of Life and Independence of Persons Disabled by Severe Mental Illness through Supported Employment) paper analysing predictors of employment, Catty et al. [22] found that patients with prior work history, fewer met social needs and better relationships with their vocational workers were more likely to obtain employment and work for longer. Clinical remission and swifter service uptake were associated with working more. Having an IPS service closer to the original IPS model (model fidelity) was the only service characteristic associated with greater effectiveness [22]. In another paper, Catty et al. [23] analysed the influence of the client–(clinical) key worker relationship and concluded that the impact of the client–vocational worker relationship was likely to be on the shared task of finding employment, rather than on clinical and social functioning parameters. However, good client–vocational worker relationships did not detract from client–key worker relationships. In concluding, Catty et al. [22] emphasised the importance of relational skills and high IPS fidelity to achieve optimal outcomes.

In the German EQOLISE study centre (Ulm/Günzburg), 52 patients with severe mental illness were included in the study [24], 26 patients received the IPS intervention (by a local, trained IPS worker at the study centre) while 26 patients were recruited into the VR comparison group. Two vocational services (RPK Kempten, RKU Ulm) provided the control intervention, but no study resources were available for the vocational intervention. Thus, access and funding had to be organised according to the rules of German social legislation and regional funding practice (by social services and the disability pension system). At study entry, 40 (77%) study participants received some form of state/public subsidy. A total of 259 patients were screened by study staff, and 52 patients gave written informed consent.

Data analysis, in the EQOLISE study, followed the intention-to-treat approach. At the German study site, only nine study participants in the control group actually started the VR intervention. The duration of the control intervention, on average, was 7.4 months (at RPK Kempten) and 1.5 months (at RKU Ulm), respectively. One patient in either control service dropped out prematurely. There was a clear preference, among study participants (who were informed about the RCT design), for the IPS intervention. There was differential study dropout, and some study participants in the control arm dropped out because they were either worried the intervention would take too long or afraid they might lose their monthly disability allowance. Some study participants decided, in the course of the procedure, to apply for a disability pension which prevented them from being enrolled in a VR intervention, and some patients had their application for VR transformed into a pension request which, again, prevented them from starting the VR intervention.

Overall, there were 17 study dropouts in the VR control group (service dropouts), but these patients were prepared to participate in all the follow-up study interviews/appointments. In the IPS group, there was one intervention and study dropout, and one study participant deceased during the study follow-up period (death being considered unrelated to the EQOLISE study). In the SE group, IPS worker support began with a detailed initial interview focusing on school training, professional background, working experience and job record, and the intervention then consisted mostly in the (joint) preparation of job applications, counselling with regard to job application and job interview, generic advice and accompanying the patient to the interview (however, at the German study site no IPS worker sat in on any of the interviews as patients preferred to be unaccompanied). About 60% of all appointments were in patients' flats or other private accommodation, and there were appointments in parks or cafes (about 10%) or in the IPS worker office (about 30%). Comparison of the two study groups, in the Ulm/Günzburg study site, resulted in no significant between-group difference, with job integration rates, however, being relatively high in both study groups (53.8% and 42.3%, respectively).

There was, however, a significant difference with longer job tenure in the IPS group. Patients who received state subsidies generally retained those whether or not they found (and sometimes held) low-paid part-time jobs. The IPS fidelity score was satisfactory at the Ulm/Günzburg site, and so was the contrast between the two interventions (both IPS and VR being rated on the IPS fidelity scale). Thus, there were substantial problems in conducting the RCT in the specific German social system context with high 'service dropouts' (not study dropouts) and a higher proportion of dropouts in the control group. Preference for one of the interventions, in trials testing complex interventions, can lead to selection effects and compromise the internal (and possibly external) validity of trials. At the German EQOLISE centre, there was a 'bias' against the control intervention. However, as this applied to a centre with a finding of non-superiority, there were no difficulties in interpreting study findings. At the Ulm/Günzburg site, the rules governing recruitment into and participation in the EQOLISE trial are likely to have led to a selection effect favouring patients with a very high motivation to go back to work. In future similar situations, patient preference randomised controlled trials (PPRCT) could be an option in this kind of situation, and they have been proposed by some authors [7, 25].

NODPAM: 'A discharge planning intervention that failed'

Continuity of care and the quality of hospital discharge planning are considered important process quality indicators, and they are likely to be related to patient outcome. Steffen et al. [26] conducted a systematic review of the recent literature to determine and estimate the efficacy of discharge planning interventions on patient outcome, ensuring community tenure, and saving costs. Studies published until January 2008 were identified and screened, and 11 studies were included. Discharge planning strategies varied; most were limited to preparing discharge during inpatient treatment. Pooled risk ratios were 0.66 for hospital readmission rate and 1.25 for adherence to outpatient treatment. Effect sizes were negative for mental health outcome, and non-significantly positive for quality of life. The authors concluded that discharge planning interventions are effective in reducing rehospitalisation and improving adherence with aftercare among people with mental disorders.

The NODPAM (Needs-Oriented Discharge Planning And Monitoring) study was a multisite RCT conducted in five psychiatric hospitals across Germany in the target group of people with severe mental illness with defined high utilisation of inpatient psychiatric care during two years prior to the current admission. Data of 491 study participants were collected, and the manualised intervention applied key principles of needs-led care and focused on the inpatient–outpatient transition. A trained intervention worker provided two intervention sessions of (a) needs-led discharge planning just before discharge (with patient and responsible clinician) and (b) a monitoring session following the same procedure as the first session three months after discharge (with patient and outpatient clinician present). A written treatment plan was signed by all participants after each session. The primary endpoint was reduction in hospital days in the intervention group. Secondary endpoints included the compliance with aftercare, clinical outcome and quality of life as well as cost-effectiveness and cost-utility [27]. The follow-up period was 18 months. The NODPAM intervention was described by von Rad et al. [28]. A series of papers has analysed different aspects of this trial. Intention-to-treat analyses showed no effect of the intervention on both primary and secondary outcomes [29]. The authors concluded that, with process evaluation pending, the intervention could not be recommended for implementation in routine care. Other approaches, for example, team-based community care, might be more beneficial for people with severe and persistent mental illness.

In a first process evaluation paper, Steffen et al. [30] analysed data of $n=241$ participants allocated to the intervention group (at three-month follow-up) with regard to quality of intervention implementation, acceptance and changes in care needs. The intervention was accepted well among both patients and staff. In a sub-group of participants, there were manual violations. Total and unmet needs decreased between baseline and follow-up. Numbers of care needs (and change in needs) varied by centre, and there was a trend towards variation of effect by dose. The authors concluded that the NODPAM intervention was feasible and that there might be scope for an effect if the intervention were altered or 'enhanced'. In a second process paper, Bäuerle et al. [31] analysed (a) differences of intervention dropouts versus adherent intervention group patients and (b) the impact of intervention process variables on unmet needs (over time). Patients with more severe forms of illness (schizophrenia, longer inpatient treatment duration) were more likely to be among intervention dropouts, a relatively high proportion of unmet needs persisted in intervention participants. Good intervention implementation and high patient satisfaction with the intervention received were associated with a reduction of unmet needs. Thus, the NODPAM intervention failed to reach patients with high service use and more severe forms of illness, and the intervention process appeared to be related to outcome. The intervention, according to the authors, was not well integrated in routine treatment and was experienced as extraneous to routine care.

The following might be reasons for the lack of effectiveness of the NODPAM discharge planning intervention:

- One hypothesis is that the intervention was too 'weak' to improve the transition process from inpatient to outpatient mental health care in the high utiliser target group; the NODPAM study process evaluation suggests that this may have been the case [30].
- It could also be that the German mental health-care system makes it difficult for this type of intervention to succeed. Improvement in discharge planning will only lead to a reduction in readmission rates among patients with severe mental illness *if* outpatient and community care meet the care needs of discharged patients; this includes crisis intervention and low-threshold psychosocial support measures. If such services are lacking (as appeared to be the case in the NODPAM sites), even a high-quality discharge planning intervention will be of limited use.
- Also, lead clinicians in inpatient services participating in the NODPAM study did not take steps to reduce inpatient admissions (there were no incentives to admit *fewer* patients) and to reduce readmissions to inpatient care; there were no incentives for clinicians to 'test' or develop new pathways of care for high-utilising or revolving-door patients.

Irrespective of whether these factors contributed to non-effectiveness in this trial, the NODPAM study results point to the role of institutional and service context in influencing the effects of interventions that target the care process.

QUATRO: 'An adherence intervention that failed'

Non-adherence rates for prescribed antipsychotic medication have been estimated to be about 50% [32–34]. The QUATRO study aimed at evaluating the effectiveness of adherence therapy, a brief cognitive-behavioural approach to improving adherence with antipsychotic medication, in improving quality of life for people with schizophrenia [35–37]. A 52-week, single blind, multicentre RCT of the effectiveness of adherence therapy was performed. Participants were individually randomised to receive either eight sessions of adherence therapy or health education, a control condition with no focus on adherence controlling for time spent with the therapist. Assessments were undertaken at baseline and at 52-week follow-up. $N=409$ patients were randomised (204 to adherence therapy and 205 to health education), and baseline and follow-up data for the core outcome measures were collected for 349 (85.3%) participants.

Adherence therapy was found to be no more effective than health education in improving quality of life. Thus, the QUATRO effectiveness trial provided evidence for the lack of effect of adherence therapy in people with schizophrenia with recent clinical instability, treated in ordinary clinical settings. This applied to primary and secondary outcome measures (treatment adherence, psychopathology and quality of life). Considering that over two-thirds of patients referred to the QUATRO trial meeting inclusion criteria were excluded and not randomised, the authors discuss that QUATRO might have been biased towards a subsample of more cooperative and adherent people who were unlikely to benefit from adherence therapy [32]. Therefore, the authors consider a potential 'ceiling effect' with little room for further adherence improvement. One potential confounder of the QUATRO study results might be that adherence therapy is effective only when delivered by staff who are already members of a multidisciplinary clinical team, or that it might be selectively effective only in those patients who are least treatment adherent (who were likely not to be randomised or dropped out of the QUATRO trial).

Puschner et al. [38] aimed to develop a meaningful model of the relationship between quality of life and adherence including mediating variables. They used graphical modelling to investigate the relationships between the variables. No direct relationship could be discerned between subjective quality of life and adherence to medication. Mediating variables, most importantly symptoms, global functioning and medication side effects, were identified, and the authors concluded that, when aiming at improving quality of life in people with schizophrenia, variables other than adherence, that is, symptomatic impairment, global functioning levels and medication side effects, should be targeted. One conclusion, on the basis of the QUATRO trial, could be that limitations in our understanding of adherence are likely to hamper the design of interventions to improve compliance.

Discussion

In summary, we have reported (some of) the results of a number of effectiveness trials of complex mental health interventions with two (DIALOG and EQOLISE) showing superiority over the comparator condition and with the remainder (EMM, NODPAM and QUATRO) not coming out in favour of the innovative interventions studied. In considering plausible explanations for these findings, the following issues should be borne in mind:

- In the OM (EMM) RCT, there was no clear determination (in the study design and practical roll-out) to make the intervention a success; that is, with hind-sight, the intervention was too weak.
- In the NODPAM study, a discharge planning intervention was found not to be effective, and the authors thought that this was due to a lack of determination among lead clinicians and service management to change incentives, to reduce the level of hospitalisation and ensure the availability of post-discharge community services.
- In QUATRO, an adherence intervention focusing on compliance with anti-psychotic drug treatment failed to make any major difference; ceiling effects and the non-integration of QUATRO intervention staff with the routine clinical teams were discussed.
- DIALOG and EQOLISE, on the other hand, are RCTs that showed the inno-vative interventions to be effective. In these European multisite randomised trials, structuring patient–key worker communication improved quality of life and reduced needs (in DIALOG), and SE was superior to VR with regard to vocational outcomes (in EQOLISE).

There is converging evidence that the evaluation of complex mental health interventions requires attention to study context. Burns et al. [39] and Harvey et al. [40] found that more recent studies of assertive community treatment (ACT) showed smaller advantages over treatment as usual when compared with older studies, and that this could be due to (a) the control condition being 'too good' or 'too strong' or 'too similar' in more recent studies, (b) fidelity to treatment having deteriorated and/or (c) effects on reduction in bed use depend-ing on the level of hospitalisation in the given service context. Also, studies of home treatment (HT) in Europe showed HT to be less superior to treatment as usual than did studies in the United States, and there were findings suggesting that this could be due to control services in Europe being closer to HT than was the case in the United States [41]. Therefore, Burns [42] argued that there were methodological problems associated with 'treatment-as-usual' studies and that 'head-to-head' comparisons were generally to be preferred.

The trials discussed in this chapter suggest that it is important to closely examine all the aspects related to the implementation of novel interventions and to focus on the patient/user *and* clinician perspectives. New treatment strategies should aim to address core elements of the clinical problem targeted. New service models should impinge on patients' living conditions and social lives, and a strong theory or rationale underpinning a novel intervention may help to achieve a positive outcome. Service and treatment concepts change along with culture, science and the socioeconomic context. Currently, cognitive-behavioural theory, motivational interviewing and the concepts of 'empowerment' and 'recovery' are examples of underlying concepts or frameworks that can lead to innovative practice and interventions.

Conclusion

In drawing on the results of the complex mental health intervention trials discussed earlier, the following can be concluded:

- The DIALOG study (and non-superiority found in other trials) suggests that for interventions in community mental health care to work, it is important to aim at changing actual behaviour of both clinicians and patients. In addition, DIALOG is a trial that points to the potential of achieving behavioural change in patient–key worker interactions.
- The EQOLISE study, in turn, points to the importance of developing new interventions that are truly different from earlier models, subscribe to new intervention paradigms, manage to 'depart' from the previous care model and strive for behavioural change.

If the wealth of the evidence in mental health services research is matched by critical discussion at a high level, this is one of the most exciting areas of scientific inquiry in the attempt to develop and improve mental health care for people with severe mental disorders.

Acknowledgement

Professor Stefan Priebe, London, is gratefully acknowledged for comments on the manuscript.

References

[1] Andrews G, Peters L, Teesson M. (1994) *The Measurement of Consumer Outcome in Mental Health: A Report to the National Mental Health Information Strategy Committee.* Sydney: Clinical Research Unit for Anxiety Disorders.
[2] Eagar K. (2002) An Overview of Health Outcomes Measurement in Australia. *Mental Health Research and Development Strategy: Outcomes Conference,* Wellington.
[3] Trauer T. (ed.) (2010) *Outcome Measurement in Mental Health. Theory and Practice.* Cambridge: Cambridge University Press.
[4] Green J. (2006) The evolving randomised controlled trial in mental health: studying complexity and treatment process. *Advances in Psychiatric Treatment* **12**: 268–279.

[5] Oakley A, Strange V, Bonell C et al. (2006) Process evaluation in randomised controlled trials of complex interventions. *BMJ* **332**, 413–416.

[6] Slade M, Gask L, Leese M et al. (2008) Failure to improve appropriateness of referrals to adult community-mental health services – lessons from a multi-site cluster randomized controlled trial. *Family Practice* **25**: 181–190.

[7] Howard L, Thornicroft G. (2006) Patient preference randomised controlled trials in mental health research. *British Journal of Psychiatry* **188**: 303–304.

[8] King M, Nazareth I, Lampe F et al. (2005) Conceptual framework and systematic review of the effects of participants' and professionals' preferences in randomised controlled trials. *Health Technology Assessment* **9**: 1–186.

[9] Pawson R, Tilley N. (1997) *Realistic Evaluation.* London: Sage.

[10] Ahmed M, Boisvert C. (2006) Using computers as visual aids to enhance communication in therapy. *Computers in Human Behavior* **22**: 847–855.

[11] Van Os J, Altamura AC, Bobes J et al. (2004) Evaluation of the two-way communication checklist as a clinical intervention: results of a multinational, randomised controlled trial. *British Journal of Psychiatry* **184**: 79–83.

[12] Priebe S, McCabe R, Bullenkamp J et al. (2007) Structured patient-clinician communication and 1-year outcome in community mental healthcare. *British Journal of Psychiatry* **191**: 420–424.

[13] van den Brink R, Wiersma D, Wolters K et al. (2011) Non-uniform effectiveness of structured patients-clinician communication in community mental healthcare: an international comparison. *Social Psychiatry and Psychiatric Epidemiology* **46**: 685–693.

[14] Hansson L, Svensson B, Björkman T et al. (2008) What works for whom in a computer-mediated communication intervention in community psychiatry? Moderators of outcome in a cluster randomized trial. *Acta Psychiatrica Scandinavica* **118**: 404–409.

[15] Kordy H, Bauer S. (2003) The Stuttgart-Heidelberg model of active feedback driven quality management: means for the optimization of psychotherapy provision. *International Journal of Clinical and Health Psychology* **3**: 615–631.

[16] Lambert MJ, Hansen NB, Finch AE. (2001) Patient-focused research: using patient outcome data to enhance treatment effects. *Journal of Consulting and Clinical Psychology* **69**: 159–172.

[17] Knaup C, Koesters M, Schoefer D et al. (2009) Effect of feedback of treatment outcome in specialist mental healthcare: meta-analysis. *British Journal of Psychiatry* **195**: 15–22.

[18] Puschner B, Schöfer D, Knaup C et al. (2009) Outcome management in in-patient psychiatric care. *Acta Psychiatrica Scandinavica* **120**: 308–319.

[19] Bond GR, Drake RE, Becker DR. (2012) Generalizability of the Individual Placement and Support (IPS) model of supported employment outside the US. *World Psychiatry* **11**: 32–39.

[20] Burns T, Catty J, Becker T et al. (2007) The effectiveness of supported employment for people with severe mental illness: a randomised controlled trial. *Lancet* **370**: 1146–1152.

[21] Burns T, Catty J, White S et al. (2009) The impact of supported employment and working on clinical and social functioning: results of an international study of individual placement and support. *Schizophrenia Bulletin* **35**: 949–958.

[22] Catty J, Lissouba P, White S et al. (2008) Predictors of employment for people with severe mental illness: results of an international six-centre randomised controlled trial. *British Journal of Psychiatry* **192**: 224–231.

[23] Catty J, Koletsi M, White S et al. (2010) Therapeutic relationships: their specificity in predicting outcomes for people with psychosis using clinical and vocational services. *Social Psychiatry and Psychiatric Epidemiology* **45**: 1187–1193.

[24] Kalkan R, Dorn W, Ehiosun U et al. (2009) Unterstützte Beschäftigung bei Menschen mit schweren psychischen Erkrankungen [Supported employment for people with severe mental illness]. *Sozialpsychiatrische Informationen* **39**: 40–45.

[25] Muche R, Imhof A, SARAH-studygroup. (2003) Das Comprehensive Cohort Design als Alternative zur randomisierten kontrollierten Studie in der Rehabilitationsforschung: Vor- und Nachteile sowie Anwendung in der SARAH-Studie [The Comprehensive Cohort Design as alternative to the randomized controlled trial in rehabilitation research: advantages, disadvantages, and implementation in the SARAH study]. *Rehabilitation* **42**: 343–349.

[26] Steffen S, Kösters M, Becker T et al. (2009) Discharge planning in mental health care: a systematic review of the recent literature. *Acta Psychiatrica Scandinavica* **120**: 1–9.

[27] Puschner B, Steffen S, Gaebel W et al. (2008) Needs-oriented discharge planning and monitoring for high utilisers of psychiatric services (NODPAM): design and methods. *BMC Health Services Research* **8**: 152.

[28] Von Rad K, Steffen S, Kalkan R et al. (2010) Randomised controlled multicenter trial on discharge planning in high utilisers of mental health care. *Psychiatrische Praxis* **37**: 191–195.

[29] Puschner B, Steffen S, Völker KA et al. (2011) Needs-oriented discharge planning for high utilisers of psychistric services: multicentre randomised controlled trial. *Epidemiology and Psychiatric Sciences* **20**: 181–192.

[30] Steffen S, Kalkan R, Völker K et al. (2011) RCT on discharge planning for high utilisers of mental health care: conduct and quality of the intervention. *Psychiatrische Praxis* **38**: 69–76.

[31] Bäuerle S, Loos S, Puschner B et al. (2013) Umsetzung einer bedarfsorientierten Entlassplanungsintervention bei Patienten mit hoher Inanspruchnahme des psychiatrischen Versorgungssystems: eine Prozessevaluation [Process evaluation of a Needs-Oriented Discharge Planning and Monitoring (NODPAM) intervention for patients with severe mental illness with high utilisation of inpatient psychiatric care]. *Psychiatrische Praxis* (in press).

[32] Gray R, Leese M, Bindman J et al. (2006) Adherence therapy for people with schizophrenia. European multicentre randomised controlled trial. *British Journal of Psychiatry* **189**: 508–514.

[33] Nosé M, Barbui C, Tansella M. (2003) How often do patients with psychosis fail to adhere to treatment programmes? A systematic review. *Psychological Medicine* **33**: 1149–1160.

[34] Nosé M, Barbui C, Gray R et al. (2003) Clinical interventions for treatment non-adherence in psychosis: meta-analysis. *British Journal of Psychiatry* **183**: 197–206.

[35] Kemp R, David A. (1996) Compliance therapy: an intervention targeting insight and treatment adherence in psychotic patients. *Behavioral and Cognitive Psychotherapy* **24**: 331–350.

[36] Kemp R, Kirov G, Everitt B et al. (1998) Randomised controlled trial of compliance therapy. 18-month follow-up. *British Journal of Psychiatry* **172**: 413–419.

[37] Gray R, Wykes T, Edmonds M et al. (2004) Effect of a medication management training package for nurses on clinical outcomes for patients with schizophrenia: cluster randomised controlled trial. *British Journal of Psychiatry* **185**: 157–162.

[38] Puschner B, Born A, Gießler A et al. (2006) Adherence to medication and quality of life in people with schizophrenia. Results of a European Multicenter Study. *Journal of Nervous and Mental Disease* **194**: 746–752.

[39] Burns T, Catty J, Dash M et al. (2007) Use of intensive case management to reduce time in hospital in people with severe mental illness: systematic review and meta-regression. *BMJ* **335**: 336–340.

[40] Harvey C, Killaspy H, Martino S et al. (2011) A comparison of the implementation of assertive community treatment in Melbourne, Australia and London, England. *Epidemiology and Psychiatric Sciences* **20**: 151–161.

[41] Burns T, Catty J, Watt H et al. (2002) International differences in home treatment for mental health problems. The results of a systematic review. *British Journal of Psychiatry* **181**: 375–382.

[42] Burns T. (2009) End of the road for treatment-as-usual studies? *British Journal of Psychiatry* **195**: 5–6.

CHAPTER 10

The feasibility of applying the clinical staging paradigm to the care of people with mental disorders

Javier Vázquez-Bourgon[1], *Luis Salvador-Carulla*[2,3],
Benedicto Crespo-Facorro[1] *and José Luis Vázquez-Barquero*[1]

[1] Department of Psychiatry, Psychiatric Research Unit of Cantabria, University Hospital "Marqués de Valdecilla", IFIMAV, CIBERSAM, Santander, Spain
[2] Centre for Disability Research and Policy, Faculty of Health Sciences, University of Sydney, Australia
[3] Spanish Research Network on Mental Health Prevention and Promotion (Spanish IAPP Network)

Clinical staging: A new paradigm for intervention in mental health

Medical specialists have long been aware of the advantages of prevention over treatment, and the benefits of early diagnosis and treatment of disease. This model has been successfully applied to oncological and other serious physical diseases. This has not been the case, however, in mental disorders, where both psychiatric knowledge and practice has been historically derived from selected sub-samples of patients with well-established, often chronic, disorders. In these circumstances, the intrinsic nature of the illness tends to be confounded with variables related to long-term treatment and clinical course. This has affected the understanding of key elements of mental disorders, such as their aetiological basis, and more specifically their clinical manifestations and susceptibility to treatment. This is also true of the ways in which we evaluate and classify these disorders. Thus, there is a compelling need to adopt the early intervention paradigm in mental health.

A well-recognised fact is that most adult mental disorders have their onset between late childhood and early adult life [1]. This means that the implementation of the early-stage paradigm should have its maximum focus on these age groups. However, the onset of mental disorders is often difficult to distinguish from transitory and benign psychopathological and emotional dysfunctions. The situation is made even more complex as we are still lacking clear operational criteria for establishing the threshold for 'caseness' and for delineating the clinical 'entities' that

Improving Mental Health Care: The Global Challenge, First Edition.
Edited by Graham Thornicroft, Mirella Ruggeri and David Goldberg.
© 2013 John Wiley & Sons, Ltd. Published 2013 by John Wiley & Sons, Ltd.

precede the onset of mental disorders. An example of this difficulty is found in the data provided by Van Os Hanssen et al. [2], demonstrating in a normal community sample the presence of psychopathological experiences which tend to be associated with psychosis. The same could be said for other psychopathological experiences such as depression or anxiety, in which it is not always possible to establish the precise limits between normality and psychopathology.

Although the application of the clinical staging model has proved to be very useful in medical care, it is only recently that it has been extended to the field of mental health. In fact, clinical staging in psychiatry was initially proposed in 1993 by Fava and Kellner [3], and it rapidly became focused on early signs of psychosis. As a result of this, we have seen a significant spread of 'early intervention services for psychosis' worldwide [4]. Despite this, there have not been up until now significant initiatives to apply the model to other mental disorders. Thus, the objective of this chapter is to consider, based on the experience acquired with its implementation in psychosis, the feasibility of extending the paradigm to other major mental disorders.

Principles underlying the application of the clinical staging model to mental disorders

The application of the clinical staging model is based on the idea that the longitudinal course of a disease is likely to progress from an 'at-risk' to a prodromal status, and finally to a fully developed diagnostic entity. It also implies that the disease progresses through different stages that are characterised by phase-specific clinical manifestations. From a clinical perspective, it also assumes that earlier stages have better prognosis, require less intensive treatments and tend to respond better to interventions. In this context, it offers a framework to integrate appropriate phase-specific therapeutic and preventive strategies and may also assist in developing innovative early intervention services. A series of key concepts are incorporated into the model, the most relevant of which will be reviewed in this chapter, making special emphasis on their application to different mental disorders.

New perspectives in mental health prevention

Based on the successful implementation of preventive strategies in infectious disease, preventive interventions have been extended to non-infectious and chronic diseases, including mental illness. In this context, the traditional classification system for prevention differentiating the three levels of Primary, Secondary and Tertiary Prevention has been regarded as unsatisfactory. To resolve the situation, in the early 1990s, the Committee on Prevention of Mental Disorders of the Institute of Medicine proposed a new model of preventive intervention describing the three levels of *Universal*, *Selective* and *Indicated* prevention [5]. At the *Universal*

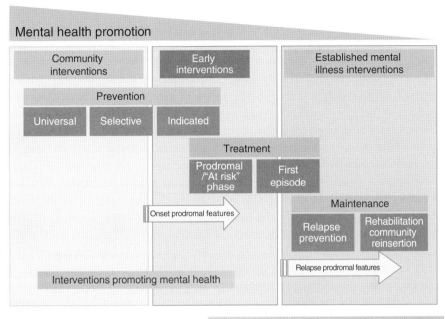

Figure 10.1 Integrating the new prevention model with the staging paradigm.

level, preventive interventions are targeted to the general public or to a whole population group that has not been identified on the basis of individual risk. At the *Selective* level, interventions are directed to asymptomatic populations, with a higher risk of a particular disorder. Finally, at the *Indicated* level, preventive interventions are targeted to high-risk individuals who are identified as having minimal, but detectable, signs or symptoms foreshadowing mental disorders, but who do not meet the diagnostic criteria for the disease.

The relevance of this new model of prevention is due to the fact that it allows integrating the clinical manifestations into a comprehensive construct belonging to the different stages of the illness, with interventions directed to promoting mental health and preventing and treating mental illness (Figure 10.1). Thus, the concept of *Indicated* prevention is the basis for the early intervention paradigm. In this context, *Indicated* prevention pursues the objectives of (a) improvement of the burden of the early pre-clinical syndromes and (b) prevention of the development of the illness.

The duration of untreated mental illness and its consequences

There is increasing evidence that, even in countries with sophisticated health-care systems, there is usually a long period between the time a person develops a mental disease and it is correctly identified and treated (Figure 10.2). This was initially demonstrated for non-affective psychosis, where the duration of untreated psychosis ranged from several weeks up to six years [6–8]. The duration of untreated mental illness (DUMI) reported for other major mental disorders is also similar. This is the case, for example, for bipolar disorders (delay ranged from five to ten years) [9, 10], unipolar depression (mean delay seven years) [11], anxiety disorders (up to four years) [12] and also for eating disorders, where the DUMI ranged from one to four years [13].

The relevance of this long period of untreated mental illness is derived from its supposed association with a poorer outcome and treatment response. This has, for example, been demonstrated, although not in a very conclusive way, for non-affective psychosis [7, 14, 15]. Also in bipolar disorders, long duration of untreated illness appears to be associated with poor response to treatment [9, 16], poorer psychosocial adjustment, higher number of hospitalisations and an increased risk of suicide [17, 18]. Similar findings have been reported for other mental disorders, such as unipolar depression [11, 19], anxiety disorders [20] and eating disorders [21]. This sort of association, however, would have to be replicated for the other major mental disorders in future prospective studies.

Brain imaging studies have also shown in certain major mental disorders, typically psychosis, bipolar disorders and unipolar depression, an association of longer duration of illness with third and fourth ventricle enlargements and also with reduced grey matter in the temporal lobe, hippocampus, cerebellum and in some areas of prefrontal cortex [19, 22–24]. In a similar way, brain alterations

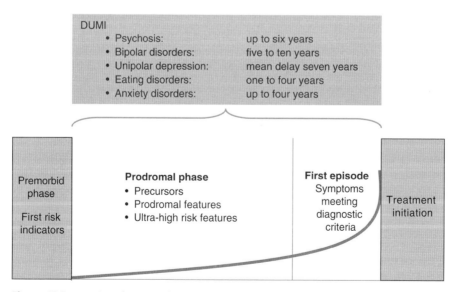

Figure 10.2 Duration of untreated mental illness (DUMI) in different mental disorders.

have also been reported for other psychiatric diseases such as eating and anxiety disorders [25, 26]. Furthermore, it has been suggested that the chronic presence of the disorder, or the development of multiple episodes, may lead to permanent alterations in neural activity which in turn results in poorer response to treatment or on greater liability to relapse [22, 27, 28]. Based on these findings, a neurotoxic effect of the untreated illness has been postulated for psychosis [29]. This concept has also been extended to other major mental disorders such as bipolar disorders [8, 22] or depression [11]. In addition to this neurotoxic component, psychotoxic and sociotoxic effects of the untreated illness have also been postulated to account for the consolidation of the altered patterns of behaviour and for the crystallisation of sick social roles at the community and family level [29].

The critical period in mental illness

The critical period hypothesis was originally formulated for psychosis and proposes that the early phase of mental disorders constitutes a 'critical period' during which symptomatic and psychosocial deterioration progresses rapidly. It also supposes that the progression of morbidity slows or stops afterwards and the level of the recovery attained by the end of the critical period endures into the long term [30]. In addition, Crumslish et al. [31] have indicated that the critical period should also include the prodrome as well as all the initial sub-clinical stages of the illness. Thus, the general consensus is that the critical period extends from three up to five years [32, 33].

There is now increasing evidence supporting that a similar critical period could be postulated for other major mental disorders such as depression or bipolar disorders. In the case of depression, for example, it has been reported that the absence of treatment during the early stages of the illness appears to be associated to deleterious effects on the psychosocial adjustment of patients as well as to neuroanatomical abnormalities in brain regions [11, 19, 23]. In bipolar disorders, it has been postulated that the timing of neurobiological changes suggests that the early stages of the illness constitute a critical period. Salvadore et al. [34] have suggested that in bipolar disorders, the optimal period for neuroprotective interventions is either the prodromal phase or during the early stages of the illness.

In conclusion, the available information supports the opinion that in most major mental disorders, effective early intervention procedures should be implemented during the stage of maximum susceptibility to the illness's noxae and also to the neuropsychosocial protective effects of interventions. It also provides evidence that therapeutic and preventive interventions should be maintained during the whole critical period.

Table 10.1 Main objectives of the staging paradigm.

Clinical objectives	To identify persons at risk (ultra-high risk) of developing the illness
	To reduce or minimise disruption of normal developmental processes
	To prevent or postpone the transition to full-blown disorder
	To provide early identification and treatment of the first episode
	To identify persons at risk of relapse and to prevent the development of a relapse
	To stimulate the acquisition of insight into the nature of the illness
	To promote the development of treatment adherence
	To prevent the development of psychiatric comorbidity
	To reduce social and personal costs associated to the disorder
	To promote quality of life and social integration and to prevent stigma
Research objectives	To elucidate the biological and psychosocial basis of mental disorders
	To clarify the psychopathological and clinical structure of the early stages of the disorders
	To identify predictors of transition from one stage to the next and predictors of relapse
	To investigate the efficacy and cost-efficacy of early intervention strategies
Health service objectives	To develop novel phase-specific mental health services and programmes for the early phases of mental disorders, exploring their effective integration in the mental health service structure
	To investigate the cost-efficacy of the early intervention services

Objectives of early intervention

We postulate that in mental disorders, the objectives of early intervention extend to the clinical, research and service provision areas. As outlined in Table 10.1, the clinical objectives include both early detection of patients at risk and the initial outbreak of the illness and also the optimal early treatment. In addition, the prevention of relapses and of development of comorbidity and of disability constitutes an important task. At the same time, the early intervention model provides a useful framework for implementing research. The aims here will be directed to (a) acquire precise information on the origin and natural course of the disease, (b) clarify the psychosocial and biological bases of the disorders, (c) identify the predictors of transition from one stage to the other and (d) develop and test effective interventions. Finally, the staging paradigm should also integrate objectives directed to the development and verification of novel early intervention strategies and health-care services.

Operational criteria for the early stages of mental disorders

A key element of the staging paradigm is to establish operational criteria for the sequence of the pre-diagnostic and diagnostic stages of the illness (Table 10.2). Since we do not have biological markers to define the different stages, these

Table 10.2 The application of McGorry's 'Clinical Staging Model' to mental disorders [63].

Stage	Clinical definition	Target population	Potential interventions
0	Increased risk of disorder No symptoms currently	Young age first-degree relatives of probands	Psychoeducation for young persons and family Promotion of healthy lifestyles Resilience training
1a	Mild or non-specific symptoms of the disorder. Mild functional change or decline Psychosocial deficits (including cognition)	Screening of young population. Referred from school, primary care, social welfare and so on	Psychoeducation for young persons and family Promotion of healthy lifestyles Simple CBT skill training
1b	Presence of 'ultra-high risk' syndrome: moderate but sub-threshold symptoms. Slight functional decline (GAF < 70). Possible moderate neurocognitive deficits	Screening of at-risk young population. Referred from school, primary care, social welfare and so on	Psychoeducation for young persons and family CBT skill training Problem solving Prevention of risk factors for transition Promotion of healthy lifestyles Identification of early signs of illness
2	First episode. Full-threshold disorder. Moderate to severe typical symptoms. Marked functional decline (GAF: 30–50). Possible cognitive deficits	Referrals from primary care, specialist care agencies, emergency department, welfare agencies	Pharmacological treatment Psychological treatment (CBT) Psychoeducation including promotion of treatment adherence, relapse prevention and identification of early signs of relapse
3a	Incomplete remission from first episode	Referrals from primary care, specialist care agencies	As in Stage 2. Emphasising pharmacological treatment Promotion of social integration
3b	Recurrence or relapse of the disorder which stabilises with treatment. Residual symptoms or psychosocial decline (GAF, cognition functioning and so on below the best level of improvement at remission from first episode)	Referrals from primary care, specialist care agencies	Emphasis on long-term pharmacological treatment Maintenance of social integration
3c	Multiple relapses	Referrals from primary care, specialist care agencies	Emphasis on long-term pharmacological treatment Maintenance of social integration
4	Failure to respond to treatment and/or severe, persistent symptoms. Marked psychosocial deficits as indicated in GAF, neurocognition, functioning and so on	Referrals from primary care specialist care agencies	Emphasis on long-term pharmacological treatment Maintenance of social integration

GAF, global assessment of functioning; CBT, cognitive-behavioural therapy.

should be mainly identified by the patient's psychopathology. The stages so defined may in turn correlate with prognosis and treatment, and hopefully in the future with a specific pathophysiology from which we could derive reliable and phase-specific biological markers. To guide clinicians in identifying the stages at which the individuals are at a particular point in time, different concepts have been proposed. Although they were originally developed for psychosis, the fact is that they are now in the process of being applied, with certain adaptations, to other mental disorders.

Stage 0: 'At-risk asymptomatic'

The first stage in the model (Stage 0) is defined as *at-risk asymptomatic* where a range of risk factors may be operating. In the case of psychosis, several risk factors have been identified. These include a family history of mental illness, substance abuse and premorbid personality traits. Factors relating to premorbid predisposition include poor communication, lack of social behaviour and a higher tendency to show sensitivity feeling. They are associated with a higher relative risk of developing mental illness, especially psychosis, during adulthood [7, 35, 36]. Similarly, in patients who develop depression, anxiety or bipolar disorders, it has also been demonstrated that long before the disorder appears, during childhood and adolescence, it is possible to detect certain premorbid features, typically functional deficits, irritability, sensitivity or poor psychosocial adjustment [10–12, 17, 19]. The specificity and predictive capacity of these features are, however, in need of verification.

Stage 1: The prodrome

In the process of illness development, individuals may start to exhibit a range of mild, non-specific, sub-threshold symptoms (Stage 1). They have been tradition- ally defined as 'prodrome' or 'precursor' of a full-threshold disorder [37]. The idea that prodromal manifestations started to appear long before the onset of a disorder, or before a relapse, has been in common use in medicine for a long time. It was applied to psychosis as early as 1938 by Cameron [38]. Since then, its clinical use in psychosis has grown significantly in parallel with the development of early intervention clinics [39, 40]. Based on the success of its application to psychosis, in recent years, the extension of this concept to other psychiatric disorders has been attempted. In particular, a prodromal phase for bipolar disorders has been proposed by different authors [8, 17, 22, 41, 42]. In the case of depression, several authors have asserted that the presence of sub- syndromal depression, minor depressive symptoms or brief depressive experiences could be regarded as a prodrome and tends to be associated to a higher risk of developing major depressive disorders at a later age [19, 43–45]. In addition, a recent review of the literature by Fava and Tossani [46] conclude that anxiety and irritability were frequently found as a prodrome for depression. Similarly, prodromal features and precursor indicators have also been described for other mental disorders such as eating and anxiety disorders [47–50].

We have to point out that even in the case of psychosis, not to mention other psychiatric disorders, the application of the concept of prodrome to routine clinical practice still has limitations. The more relevant limitation lies in the fact that this clinical entity is mainly composed of non-specific features, which tend to overlap from one disorder to another. In this respect, the data from Häfner's Schizophrenia and Depression Study (ABC study) indicate that depression and schizophrenia shared 8 of the 11 most frequent prodromal symptoms, these being non-specific depressive symptoms and indicators of functional impairment [7]. Much the same could be said for the overlap of prodromal features in other mental disorders. It may even be that the concept of the prodrome may be thought of as a non-specific precursor for the development of mental disturbances in general. In line with this view, in a recent paper, McGorry [51] proposed the possibility that in phenotypically similar disorders, it would tend to appear as a 'pluripotential prodrome' characterised by common features which at later stage may develop into one of a range of disorders, which may include psychotic disorders, bipolar and unipolar depression, anxiety disorders and substance use disorders. So, the question here is to establish which other end-stage disorders may have a common 'pluripotential' prodromal component. A solution to this question has to be found at the psychopathological and the biological level in future studies.

The second limitation is related to the fact that the concept of prodrome can only be, at present, applied retrospectively once the person has developed the illness. This is due to the practical difficulties in detecting a clinical entity prospectively. To do this, it would be necessary to define the clinical frontier between a particular clinical entity and normal human experiences, and, what is undoubtedly more difficult, to distinguish the prodrome from earlier premorbid components. It would also be necessary to identify, in a reliable way, the point at which the clinical manifestations start to meet the diagnostic criteria.

The ultra-high-risk criteria

To resolve the limitations inherent in the concept of the prodrome, in the case of psychosis, the concept of 'ultra-high risk' was developed incorporating a more specific operational definition. The criteria adopted combined the following elements: (a) attenuated positive symptoms, (b) brief intermittent psychotic symptoms and (c) combination of one or more risk factors (always including genetic risk) and functional decline. Unfortunately, this concept still generates a 60–80% false positive rate of transition to psychosis, though interestingly enough its presence tends to anticipate the development of other mental disorders, specially depression and anxiety.

The concept of 'ultra-high risk' has also been applied in the staging models proposed for other mental disorders. Such is the case of the models proposed for bipolar disorders [10, 22], depression [11, 19] or anxiety disorders [12]. The clinical formulation of these proposals is, however, in a preliminary stage, so their operational criteria have to be improved and validated by empirical research in future studies.

Improvement of risk criteria

Although advances have been made in developing operational criteria for the concepts used at this stage (Stage 1) of mental disorders, currently recognised risk indicators for the development of these diseases are not sufficiently predictive to correctly identify persons at risk who later will develop the illness. Thus, further progress is needed in improving the predictability of the risk criteria used for the different disorders. For this, as Klosterkötter et al. [52] have recently suggested in relation to psychosis, we should in the future strive for improving the risk criteria by, first, risk enrichment with the inclusion of biological risk factors and, second, stronger individualisation of the risk estimation by stratification.

Among the risk enrichment strategy we could, for example, expect that in psychosis, the incorporation of brain morphological changes, genetic markers and specific cognitive impairments may play a significant role in the future. In a similar way, the initial staging model proposed by Berk et al. [41] concerning bipolar disorders has been further developed by Kapczinski et al. [53], incorporating a longitudinal appraisal of clinical variables as well as functioning, neurocognition and biomarkers. We have to point out, however, that the success of this strategy is dependent on the future progress of research on the impact of biological and environmental risk factors and their interaction in the development of mental disorders.

Regarding the risk stratification, we could argue that in psychiatry as it has happened in other medical disciplines, such as oncology, it would be desirable to establish risk modelling strategies to define sub-groups of population with progressive prognostic indices of transition to particular disorders. This approach has been introduced, for example, in the European Prediction of Psychosis Study (EPOS) in which a multivariate prognostic index, with four risk levels, was constructed for the stratification of the risk of transition to psychosis from a prodromal stage [54].

Further research will be needed to explore whether these strategies of improving the risk criteria could be adopted for the different mental disorders, and whether their application could derive in a precise early identification of those individuals who would later develop a specific mental disorder.

Evaluation procedures for identifying the at-risk status

A key element in the process of identifying preclinical syndromes is the availability of reliable and valid evaluation instruments. To satisfy this need, several instruments and procedures have been developed for psychosis: such is the case, for example, of the comprehensive assessment of at-risk mental states [55], the Structured Interview for Prodromal Syndromes (SIPS) and the Scale of Prodromal Symptoms (SOPS) [56] and the Hillside Recognition and Prevention Procedure [57]. However, the predictive accuracy of such instruments for the transition to a full-blown disorder is still limited [52]. Unfortunately, the situation is even more unsatisfactory in the case of other major mental disorders, where there are no specific instruments. Thus, there is an impending need to continue developing reliable phase-specific instrument for the identification and evaluation of the syndromes which define the different early pre-clinical stages of major mental disorders.

Stage 2: The first episode of a full-threshold disorder

The second stage involves a clinical focus on the period following the onset of a fully fledged first episode of the disorder. It includes early detection and treatment, and the goal is to minimise the duration of the untreated mental illness. For this, specialised early intervention services and clinical programmes have extensively been developed for psychosis all around the world, following the guide set by the Early Psychosis Prevention and Intervention Centre [4]. Based on this experience, in the last few years, there have been attempts to implement early intervention services for other mental disorders, such as bipolar disorders [17, 22, 58], depression [59] and anxiety disorders [60]. However, we are still lacking reliable evidence regarding the efficacy and cost-efficacy of these new services.

Stages 3 and 4: Incomplete recovery, relapse and treatment resistance after the first episode

Stage 3 includes the first few years following the onset of the disorder. This has been designated as the 'critical period', and it is generally assumed that during this period the parameters for the long-term outcome of the disorder are established [61]. As indicated in Table 10.2, several sub-stages have been defined in this critical period depending on the characteristics of the remission process. It has been suggested that during this phase, that tends to last between three and five years, the patient's and family's insight into the illness is reinforced. The development of comorbidities, relapses and suicide can also be prevented and better adherence to treatment consolidated. Finally, Stage 4 is defined by a failure to respond to treatment and by the presence of severe persistent symptoms and marked psychosocial deficits.

Strategies of mental health care in the clinical staging model

The staging paradigm provides a useful framework for implementing in most major mental disorders phase-specific therapeutic and preventive actions (see Table 10.2). However, in implementing intervention strategies for the early stages of mental disorders, a prerequisite is that individuals at risk should establish contact with mental health-care services. Thus, as the general population, and especially young people, tends to be reluctant to seek help for mental disorders, it is necessary to encourage individuals at risk to access mental health services, thus making possible the process of early identification and treatment. For this, specific educational and help-seeking facilitative actions, at the level of general population and of primary care units, should be implemented for all mental disorders [62].

During the 'at-risk' stage (Stage 0), promotion of healthy lifestyles, resilience training and psychoeducation for the general population, and more so for young persons, have proven to be beneficial for optimising mental health and quality of life. They may also be useful to prevent, in young people 'at risk', the transition to subsequent symptomatic stages. Therefore, irrespective of the mental disorder considered, they should be of general use in mental health, but more so in primary care, social welfare and educational services.

The clinical relevance of this symptomatic, yet pre-clinical, stage (Stage 1) is derived from the fact that it constitutes the earliest point at which preventive clinical interventions could be initiated to avoid or ameliorate the transition to a full-blown disorder. At this stage, great emphasis should be made on psychoeducation for persons at risk and their families and promotion of healthy lifestyles, cognitive-behavioural therapy (CBT) skill training and vocational rehabilitation. More specific psychosocial interventions have also been extensively used at this stage with very good results in psychosis, bipolar disorders, unipolar depression and anxiety [17, 59, 63–65]. A potential benefit of early identification of individuals 'at risk' or in a 'prodromal' state, for example, in psychosis, is that it allows, in certain circumstances, the early implementation of effective and safe antipsychotic treatments. In addition to their neuroprotective effect, antipsychotics will hopefully ameliorate, delay or prevent the onset of a fully fledged psychotic disorder. And the same could be postulated for the instauration of appropriate pharmacological treatment for the prevention of the transition to other major mental disorders. Thus, the combined use of pharmacological and psychosocial interventions is becoming increasingly important for the treatment of the early phases of major mental disorders.

The model of a 'pluripotential prodrome' describing a common constellation of symptomatic features could also apply to interventions. This means that the intervention required at this clinical stage should prove to be equally beneficial in preventing the transition to any of the possible alternative forms of mental disorders. It remains, however, to establish, by naturalistic and randomised trials, the efficacy of these 'pluripotential' interventions in preventing the transition from this clinical stage to the different target disorders.

At the onset of a frank first episode of the disorder (Stage 2), in addition to psychological treatments in the form of psychoeducation and CBT, appropriate pharmacological treatment is usually required. In using pharmacological treatment at this stage, we should be guided by the principle of prescribing the lower effective dose, thus looking for a maximum efficacy with minimum side effects. In combining the different therapeutic strategies, we should be aiming at not only the resolution of symptoms but also the promotion of social integration and the prevention of comorbidities and relapses. For this, the attainment of adequate levels of insight and of treatment adherence is essential.

Similarly, in other mental disorders, such as depression, anxiety and bipolar illness, the combination of pharmacological treatment with psychological interventions, such as psychoeducation, self-help or physical exercise, should be regarded as the appropriate treatment in the early stages of the disorders [19, 34, 65–67].

In Stage 3, the therapeutic emphasis should be on long-term pharmacological and psychosocial interventions, aiming at maintaining the remission of symptoms or at resolving the remaining symptoms and deficits. Reinforcing the insight and the adherence, preventing, and if necessary treating, relapses, co-morbidities and disabilities, becomes an additional main target for intervention at this stage. At the same time, psychological and social interventions should also be contemplated for the promotion of social integration and social recovery [68].

Finally, at Stage 4, the emphasis has to be made on finding the most effective combinations of intensive pharmacological and psychosocial interventions to deal with the refractory symptoms. In addition, the incorporation of strategies directed to rehabilitate persistent psychosocial deficits should be necessary. For this, specific 'early-rehabilitation services' should be ideally developed.

Repercussions of the application of clinical stage paradigm

The application of the clinical staging paradigm should impact both at the theory and practice of psychiatry. This is important as it is well known that, at present, not only the diagnostic and evaluation systems but also the intervention programmes and the health-care services available are not well adapted to the early phases of mental disorders.

From a theoretical perspective, the staging paradigm will allow to investigate the origin and nature of mental diseases without the spurious contamination of the illness chronicity and long-term treatment. This will promote a more precise clarification of the mechanisms and factors underlying the origin and clinical course of the disorder. In fact, the possibility to differentiate the key biological and psychological processes underlying the origin and course of the disorder from epiphenomena, and clinical sequel, should allow a more precise understanding of the intrinsic nature of illness. In this respect, recent studies conducted in psychosis as well as in bipolar disorder and depression indicate that clinical staging might be useful to improve the process of early diagnosis and to facilitate research into the evolution of the disorder in subjects at risk [19, 51, 69]. Moreover, the information achieved on the way in which social and biological factors may condition the transition of the illness from one stage to the other should also facilitate the development of more effective interventions.

Furthermore, the new paradigm should also allow refining the present diagnostic system. In psychiatry, the traditional diagnostic system is derived from a categorical delimitation of illness based on the combination of well-established psychopathological manifestations organised through syndromes and symptoms' dimensions. This strategy, however, conceals the nature of the different stages of the flow of the illness and pays no attention to the dimensions of time and sequence which characterised the process of developing the illness. This implies that consideration should be given to establishing the diagnosis of a particular disease to the symptoms' dimensions at different points of time presentation. Thus, a new conceptualisation is needed about mental illness that integrates the clinical features of the early phases of mental illness. Indeed, recently, staging has been promoted by different authors as a course specified for future mental illness classificatory systems [70, 71]. It is expected that by incorporating this information on future classificatory systems, it would also be possible to develop more precise and phase-specific evaluation procedures.

From the perspective of clinical practice, the new paradigm would also provide a framework for optimal treatment according to the stages of other disorders such as bipolar disorders, depression and anxiety disorders. A key element of this will be to obtain more accurate information regarding the factors acting on the transition from one stage to another and the ways to intervene in this process. In fact, delimitating discrete stages according to the natural history of the disease facilitates the development of a prevention-orientated framework.

Finally, from a mental health service perspective, the early intervention model will set the theoretical basis for the reform of traditional mental health services and for integrating into the mental health system new and more efficient phase-specific services [72, 73]. It is well recognised that these new services will maximise the chances of treatment engagement, continuity of care, family and social support, vocational recovery and ultimately the disappearance of stigma attached to mental illness and its treatment.

References

[1] Kessler RC, Berglund P, Demler O et al. (2005) Life time prevalence and age-of-onset distribution of DSM-IV disorders in the National Comorbidity Survey Replication. *Archives of General Psychiatry* **62** (6): 593–602.

[2] Van Os Hanssen M, Bijl RV, Ravelli A. (2000) Strauss revisited: a psychosis continuum in the general population. *Schizophrenia Research* **45**: 11–20.

[3] Fava G, Kellner R. (1993) Staging: a neglected dimension in psychiatric classification. *Acta Psychiatrica Scandinavica* **87**: 225–230.

[4] Edwards J, McGorry PD. (2002) *Implementing Early Intervention in Psychosis: A Guide to Establishing Early Psychosis Services.* London: Dunitz.

[5] Mrazek PJ, Haggerty RJ (eds.). (1994) *Reducing Risks for Mental Disorders: Frontiers for Preventive Intervention Research.* Washington, DC: National Academy Press.

[6] Marshall M, Harrigan S, Lewis S. (2009) Duration of untreated psychosis: definition, measurement and association with outcome. In: Jackson J, McGorry PD (eds.), *The Recognition and Management of Early Psychosis: A Preventive Approach.* Cambridge: Cambridge University Press, pp. 125–145.

[7] Häfner H, Maurer K. (2005) Podromal symptoms and early detection of schizophrenia. In: Maj M, Lopez-Ibor JJ, Sartorius N et al. (eds.), *Early Detection and Management of Mental Disorders.* Chichester: John Wiley & Sons, Ltd, pp. 1–50.

[8] Vázquez-Barquero JL, Artal Simón J. (2005) The early phases of psychosis. In: Vázquez-Barquero JL, Crespo-Facorro B, Herran A (eds.), *Las fases Iniciales de las Enfermedades Mentales: Psicosis.* Barcelona: Masson Edit, pp. 3–7.

[9] Baethege C, Smolka, MN, Grushka P. (2003) Does prophylaxis-delay in bipolar disorder influence outcome? Results from a long-term study of 147 patients. *Acta Psychiatrica Scandinavica* **1007**: 260–267.

[10] Vázquez-Barquero JL, Artal Simón J, Vázquez-Bourgon J et al. (2007) The instauration of the early phase paradigm to the early phases of the bipolar spectrum disorders. In: Vázquez-Barquero JL, Artal-Simon J, Crespo-Facorro B (eds.), *Las fases Iniciales de las Enfermedades Mentales: Trastornos Bipolares.* Barcelona: Elsevier-Masson Edit, pp. 3–15.

[11] Vázquez-Barquero JL, Gaite L, Vázquez-Bourgon J et al. (2008) Feasibility and justification of applying the early phase paradigm to depressive disorders. In: Vázquez-Barquero JL, Ayuso Mateos JL, Artal-Simon J (eds.), *Las fases Iniciales de las Enfermedades Mentales: Trastornos Depresivos.* Barcelona: Elsevier-Masson Edit, pp. 4–16.

[12] Vázquez-Barquero JL, Herran Gómez A. (eds.). (2007) Feasibility of applying the early phase paradigm to the early phases of anxiety disorders. In: *Las fases Iniciales de las Enfermedades Mentales: Trastornos de Ansiedad.* Barcelona: Elsevier-Masson Edit, pp. 1–7.

[13] Schoemaker C. (1997) Does early intervention improve the prognosis in anorexia nervosa? A systematic review of the treatment outcome literature. *International Journal of Eating Disorders* **21** (1): 1–15.

[14] Perkins DO, Gu H, Boteva K et al. (2005) Relationship between duration of untreated psychosis and outcome in first-episode schizophrenia: a critical review and meta-analysis. *American Journal of Psychiatry* **162** (10): 1785–1804.

[15] Marshall M, Lewis S, Lockwood A et al. (2005) Association between duration of untreated psychosis and outcome in cohorts of first-episode patients: a systematic review. *Archives of General Psychiatry* **62** (9): 975–983.

[16] Baldessarini RJ, Tondo L, Hennen J. (2003) Treatment-latency and previous episodes: relationships to pretreatment morbidity and response to maintenance treatment in bipolar I and II disorders. *Bipolar Disorders* **5** (3): 169–179.

[17] Conus P, Berk M, Lucas N et al. (2009) Preventive strategies in bipolar disorders: identifying targets for early intervention. In: Jackson E, McGorry P (eds.), *The Recognition and Management of Early Psychosis: A Preventive Approach*. Cambridge: Cambridge University Press, pp. 223–239.

[18] Conus P, Berk M, McGorry PD. (2006) Pharmacological treatment in the early phase of bipolar disorders: what stage are we at? *Australian and New Zealand Journal of Psychiatry* **40**: 199–207.

[19] Hetrick SE, Parker AG, Hickie IB et al. (2008) Early identification and intervention in depressive disorder: towards a clinical staging model. *Psychotherapy and Psychosomatics* **77**: 263–270.

[20] Slaap BR, de Boer JA. (2001) The prediction of nonresponse to pharmacotherapy in panic disorder: a review. *Depress Anxiety* **14** (2): 112–122.

[21] Willi J, Limacher B, Grossmann S et al. (1989) Long-term study of the incidence of anorexia nervosa. *Nervenarzt* **60** (6): 349–354.

[22] Vieta E, Reinares M, Rosa AR. (2011) Staging bipolar disorder. *Neurotoxicity Research* **19**: 279–285.

[23] Campbell S, Marriott M, Nahamias C et al. (2004) Lower hippocampus volume in patients suffering from depression: a meta-analysis. *American Journal of Psychiatry* **161**: 598–607.

[24] Pantelis C, Velakoulis D, McGorry PD et al. (2003) Neuroanatomical abnormalities before and after onset of psychosis: a cross-sectional and longitudinal MRI comparison. *Lancet* **361**: 281–288.

[25] Connam F, Campbell IC, Katzman M et al. (2003) Neurodevelopmental model for anorexia nervosa. *Physiology & Behavior* **79**: 13–24.

[26] Massana Montejo G. (2007) Imagen Cerebral en el Trastorno de Pánico: una visión desde las fases tempranas. In: Vázquez-Barquero JL, Herran Gomez A (eds.), *Las fases Iniciales de las Enfermedades Mentales: Trastornos de Ansiedad*. Barcelona: Elsevier-Masson Edit, pp. 73–82.

[27] Moorhead TW, McKirdy J, Sussmann JE et al. (2007) Progressive grey matter loss in patients with bipolar disorder. *Biological Psychiatry* **62**: 894–900.

[28] Post RM. (1992) Transduction of psychosocial stress into the neurobiology of recurrent affective disorder. *American Journal of Psychiatry* **149**: 999–1010.

[29] McGlashan TH. (2006) Is active psychosis neurotoxic? *Schizophrenia Bulletin* **32**: 609–613.

[30] Birchwood M, Fowler D, Jackson C. (1998) Early intervention in psychosis. The critical period hypothesis. *British Journal of Psychiatry* **172** (Suppl. 33): 53–59.

[31] Crumslish N, Whitty P, Clarke M et al. (2009) Beyond the critical period: longitudinal study of 8-years outcome in first-episode non affective psychosis. *British Journal of Psychiatry* **194** (1): 18–24.

[32] McGorry PD. (2002) The recognition and optimal management of early psychosis: an evidence-based reform. *World Psychiatry* **1**: 76–83.

[33] Harrison G, Hopper K, Craig T. (2001) Recovery form psychotic illness: a 15 and 25 year international follow-up. *British Journal of Psychiatry* **178**: 5006–5017.

[34] Salvadore G, Drevets WC, Henter ID et al. (2008) Early intervention in bipolar disorder, part II: therapeutics. *Early Intervention Psychiatry* **2**: 136–146.

[35] Malmberg A, Lewis G, David A et al. (1998) Premorbid adjustment and personality in people with schizophrenia. *British Journal of Psychiatry* **172**: 308–313.

[36] Davidson M, Reichenberg A, Rabinowitz J et al. (1999) Behaviour and intellectual markers for schizophrenia in apparently health male adolescents. *American Journal of Psychiatry* **156**: 1328–1335.

[37] Eaton WW, Badawi M, Badap P. (1995) Prodromes and precursors: epidemiologic data for primary prevention of disorders with slow onset. *American Journal of Psychiatry* **152** (7): 967–972.

[38] Cameron DE. (1938) Early schizophrenia. *American Journal of Psychiatry* **93**: 567–578.

[39] McGorry PD, Yung AR, Phillips L. (2003) The "close in" or "ultra high-risk" model: a safe and effective strategy for research and clinical interventions in prepsychotic mental disorder. *Schizophrenia Bulletin* **29** (4): 771–790.

[40] Hafner H and der Heiden JA. (1999) The course of schizophrenia in the light of modern follow-up studies: The ABC and WHO studies. *European Archives of Psychiatry and Clinical Neuroscience* **249** (4): 14–16.

[41] Berk M, Conus P, Lucas N et al. (2007) Setting the stage: from prodrome to treatment resistance in bipolar disorder. *Bipolar Disorders* **9**: 671–678.

[42] Kapczinski F, Vasco D, Kauer-Sant'Anna M et al. (2009) Clinical implications of a staging model for bipolar disorders. *Expert Review of Neurotherapeutics* **9**: 957–966.

[43] Wilcox HC, Anthony JC. (2004) Child and adolescent clinical features as forerunners of adult onset major depressive disorder: retrospective evidence from an epidemiological sample. *Journal of Affective Disorders* **82**: 9–20.

[44] Cuijpers P, Smit F, Willemse G. (2005) Predicting the onset of major depression in subjects with subthreshold depression in primary care: a prospective study. *Acta Psychiatrica Scandinavica* **111**: 133–138.

[45] Fergusson DM, Horwood J, Rider EM et al. (2005) Subthreshold depression in adolescent and mental health outcomes in adulthood. *Archives of General Psychiatry* **62**: 66–72.

[46] Fava G, Tossani E. (2007) Prodromal stage of major depression. *Early Intervention in Psychiatry* **1**: 9–18.

[47] Casper RC. (2005) Precursors, prodromes and early detection of eating disorders. In: Maj M, Lopez-Ibor JJ, Sartorius N et al. (eds.), *Early Detection and Management of Mental Disorders*. Chichester: John Wiley & Sons, Ltd, pp. 211–229.

[48] Jacobi C, Hayward C, de Zwaan M et al. (2004) Coming to terms with risk factors for eating disorders: application of risk terminology and suggestions for a general taxonomy. *Psychological Bulletin* **130**: 19–65.

[49] The Mcknight Investigators. (2003) Risk factors for the onset of eating disorders in adolescent girls: results of the Macknight Longitudinal Study. *American Journal of Psychiatry* **160**: 248–253.

[50] Stein DJ, Seedal S, Carey P et al. (2005) Precursors, early detection and prevention of anxiety disorders. In: Maj M, Lopez-Ibor JJ, Sartorius N et al. (eds.), *Early Detection and Management of Mental Disorders*. Chichester: John Wiley & Sons, Ltd, pp. 231–248.

[51] McGorry PD. (2010) Staging in neuropsychiatry: a heuristic model for understanding, prevention and treatment. *Neurotoxicity Research* **18** (3): 244–255.

[52] Klosterkötter J, Schultze-Lutter F, Bechdolf A et al. (2011) Prediction and prevention of schizophrenia: what has been achieved and where go next? *World Psychiatry* **10** (3): 165–174.

[53] Kapczinski F, Dias VV, Kauer-Sant'Anna M et al. (2009) The potential use of biomarkers as an adjunctive tool for staging bipolar disorders. *Progress in Neuropsychopharmacology* **33**: 1366–1371.

[54] Ruhrmann S, Schultze-Lutter F, Salokangas RK et al. (2010) Prediction of psychosis in adolescents and young adults at high risk: results from the prospective European Prediction of Psychosis Study (EPOS). *Archives of General Psychiatry* **67**: 241–251.

[55] Yung AR, Yuen HP, McGorry PD et al. (2005) Mapping the onset of psychosis: the comprehensive assessment of at-risk mental states. *Australian and New Zealand Journal of Psychiatry* **39**: 964–971.

[56] McGlashan T, Walsh B, Woods S. (2010) *The Psychosis-Risk Syndrome. Handbook for Diagnosis and Follow-Up*. New York: Oxford University Press.

[57] Cornblatt B. (2002) The New York High-risk Project to the Hillside Recognition and Prevention RAP Program. *American Journal of Medical Genetics* **114**: 956–966.

[58] Conus P, McGorry PD. (2002) First Episode Mania: a neglected priority for early intervention. *Australian and New Zealand Journal of Psychiatry* **36**: 158–172.

[59] Davey CG, Allen N, Koutsogiannis J et al. (2008) El Programa ORYGEN como tratamiento de las fases tempranas de los trastornos depresivos. In: Vázquez-Barquero JL, Ayuso Mateos JL, Artal-Simon J (eds.), *Las fases Iniciales de las Enfermedades Mentales: Trastornos Depresivos*. Barcelona: Elsevier-Masson Edit, pp. 157–161.

[60] Herran-Gomez A, Ramirez ML, Ayestaran A et al. (2007) El Programa de Fases Tempranas del Trastorno de Angustia del Hospital Universitario Marques de Valdecilla. In: Vázquez-Barquero JL, Herran Gomez A (eds.), *Las fases Iniciales de las Enfermedades Mentales: Trastornos de Ansiedad*. Barcelona: Elsevier-Masson Edit, pp. 181–187.

[61] Birtwood M, Fiorillo A. (2000) The critical period for early intervention. *Psychiatric Rehabilitation Skills* **4**: 182–198.

[62] Sayal K, Coope C, Ashworth M et al. (2010) Parental help-seeking in primary care for child and adolescent mental health concerns: qualitative study. *British Journal of Psychiatry* **197**: 476–481.

[63] McGorry PD, Hickie IB, Yung AR et al. (2006) Clinical staging of psychiatric disorders: a heuristic framework for choosing earlier, safer and more effective interventions. *Australian and New Zealand Journal of Psychiatry* **40**: 616–622.

[64] Lambert M. (2009) Initial assessment and initial pharmacological treatment in the acute phase. In: Jackson E, McGorry P (eds.), *The Recognition and Management of Early Psychosis: A Preventive Approach*. Cambridge: Cambridge University Press, pp. 177–200.

[65] Carrera-Arce M, Hoyuela F, Rodriguez-Cabo B. (2007) Tratamiento Psicológico en las fases tempranas del trastorno de Angustia. In: Vázquez-Barquero JL, Herran Gomez A (eds.), *Las fases Iniciales de las Enfermedades Mentales: Trastornos de Ansiedad*. Barcelona: Elsevier-Masson Edit, pp. 125–131.

[66] Dowrick C, Dunn G, Ayuso-Mateos JL et al. (2000) Problem solving treatment and group psychoeducation for depression: multicentre randomised controlled trial. Outcomes of Depression International Network (ODIN). *BMJ* **321**: 1450–1454.

[67] Nutt D. Fundamentos biologicos del tratamiento farmacologico de los trastornos de angustia. In: Vázquez-Barquero JL, Herran Gomez A (eds.), *Las fases Iniciales de las Enfermedades Mentales: Trastornos de Ansiedad*. Barcelona: Elsevier-Masson Edit, pp. 103–111.

[68] Fowler D, Hodgekins J, Paintr M et al. (2009) Cognitive behaviour therapy for improving social recovery in psychosis: a report from the ISREP MRC Trial Platform Study (Improving social recovery in early psychosis). *Psychological Medicine* **39** (10): 1627–1636.

[69] Duffy A, Alda M, Hajet T et al. (2010) Early stages on the development of bipolar disorder. *Journal of Affective Disorders* **121**: 127–135.

[70] Colom F, Vieta E. (2009) The road to DSM-V: bipolar disorder episode and course specifiers. *Psychopathology* **42**: 209–218.

[71] McGorry PD. (2007) Issues for DSM-V. Clinical staging: a heuristic pathway to valid nosology and safer, more effective treatment in psychiatry. *American Journal of Psychiatry* **164**: 859–860.

[72] McGorry PD. (2005) Evidence based reform of mental health care. *BMJ* **331**: 586–587.

[73] Horton R. (2007) Launching a new movement for mental health. *Lancet* **370**: 806.

CHAPTER 11

Work, mental health and depression

Aart Schene[1], Hiske Hees[1], Maarten Koeter[1] and Gabe de Vries[2]
[1] Department of Psychiatry, Academic Medical Center, University of Amsterdam, Amsterdam, The Netherlands
[2] Department of Occupational Therapy, Arkin, Amsterdam, The Netherlands

Introduction

People with mental health problems, or in more severe cases mental disorders, want to be normal citizens just as much as others do. They like to participate in social life, to have friends and leisure time activities and, important for our theme, to have jobs. Certainly, they also have their peculiarities, their symptoms, symptomatic behaviours and disabilities. However, these characteristics do not mean that they, like the rest of us, do not have their particular requirements concerning both lifestyle and living conditions. Although stigmatised and excluded for centuries, people with mental disorders living in modern societies ask to be accepted as normal people as much as possible.

Their wish to be integrated into society, in particular with regard to having a job, has become more problematic, especially during the last few decades of the twentieth century. Their increasing cry for emancipation is better understood when seen in relation to more recent changes in the labour market, where, as a result of rapid economic developments, the percentage of relatively simple jobs decreased, while the percentage of high-education/high-skill jobs increased. Of those with schizophrenia, for instance, around 40% were able to participate in the labour market in 1955 as compared to a mere 8% in 2001. Modern service-oriented economies need motivated, independent employees who are able to deal with complex interpersonal as well as high cognitive demands in the workplace. Workload has shifted from physical to mental demands, and so modern workers are increasingly selected on their psychological and mental, rather than their physical, capacities.

During the 1990s, there was a renewed interest in the theme of mental illness and work following the impact of a small-scale (when compared to English-speaking

Improving Mental Health Care: The Global Challenge, First Edition.
Edited by Graham Thornicroft, Mirella Ruggeri and David Goldberg.
© 2013 John Wiley & Sons, Ltd. Published 2013 by John Wiley & Sons, Ltd.

countries) deinstitutionalization process in the Netherlands. With an increasing number of patients living outside hospital settings, recovery and (vocational) rehabilitation became major topics. Within this context, we organised the Fifth World Congress for Psychosocial Rehabilitation in the Netherlands in 1996 entitled 'Towards full citizenship of the person with mental illness through Psychosocial Rehabilitation'. Here, full citizenship was connected to quality of life, defined as the qualitative evaluation of the different social roles a person has. Work was certainly one of the important roles that received a lot of attention.

However, the topic 'work and mental disorders' was not only of interest in relation to the more traditional severe and chronic mental illnesses. In fact, during the same period, many of the Western countries saw themselves confronted with new statistics showing that sickness absence and long-term disability pensions were increasingly and highly related to a broad spectrum of mental problems. The public costs of short-, medium- and long-term sickness absence all increased, and during the turn of the century, the role of occupational physicians, but also of mental health workers, was openly debated with one conclusion: they all should have a greater responsibility in reducing sickness absence related to mental illnesses.

A local reason to be more interested in the connection between mental disorders and work was a clinical one. In our programme for mood disorders in the Academic Medical Centre in Amsterdam, we learnt that the phase during which patients had to return to their jobs after a period of absenteeism because of depression was a vulnerable one. In this phase, many patients showed a recurrence of their symptoms, or sometimes relapsed into depression. It became clear that an effective treatment should also focus, preferably from the earliest moment onwards, on the re-integration of patients to their jobs. This point of view was new in the Netherlands, and was at least debatable. For many years, medical professionals did not want to be included in discussions in which they had to give medical expert opinions about the work capacity of their patients. As a consequence, they also abstained from including work-focused treatments in their therapeutic arsenal.

In this chapter, we first discuss the meaning of work for mental health, changes in the workplace over the last few decades and their consequences for those with mental illness, and the impact of mental disorders (in particular unipolar and bipolar disorder) on the capacity to work. We then describe a set of studies from our own group, focusing on common mental disorders, severe mental illness and depression.

Work and mental health

Our theme considers one of the main sociological roles people have in life: their work role. Each week has 168 hours, of which about one-third are used for sleeping. Of the remaining 110–120 hours, about a third is spent at work and the other two-thirds on private life and leisure activities. Within these life areas, most people consider private or family life to be the most important, but work certainly follows as a close second, and for quite a few people, work is even more important than private life.

Why is work such an important aspect of peoples' lives? Work helps us to define ourselves, both in relation to other people and in relation to our direction and purpose in life. It provides us with an opportunity to train and develop new skills and to achieve goals. In addition, work provides an identity and a position in society. It defines who we are, how 'good' and masterful we are and, in some way, how economically strong and independent we are. Having no job, losing your job, being threatened with losing your job or having problems at work may all have a great impact on work identity and, consequently, on mental health.

However, the extent of this impact is greatly influenced by the relationship one has with his or her work, and these relationships vary widely. Work, for some, may be therapeutic, while it may cause or contribute to illness, disability and/or low quality of life in others [1]. For some, having a job that contributes to societal appraisal may be the main determinant of self-esteem, while for others, a job may just be a means to earn money in order to participate in private and leisure activities. Their self-esteem may be only loosely related to achievements at work.

Work is a goal-oriented activity that requires planning, organisation and concerted action and produces results that are valued by society. At the same time, it is a social activity that brings people together, creating social networks and enhancing contacts. Work always exceeds individual goals and needs, creating social duties and responsibilities. During their development, people learn step by step to socialise into these complex work roles and conditions, and by doing so create their own work personality and earn a respectable position in society [2]. Interacting and working closely with others make work a learning opportunity to develop coping strategies to deal with power and influence.

Work helps us create vital conditions for the maintenance of overall physical and mental health. The income from work not only offers us an opportunity to lead an active and healthy life, but also allows us to indulge in luxury, helping us define our position and identity in society. Loss of job is thus related to feelings of guilt and reduced self-esteem, to financial debt and to disturbed social role patterns and diminished social status [3].

Changes in the workplace

Over the last century, there have been impressive changes in the workplace – for example, type of work, work conditions, skills needed, speed with which changes are implemented, and the number of reorganisations. The current field of work activities is now mainly characterised by services, while agriculture and industries have declined. The introduction of information and communication technologies, globalisation, new production concepts, high-tech quality standards and the proliferation of highly skilled jobs require well-trained and thoroughly skilled workers.

People not only have to be flexible and proactive, they also need employability. Working security has also reduced. People are no longer their own masters but have to adapt to social hierarchies, which, because of reorganisations, can change rapidly. Because of all these changes and high demands, people who lack the requisite characteristics are in danger of being left out, thereby being deemed incapable and unfit.

With this change from physical work to intellectual work, from being your own boss to working in highly dependent conditions, from having stable lifelong jobs to a long row of relatively short-term contracts and from ever-increasing levels of efficiency and job performances, it is not surprising that those with mental health problems, vulnerable personalities or real mental disorders are high on the list of those who do not survive this struggle to be among the fittest. Workers in the European Union reported symptoms such as fatigue, stress, headaches and irritability as the most important health problems after musculoskeletal symptoms [4].

Socio-political context

Among people of working age, chronic diseases are increasingly prevalent [5]. Diabetes, cancer and gastrointestinal, respiratory, musculoskeletal, cardiovascular and mental disorders are common [6]. Chronic conditions require self-management, regular medical care, but also occupational interventions to reduce the consequences for the worker and the workplace in terms of sickness days, early retirement and job loss. All of these do not only have a tremendous impact on the person and his or her relatives but also on employers and society. To prevent these negative consequences, recent policies that encourage continued employment for employees with long-term health problems and disabilities have been developed [7].

In the Netherlands, before 2002, the state was responsible for the provision of work disability benefits. From 2002 onwards, employers became responsible, and over the next few years, organisations started to create social medical teams which had the responsibility to monitor organisational health and safety policies and procedures. One of their main targets was to promote job retention for employees who were ill. During that first decade of the millennium, responsibilities shifted from the state to the companies and organisations. In these companies, this change included a shift from being responsible for health and safety to one that included job retention. For occupational physicians and occupational health services, this meant a shift towards integrated social medical teams, which besides occupational physicians also included line managers and human resource managers.

Different mental disorders and work

The impact of mental disorders on the capacity to work is to a large extent determined by three factors: the age of onset, the longitudinal course and the current type and severity of symptoms and related disabilities. Adjustment disorders, for instance, are of limited duration and mostly not severe in terms of symptoms and disabilities. Although people may have these disorders at an early age, the low severity, the short duration and the (mostly) full recovery categorise adjustment disorders in the 'low-impact' category in terms of consequences for work.

At the other side of the spectrum are mostly chronic and disabling conditions like autism, schizophrenia, severe personality disorders and severe mood disorders. These disorders have an early or very early age of onset, mostly interrupting school, study or early work careers. Schizophrenia, for instance, with its peak onset between the age of 15 and 25, interrupts the life of adolescents, who normally do not reach the study and working level expected of them. They lose contact with peers and former school friends and are at great risk of not finding a job, and if they do find one, it is not in accordance with their own expectations or IQ level. Because of the chronic character of the disorder, there is little chance this will change in later life.

Mood disorders, unipolar depression and bipolar or manic depressive illness are medium-impact disorders. Mood disorders, more than other mental disorders, differ widely in terms of severity, course and functional outcome. Compared to psychotic disorders like schizophrenia, they occur mostly at a later age, are less disabling and less chronic. They often have a recurrent course, in many cases with low or absent symptomatology and low disabilities between episodes of illness. Both unipolar and bipolar patients are in many cases people who have been able to finish school, study and who have had a successful phase of early career. They have found a job and a position in the labour market. Many have been able to start family and lead a social life. However, episodes of depression may last for many months; some patients may not recover fully while 10–15% of patients may develop chronic conditions. In such cases, the consequences for occupational functioning need our full attention.

The impact of illness on work can roughly be divided into absenteeism and presenteeism. The latter implies that a person continues to be at the workplace, although he or she is suffering from a disease which may influence his or her working capacity. We speak of 'difficult days' or 'extra effort days' if someone's output or productivity is more or less the same; symptoms or disabilities are low or the person is able to preserve his or her normal work functioning by putting in extra effort. If, despite the extra effort productivity is low, but there is no absenteeism, terms like 'work cut back days' or 'partial days' are used. Absenteeism, on the other hand, can be incidental, frequently incidental, short term, long term or enduring, which may lead to the receipt of a disability pension.

Work and depression

Depression is among the medical conditions with the highest negative impact on work outcome. Depressed workers are at increased risk for both short-term [8] and long-term [9] sickness absence. They claim substantially more work disability pensions than their non-depressed colleagues. The impact of depression is even higher than debilitating medical conditions such as rheumatoid arthritis and ischemic heart disease [10]. Out of the ten most common chronic health conditions, depression is associated with the highest reduction in productivity in the workplace [11].

Not being able to participate fully in the labour market due to depression can lead to economic and social deprivation, which in turn has a negative impact on the course of depression. Studies have demonstrated that employees who have experienced a depression-related disability episode are seven times more likely to have another mental-health-related disability episode within 12 months [12].

The financial burden of depression-related work disability for society is substantial and will only continue to increase [13]. In 2000, in the United States, two-thirds of the total costs associated with depression were work-related ($51.5 billion out of a total of $83.1 billion). Even when depressed employees are clinically treated for depression, they still incur 3.2 times higher absenteeism-related costs when compared to non-depressed employees [14]. However, these costs do not yet include costs related to productivity loss (presenteeism) which are estimated to be three to five times higher than the costs of absenteeism and medical treatment combined. Employers have become increasingly aware of these productivity costs associated with mental disorders and the importance of fostering a mentally healthy workforce [15, 16].

In short, depression can provoke the following illness-related problems at the workplace [17]:

1 *Cognitive limitations*: problems with concentration, problems with what (and when) to plan, a limited capability to cope with complex stimuli, problems with memory and decision-making. Depression changes the capacities to engage in goal-directed use of time, energy, interest and attention. Occupation, in its broadest context, is precisely that: goal-directed use of time, energy, interest and attention.

2 *Emotional restrictions*: an inferiority complex, guilt sentiment, loss of interest and motivation, loss of initiative, apathy and loss of self-esteem are all problematic in executing daily activities at work, for example, interaction with clients or taking on more work than one can handle.

3 *Social restrictions*: difficulty in dealing with clients, colleagues and supervisors, which are caused by low mood, irritability, introverted behaviour or social anxiety of the employee with depression.

Work and bipolar disorder

Although the relationship between employment and mental disorders received far more attention in the research on schizophrenia and depression, this has also been of interest in the field of bipolar disorder. Dean [18] identified 14 quantitative studies focusing on work impairment in bipolar disorder. Rates of employment were rather low in comparison with patients with unipolar depression. Many patients worked below their expected level of employment. Dickerson [19] studied 117 patients and found that employment status was significantly associated with level of cognitive functioning (especially verbal memory), severity of symptoms, history of psychiatric hospitalisation and level of maternal education. Other researchers [20] have reported that there appears to be a marked time lag between symptomatic recovery from a mood episode and return to the workforce.

In a study using grounded theory, Tse [21] found wide variability in the manner in which individuals with bipolar disorder were able to engage in paid work. Determining whether or not a person with (levels of) persistent psychiatric disabilities can cope with a particular job is related to a complex set of different and interacting variables. In a summarising vocational integration model, he defined four interacting components:

1 *Individual component* (the way the person with bipolar disorder deals with, e.g. adverse side effects of medication, stress in the workplace, loss of confidence, the disturbances of the illness)
2 *Support component* (family, social, professional, community support systems)
3 *Work component* (meaning, value, job satisfaction, job flexibility, job structure, match between job demands and person's abilities and/or disabilities)
4 *Wider context component* (governmental policies, income support, societal attitudes, overall economic status of the country)

These four components interact with each other, in particular with the individual's current stage of recovery from mental illness. The role of the employers is crucial here: are they, given a certain level of symptomatology, willing to accommodate the employee's specific requirements, for instance, regarding flexible working hour schedules, short breaks, temporarily simplifying expected tasks and the provision of extra support. Hammen [22] also found that the presence of a strong and supportive relationship was a stronger predictor for work functioning than current symptomatology.

Mental health, mental health care and work: Own studies

During the last 10–15 years, we and our colleagues have conducted several studies on work and mental disorders, with a special focus on depression. We will summarise and discuss these in the next paragraphs.

Studies in common mental disorders

We analysed the influence of (a) personality characteristics and (b) common mental disorders on impaired work functioning. Using data from the Netherlands Mental Health Survey and Incidence Study (NEMESIS), a prospective cohort study in the adult population, higher neuroticism, more external locus of control and lower self-esteem were each significantly related to subsequent impairment in work functioning. Mental disorders like depressive, anxiety and substance abuse disorders were also significantly associated with later impairment in work functioning. However, this association was no longer significant once the influence of the personality traits was taken into account [23].

As stated earlier, occupational stress has increased rapidly in Western countries. What can be done to improve coping with work stress? In a systematic review, we evaluated what types of occupational stress interventions are most effective [24]. Most of the 48 studies used volunteer samples instead of clinically referred samples. Interventions that did not focus on the worker but on the organisation as a whole were not effective. For the individual-focused interventions, we found a moderate effect for cognitive-behavioural interventions and a minor effect for relaxation techniques. Effects were most pronounced in terms of psychological complaints, psychological resources and response and perceived quality of life. However, it was hard to tell whether these programmes really prevented illness and sick leave. The studies tended to focus on the prevention of psychological symptoms and work disability.

For employees on sick leave because of an adjustment disorder with occupational dysfunction, we compared for the first time with a controlled study design an innovative activating intervention given by occupational physicians. The new intervention was based on the graded activity approach, cognitive-behavioural treatment and stress inoculation training and aimed at the acquisition of coping skills and at regaining control [25]. It was compared with care as usual. The mean time to return to work was 53 days with usual care and 36 days for the new intervention, and the mean time to *full* return to work was 91 and 69 days. At three months, 26% and 12% of patients, respectively, had not returned to work, but after a further three months, all patients had done so. Recurrence rate was also lower with the new treatment, but interestingly there were no differences with regard to symptom reduction between both conditions. At 12 months, all patients had fully returned to work, and psychological symptoms had decreased to approximately normal levels.

Studies on patients suffering from severe mental illness

In the field of severe mental illness, we assessed predictors of employment outcome after participation of patients for at least six months in psychiatric vocational rehabilitation programmes. A systematic review [26] showed that outcome was not related to diagnosis and psychiatric history but was related to better work performance and social functioning during the programme, higher work-related self-efficacy and a longer period of education. The influence of psychiatric symptoms could not be ruled out nor confirmed definitively.

In another study, we focused on the insights of experienced professionals working in vocational rehabilitation about relevant client characteristics for the completion of vocational rehabilitation programmes, which meant that they had been successful in finding a job. Success was predicted not only by better generic work performance but also by less severe psychiatric symptoms, more self-insight, a perceived need for change and an ability to cope with work pressure. Here, work history was not related to success [27].

As good instruments were lacking, we developed two scales: the Generic Work Behavior Questionnaire, which assesses the core dimensions of work behaviour of people with severe mental illnesses in vocational rehabilitation [28], and the Illness Self-Management Assessment Instrument for Psychiatric Rehabilitation (ISM-PVR), which identifies perceived mental-illness-related barriers to achieving a vocational goal as well as coping strategies employed by the client to overcome those barriers [29].

Studies on patients suffering from depression

As mentioned earlier, depression has far-reaching consequences for work functioning and absenteeism. For patients for whom depression is related to impairment in occupational functioning, recovery may stagnate if 'work' is not part of the treatment plan. However, in a systematic review of the literature on occupational therapy (OT) and depression [30], we found that although work had been an outcome parameter in depression studies, no particular occupational intervention had been developed to improve depression or work outcome. This conclusion was supported by a later review [31].

Therefore, we started to develop occupational interventions, based on literature and clinical expertise, that focused on (a) early assessment of occupational history, current occupational problems and the possibility of returning to the workplace and (b) education and training with regard to personal performance in the workplace.

Study I: Does addition of occupational therapy to clinical treatment improve depression and work outcome?

The first intervention, provided by staff trained in the relationship between occupational impairment and mental disorders, has a duration of six months. After we found positive results in a pilot study, we conducted a randomised controlled trial (RCT) to examine whether it was possible to improve the treatment of depression by focusing on such an important life domain as work [32]. We determined the cost-effectiveness of the addition of OT to treatment as usual (TAU). We included patients with a 'work-related depression', a depressive disorder that was predominantly (greater than 50% as clinically estimated by senior psychiatrists) caused or evoked by stressful psychological circumstances in the workplace. Sixty-two adults with major depression, with a mean absenteeism of 242 days, were randomised to TAU (outpatient psychiatric treatment) or TAU + OT. The main outcome measures were depression symptoms, work resumption, work stress and costs. Assessments were conducted at baseline and at 3, 6, 12 and 42 months.

Depression improved significantly ($p < 0.001$) in both conditions between baseline and 12 months, and with a trend ($p = 0.080$) between 12 and 42 months. Although TAU and TAU + OT did not differ ($p = 0.950$) in terms of depression symptoms during the first 12 months, they did so during the next 30 months ($p = 0.032$) in favour of OT. In addition, TAU + OT patients worked significantly more hours than TAU patients ($p = 0.035$) over the first 18 months, but not over the later period (months 19–42). Furthermore, we found that patients receiving OT returned to work earlier (TAU + OT = 207 days; TAU = 299 days, $p = 0.010$), but without having more work stress. Regarding cost-effectiveness, the OT intervention showed a median economic gain of about \$4000–5000 per patient.

We concluded that the addition of OT to good clinical practice (TAU) resulted in an earlier return to work and an increased reduction in work-loss days during the first 18 months, without any negative effects on mental health (both in terms of work stress and depression symptoms). Possibly related to the fact that patients at the start of the study had already a mean absence from work of 8 months, we found a slow recovery: at 12 months still about a third fulfilled criteria for depression, at 24 months about 55% were still working less than 16 hours per week, and this did not change till the end of the study (42 months).

Like others, we found that disabilities take more time to recover than symptoms. Mintz et al. [33] explained this phenomenon by distinguishing affective impairments (e.g. adequacy, disinterest in the job, being ashamed of one's work, distress at work) and functional impairments (e.g. absenteeism, poor productivity, interpersonal problems at work). The latter are related to a more severe depression whereas the former already occur in a mild depression. Possibly, OT helped patients to start their work again at the time when functional impairments had more or less disappeared, although the affective ones were still there, while TAU patients postponed this restart just because the affective impairments were still there.

Study II: Does addition of a new and shorter version of occupational therapy to clinical treatment improve depression and work outcome?

We next developed an improved version of the occupational intervention of study I. This new module of occupational therapy (nOT) was shorter (18 instead of 36 sessions) and focused mainly on coping and behavioural change at the workplace. In addition, the nOT emphasised an early return to the workplace, even before the recovery of symptoms, reflecting a shift from the traditional 'train-and-place' model to the more recent 'place-and-train' model. When starting nOT, patients were required to (start) work at least two hours per week. In this way, patients were able to directly practise the things they learnt (e.g. new coping strategies) during therapy. In addition, they maintained contact with the work environment, which enhanced understanding and social support from colleagues and facilitated their return to work. Finally, by having so-called work visits, nOT aimed to stimulate the communication between employer and employee regarding the return-to-work process [34].

The nOT consisted of 18 sessions (9 individual sessions, 8 group sessions and a meeting with the employer) and was conducted by two experienced occupational therapists who had received extensive training in the intervention protocol. OT was started within 4–8 weeks after the start of TAU and lasted for 22 weeks. During the intervention, the occupational therapist frequently communicated with the occupational physician and the treating psychiatrist/psychiatric resident. Inclusion criteria for the study were: (a) absence from work for at least 25% of their contract hours due to their depression, (b) duration of depressive disorder of at least three months or duration of sickness absence of at least eight weeks and (c) a relationship between the depressive disorder and the work situation, that is, work was one of the determinants of depressive disorder and contributed substantially (greater than 25%), or the depressive symptoms reduced productivity or hindered return to work.

Participants in TAU + nOT showed greater improvement in depression symptoms ($p = 0.03$) and an increased probability of long-term symptom remission when compared to participants in TAU (OR = 1.8, $p = 0.05$). In addition, the percentage of patients who attained *sustainable* remission (defined as ≥ six months) was higher in TAU + OT (91.6%) than in TAU (69.0%; $p = 0.04$). However, in contrast with our previous study, we did not find that nOT resulted in earlier return to work or an increased reduction in the hours of absenteeism when compared to TAU. Nevertheless, nOT did increase the probability of long-term return to work in good health (i.e. full return to work while being remitted from depression, and with better work and role functioning; OR = 1.9; $p = 0.02$). Finally, patients in nOT needed fewer sessions with a psychiatrist and fewer days of hospitalisation than those in TAU only.

Although differences between the results of the first and second study could be related to differences in length and content of the two OT modules, an important factor that may also have contributed to the discrepancy in study findings is the rapid societal changes that have occurred in the Netherlands since our previous study. First, several legislative changes (i.e. the new disability act and an improved version of the Gatekeeper's Act) had been implemented, stipulating more (financial) incentives for both the employer and employee to achieve a fast return to work. Second, guidelines for occupational physicians and mental health professionals have increasingly emphasised the importance of an early return to work before the recovery of symptoms. These societal changes probably have led to a different TAU, resulting in a reduced contrast with TAU + OT in the second study when compared to the first study, especially with regard to work resumption.

Indeed, overall, the population in this study seemed to return to work much faster than the population in our previous study (for TAU + OT: 66 days instead of 207 days, for TAU: 80 days instead of 299 days). However, in light of these societal changes that increasingly emphasised an early return to work before the recovery of symptoms, the provision of extra therapeutic support during the return-to-work process may be needed in order to increase health recovery. Indeed, in our second study, patients in TAU + OT had more improvements in their depression recovery and more frequently returned to work in good health.

Study III: Factors that facilitate a return to work after depression: Perspectives of patients, supervisors and occupational physicians

In this study, we aimed at investigating the most important factors for facilitating a return to work after sick leave due to depression from the perspectives of patients, supervisors and occupational physicians [35]. Using purposive sampling, 32 participants representing the important stakeholders in the return-to-work process – employees, supervisors and occupational physicians – were asked to formulate statements on what facilitated a return to work for patients on sick leave due to depression. A total of 41 participants rated and grouped the statements.

Using the concept mapping method, 60 unique statements that reflected facil- itating factors for return to work were identified, which could be summarised in three meta-clusters and eight clusters. The three meta-clusters consisted of work-related, person-related and health-care-related clusters. The work-related meta-cluster comprised 'Adaptation of work' (11 statements), 'Understanding and support in the workplace' (8 statements) and 'Positive work experiences' (5 statements). The person-related meta-cluster comprised 'Positive and valid self-perception' (4 statements), 'Competence in self-management' (7 statements), 'Positive level of energy' (6 statements) and 'Supportive home environment' (6 statements). Finally, the health-care-related meta-cluster comprised 'Supportive health care' (11 statements).

Stakeholder groups differed in opinion, in what they considered most important for return to work. Employees regarded their feelings and sufficient attention for their complaints as most important (e.g. 'feeling of being taken seriously', 'pacing of your work' and 'sufficient peace of mind to resume work'), while supervisors regarded clarity regarding the possibilities of the employee as most important (e.g. 'regular communication between supervisor and employee with respect to progress', 'clarity regarding tasks and expectations at work' and 'expression of mutual trust between supervisor and employee'). In turn, occupational physicians regarded the adjustment of work tasks as most important (e.g. 'reducing stress by temporarily eliminating stressful tasks', 'adjusting the workload in relation to the tasks and/or amount of work' and 'simplifying the tasks and adjusting the responsibility at work'). These findings can provide a starting point for a checklist for coordination of the return-to-work process. Differences in perspectives regarding what stakeholders see as most important for return to work should receive special consideration.

Study IV: Predictors of long-term return to work and symptom remission in sick-listed patients with major depression

Finally, using the data from our second RCT, we aimed at examining predictors for long-term return to work in sick-listed patients with major depressive disorder (MDD), and at comparing these with predictors for long-term symptom remission [36]. Potential predictors in multiple domains (clinical, socio-demographic, personality and work-related) were assessed at baseline. Long-term return to work (working the full number of contract hours for at least four weeks) and long-term symptom remission (Hamilton Rating Scale for Depression < 7) were examined during the 18-month follow-up.

Stepwise logistic regression analyses with backward elimination ($p \leq 0.05$) resulted in a final prediction model, including depression severity (OR = 0.92, 95% CI = 0.87–0.97, $p = 0.003$), comorbid anxiety (OR = 0.21, 95% CI = 0.05–0.84, $p = 0.028$), work motivation (OR = 1.87, 95% CI = 1.18–2.96, $p = 0.008$) and conscientiousness (OR = 1.10, 95% CI = 1.02–1.18, $p = 0.012$) as predictors of long-term return to work. Long-term symptom remission was only predicted by depression severity (OR = 0.93, 95% CI = 0.89–0.98, $p = 0.005$).

We thus came to the conclusion that whereas long-term symptom remission is only predicted by a lower level of baseline depression severity, long-term return to work is predicted by multiple factors, not only in the clinical domain (symptom severity, comorbid anxiety) but also by personal (conscientiousness) and work-related (work motivation) factors. These results confirm that clinical treatment alone is insufficient to improve a return to work in depressed employees. Although more research is needed, these results suggest that clinical treatment in combination with interventions that target work motivation and planning strategies facilitate both symptom remission and long-term return to work in sick-listed patients with MDD.

Conclusions and discussion

In this chapter, we have described that in terms of the 'global challenge of improving mental health care', the relationship between work and mental health requires special attention. We have mentioned the importance of work for good mental health – Galen had already mentioned in AD 172 that 'Employment is nature's best physician and is essential to human happiness' – but also the psychological stress that work can bring and the effects this can have on the development or progression of mental illness. Work is the cause and cure of many of our ills [21]. The impact of mental health problems on the capacity to work has gained increasing importance during the last few decades in most Western and high-income countries. This can best be understood by the fact that these countries have been able to develop and implement insurance and financial regulations for those who, because of an illness, are not able to work, be it for short, medium or long time periods. Questions about if, when, how much and how long mental health problems are a legitimate reason for absenteeism are difficult to answer, and for a physical-oriented health-care system, certainly far more difficult than the same questions posed in relation to pure somatic illnesses.

Not only are these difficult questions, but the number has also been growing rapidly. The leading cause of sickness absence in most high-income countries nowadays is mental disorders. Of the time covered by sick notes, around 40% is related to these disorders, at least twice that of workers certified on physical grounds [37]. In the United Kingdom, mental health problems are also the most common reason for the GP to issue a sickness certificate [38]. We have provided a description of the changes in the type of work we are doing, which, to summarize, is a change from the physical to the mental, psychological and interpersonal.

When we consider the total cost of mental disorders, we see that besides treatment and care costs, the costs of low or lost productivity are impressive. In the most severe cases, patients with mental illness do not even enter the workforce or work only for a limited number of years. In case of, for instance, depression and substance abuse, the periods of absenteeism can be limited to weeks or months, but chronicity (and so change for enduring incapacity benefits) is a risk, which makes prevention of enduring absenteeism an important issue. The impact of depression on productivity may be moderated by the nature of work or home responsibilities, sick-leave policies, financial incentives and other characteristics of the work or home environment.

The relationship between work, mental health and return to work after sickness absence is a complex, multifactorial process that is not only determined by factors related to the disease but also by socio-demographic, personal and work-related factors. In addition, several stakeholders (e.g. employee, employer, occupational physician, mental health professional) are involved in this process, who may each hold a different view on the underlying problem and solution. Finally, the relationship between work and mental health cannot be separated from the cultural and socio-political context in which this relationship is embedded. Policy changes and societal changes have a tremendous impact on the participation and return to work of patients with mental disorders. As we have seen in our trials, the effectiveness of interventions may change according to changes in socio-political context. Although this process may have many similarities for those with physical disorders, the impact of mental disorders on work ability will only increase.

What does all of this mean for those working in mental health care? We will conclude with a few suggestions. First, the relationship between mental health, mental disorders, work characteristics, absenteeism and return to work should be given greater emphasis in the training and education of mental health workers. Second, a focus on early intervention of work-related mental health absenteeism is important. In cases where people stay passively at home and lose contact with the workplace, secondary handicap begins to evolve with characteristics of the chronic sick role (apathy, preoccupation with symptoms, avoidance of occupational health appointments) [39], which grows into enduring, long-term phases of absenteeism; when this happens, interventions to bring them back to work are increasingly less effective. Third, closer collaboration between occupational physicians, general practitioners, mental health-care workers, supervisors and employees with mental health problems is certainly needed. Fourth, a closer look at both legislation, on the one hand, and (mental) health workers' attitudes, on the other, which keep patients with mental health problems in the sick role, is also needed, while stepwise return to work would be a far better option. Finally, mental health-care workers should also take greater responsibility in informing workers, supervisors as well as laypeople about the complex relationship between mental health, mental illness and work. They must create awareness as to why, how and in what intensity mental disorders interrupt the capacity to work and what can be done to return to work, to re-integrate and to work with some minor disabilities or symptoms which do not cause conflicts, errors and accidents.

Acknowledgements

This study was financially supported by the Netherlands Foundation for Mental Health (Fonds Psychische Gezondheid) and the National Institute for Patient Benefit Schemes (UWV).

References

[1] Warr PB. (1994) A conceptual framework for the study of work and mental health. *Work Stress* **8**: 84–97.

[2] Warr PB, Jackson P. (1987) Adaptation to the unemployed role: a longitudinal investigation. *Social Science & Medicine* **25**: 1219–1224.

[3] Platt S. (1984) Unemployment and the suicidal behaviour: a review of the literature. *Social Science & Medicine* **19**: 93–115.

[4] Parent-Thirion A, Fernandez ME, Huxley J et al. (2007) *Fourth European Working Conditions Survey*. Dublin: European Foundation.

[5] OECD (2010) *Sickness, Disability and Work: Breaking the Barriers, a Synthesis of Findings Across OECD Countries*. Paris: OECD Publishing.

[6] Beatty JE, Joffe R. (2006) An overlooked dimension of diversity: the career effects of chronic illness. *Organizational Dynamics* **35**: 182–195.

[7] Waddell G, Burton AK. (2006) *Is Work Good for Your Health and Well Being?* London: The Stationary Office.

[8] Kessler RC, Barber C, Birnbaum HG et al. (1999) Depression in the workplace: effects on short-term disability. *Health Affairs* **18**: 163–171.

[9] Bultmann U, Rugulies R, Lund T et al. (2006) Depressive symptoms and the risk of long-term sickness absence: a prospective study among 4747 employees in Denmark. *Social Psychiatry and Psychiatric Epidemiology* **41**: 875–880.

[10] Collins JJ, Baase CM, Sharda CE et al. (2005) The assessment of chronic health conditions on work performance, absence, and total economic impact for employers. *Journal of Occupational and Environmental Medicine* **47**: 547–557.

[11] Goetzel RZ, Long SR, Ozminkowski RJ et al. (2004) Health, absence, disability, and presenteeism cost estimates of certain physical and mental health conditions affecting U.S. employers. *Journal of Occupational and Environmental Medicine* **46**: 398–412.

[12] Dewa CS, Chau N, Dermer S. (2009) Factors associated with short-term disability episodes. *Journal of Occupational and Environmental Medicine* **51**: 1394–1402.

[13] Henderson M, Glozier N, Holland EK. (2005) Long term sickness absence. *BMJ* **330**: 802–803.

[14] Curkendall S, Ruiz KM, Joish V et al. (2010) Productivity losses among treated depressed patients relative to healthy controls. *Journal of Occupational and Environmental Medicine* **52**: 125–130.

[15] Greenberg PE, Kessler RC, Birnbaum HG et al. (2003) The economic burden of depression in the United States: how did it change between 1990 and 2000? *Journal of Clinical Psychiatry* **64**: 1465–1475.

[16] Stuart H. (2007) Employment equity and mental disability. *Current Opinion in Psychiatry* **20**: 486–490.

[17] de Vries G, Schene AH. (2009) Reintegration to work of people suffering from depression. In: Söderback I (ed.), *International Handbook of Occupational Therapy Interventions*. Heidelberg: Springer, pp. 375–382.

[18] Dean BB, Gerner D, Gerner RH. (2004) A systematic review evaluating health-related quality of life, work impairment, and healthcare costs and utilization in bipolar disorder. *Current Medical Research & Opinion* **20**: 139–154.

[19] Dickerson FB, Sommerville J, Origoni AE et al. (2001) Outpatients with schizophrenia and bipolar I disorder: do they differ in their cognitive and social functioning. *Psychiatry Research* **102**: 21–77.

[20] Kusznir A, Scott E, Cooke RG et al. (1996) Functional consequences of bipolar affective disorder: an occupational therapy perspective. *Canadian Journal of Occupational Therapy* **63**: 313–322.

[21] Tse S, Yeats M. (2002) What helps people with bipolar affective disorder succeed in employment: a grounded theory approach. *Work* **19**: 47–62.

[22] Hammen C, Gitlin M, Altshuler L. (2000) Predictors of work adjustment in bipolar 1 patients: a naturalistic longitudinal follow-up. *Journal of Consulting and Clinical Psychology* **68**: 220–225.

[23] Michon HWC, ten Have M, Kroon H et al. (2008) Mental disorders and personality traits as determinants of impaired work functioning. *Psychological Medicine* **38**: 1627–1637.

[24] van der Klink JJL, Blonk RWB, Schene AH et al. (2001) The benefits of interventions for work related stress. *American Journal of Public Health* **91**: 270–276.

[25] van der Klink JJL, Blonk RWB, Schene AH et al. (2003) Reducing long term sickness absence by an activating intervention in adjustment disorders: a cluster randomized controlled design. *Occupational & Environmental Medicine* **60**: 429–437.

[26] Michon HWC, van Weeghel J, Kroon H et al. (2005) Person-related predictors of employment outcomes after participation in psychiatric vocational rehabilitation programmes: a systematic review. *Social Psychiatry and Psychiatric Epidemiology* **40**: 408–416.

[27] Michon HWC, van Weeghel J, Kroon H et al. (2006) Predictors of successful job finding in psychiatric vocational rehabilitation: an expert panel study. *Journal of Vocational Rehabilitation* **25**: 161–171.

[28] Michon HWC, Kroon H, van Weeghel J et al. (2004) The Generic Work Behavior Questionnaire (GWBQ): assessment of core dimensions of generic work behavior of people with severe mental illness in vocational rehabilitation. *Psychiatric Rehabilitation Journal* **28**: 40–47.

[29] Michon HWC, van Weeghel J, Kroon H et al. (2011) Illness self-management assessment in psychiatric vocational rehabilitation. *Psychiatric Rehabilitation Journal* **35**: 21–27.

[30] van Nieuwenhuizen Ch, Dorrepaal E, Schene A et al. (1999) Depressiebehandeling: richtlijnen voor psychomotorische therapie en ergotherapie. *Tijdschrift Klinische Psychologie* **29**: 99–109.

[31] Nieuwenhuijsen K, Bultmann U, Neumeyer-Gromen A et al. (2008) Interventions to improve occupational health in depressed people. *Cochrane Database System Review* **2**: CD006237.

[32] Schene AH, Koeter MWJ, Kikkert MJ et al. (2007) Adjuvant occupational therapy for work-related major depression works: randomized trial including economic evaluation. *Psychological Medicine* **37**: 351–362.

[33] Mintz J, Mintz LI, Arruda MJ et al. (1992) Treatments of depression and the functional capacity to work. *Archives of General Psychiatry* **49**: 761–768.

[34] Hees HL, de Vries G, Koeter MWJ et al. (2013) Adjuvant occupational therapy improves long-term depression recovery and return-to-work in good health in sick-listed employees with major depression: results of a randomized controlled trial. *Occupational and Environmental Medicine* **70:** 252–260.

[35] de Vries G, Koeter MWJ, Nabitz U et al. (2012) Return to work after sick leave due to depression: a conceptual analysis based on perspectives of patients, supervisors and occupational physicians. *Journal of Affective Disorders* **136**: 1017–1026.

[36] Hees HL, Koeter MWJ, Schene AH. (2012) Predictors of long-term return-to-work and symptom remission in sick-listed patients with major depression. *Journal of Clinical Psychiatry* **73**: 1048–1055.

[37] Henderson M, Lelliott P, Hotopf M. (2009) Mental health and unemployment: much work still to be done. *British Journal of Psychiatry* **194**: 201–203.

[38] Dobson R. (2010) GPs want more help and training in sicknote certification. *BMJ* **340**: c5688.

[39] Summerfield D. (2011) Metropolitan police bleus: protracted sickness absence, ill health retirement, and the occupational psychiatrist. *BMJ* **342**: d2127.

CHAPTER 12

Training mental health providers in better communication with their patients

Christa Zimmermann, Lidia Del Piccolo, Claudia Goss,
Giuseppe Deledda, Mariangela Mazzi and Michela Rimondini
Department of Public Health and Community Medicine, Section of Clinical Psychology, University of
Verona, Verona, Italy

Introduction

In this chapter, we discuss the principles and characteristics of a basic training in communication skills, which we consider of general importance for all mental health providers, independent of their professional role, the psychopathology of the patient and the different contexts in which providers meet their patients.

Since mental health care is provided by multidisciplinary teams, such minimal common denominators assure a shared communicative approach to the psychiatric patients and support the later acquisition of more complex and sophisticated skills needed for specific situations such as the hallucinating, aggressive or suicidal patient, the delivery of bad news, shared decision-making or motivational interviewing. These advanced skills, however, are not considered here.

The present contribution originates from our experience as teachers and researchers of communication in health care, with a more recent focus on mental health and mental health providers comprising psychiatric residents, nurses and social workers of the South Verona Community Mental Health Service. Our considerations are underpinned by selective literature references, without any claim of exhaustiveness. As orienting framework and key concepts for us as teachers and for trainees, we utilise (a) the three-function model of a clinical encounter as proposed by Cohen-Cole [1] and Lazare et al. [2], which is also useful for providing structure to the encounter; (b) the criteria by which to evaluate the efficacy of communication [3, 4]; (c) the concept of 'agenda' and the integration of the patient agenda into the health provider agenda as a

---

Improving Mental Health Care: The Global Challenge, First Edition.
Edited by Graham Thornicroft, Mirella Ruggeri and David Goldberg.
© 2013 John Wiley & Sons, Ltd. Published 2013 by John Wiley & Sons, Ltd.

precondition for the therapeutic alliance [5]; (d) the concept of 'cue', first proposed by Goldberg et al. [6], as one of the key features of patient talk, and later taken up in several interaction analyses and cue-dedicated coding systems [7–11]; and (e) the concepts of 'empathic communication' and 'active listening' [12]. Subsequently, we show how each of these concepts has implications for training and training evaluation.

The communication exchange with patients is important in all medical specialties, but particularly so in mental health settings where diagnostic accurateness and the effectiveness of cure and care offered to the psychiatric patient depend greatly on how mental health professionals listen, relate and talk to their patients [13–15]. Patient–provider communication in mental health settings is complicated for several reasons. It occurs in a variety of places such as wards, mental health centres, outpatient departments or the patient's home; regards patients with a wide spectrum of mental disorders; and may involve different professionals such as nurses, psychiatrists, psychologists and social workers. Patient–provider encounters may vary in length from minutes to hours and may be more or less frequent. Intake interviews with new patients need to elicit all patients' chief concerns, life experiences, core values and life aims, whereas in shorter and repeated follow-up encounters, this function is limited to updating previously obtained information. In both circumstances, the patient's concerns contribute to the agenda topic of the encounter and guide communication, while knowledge of patient's experiences, values and life aims helps providers increase the relevance of decisions.

Accordingly, the central challenge for mental health professionals is how they may best adapt their communication approach to the different contexts in which they meet their patients. Therefore, communication skills pertinent to clinical objectives in mental health care are unlikely to be taken for granted, as was shown first by Maguire [16] in 1982 and Goldberg et al. in 1984 [6], who evidenced a series of shortcomings when examining the interview performance of psychiatry trainees [16] and senior psychiatrists [6]. Psychiatrists collected incomplete and inaccurate information and lacked emotion handling and active listening skills. Maguire et al. [17] were also the first to demonstrate that desirable interviewing behaviours of psychiatrists improved after training. These first promising findings were applied and developed further in general practice and subsequently in other medical specialties such as internal medicine and oncology, whereas communication research in psychiatry became a neglected issue, until recently. Periodic observational studies and reviews commenting on the state of art regarding communication in psychiatry had to conclude that communication in this field is suboptimal [3, 18–24]. This despite the importance of communication skills in psychiatry being widely recognised by international health-care associations, such as the Committee on Quality of Healthcare in America [25], the National Institute for Health and Clinical Excellence [26] and the British Association for Psychopharmacology [27], and despite the World

Psychiatric Association and the American Board of Psychiatry and Neurology having introduced communication skills as 'core' skills in the curriculum of psychiatry [28, 29].

Meanwhile, communication research in other medical specialties has flourished. Empirical evidence demonstrates the benefits on the outcome of patient care when physicians adopt patient-centred interviewing skills such as open-ended questions, acknowledgement of patients' feelings, beliefs and values or encouragement of an active patient role [30–32]. Moreover, evidence confirmed the efficacy of communication training in increasing such skills [30, 33–38].

Communication research and training in psychiatric settings, revitalised in the last decade, has taken advantage of the conceptual and methodological expertise in communication accumulated in medical settings, given that many communication problems related to information gathering, therapeutic alliance, patient involvement and treatment adherence are also relevant for mental health providers. Research findings of efficacious solutions and educational interventions, supported by a conceptual framework, can be shared and tested and eventually complemented and adapted to the particular communication aims of the different mental health professions involved in patient care.

Key concepts

The three functions of a clinical encounter

Independent of the professional role of the providers and their specific professional agenda, the patient, the context and the available time, an effective clinical encounter, according to the three-function model proposed by Cohen-Cole [1] and Lazare et al. [2], should accomplish three goals relevant also for psychiatric consultations. These functions are in brief: (a) gathering accurate and reliable information to understand the patient's problem, (b) establishing a collaborative relationship and addressing patients' emotions and (c) informing and educating patients about their illness, negotiating a treatment plan and motivating them to action. Regarding this last function, there is ongoing debate in psychiatry on the nature of the information process, which has remained relatively unexplored in comparison to other medical specialties [39]. Psychiatric patients desire information on their illness and want to have a more active role in the information process [40–42] but appear not to get what they want [18, 43]. Psychiatrists rarely encourage patients to ask questions or to find out what patients think of the proposed treatments [21, 22]. On the other hand, greater staff attention to the involvement of patients with schizophrenia in therapeutic decisions was found to be associated with improved outcomes in terms of adherence and relapse [44].

The three functions are interdependent. How well or poorly a function is met adds or detracts from the achievement of the other two. The importance of a particular function and the dedicated time varies according to the professional role of the health provider and the nature of the encounter. While the information gathering and information providing functions (a) and (c) represent different stages of the encounter, the function referred to the therapeutic relationship has to be monitored throughout the whole encounter to uphold patients' collaboration and motivation.

The concept of 'agenda'

This concept was introduced by Tate in 1994 [5] to indicate a list of topics in the mind of the patient and the health provider which they bring with them to the encounter. The patient agenda regards current problems and related beliefs, expectations, needs and emotions, the problem's impact on patient's life quality but also possible psychosocial problems unrelated to the current problem. The agenda of the health provider instead is the sum of the theoretical and clinical knowledge needed to achieve his/her diagnostic, therapeutic, rehabilitative or educational aims. The agenda items of the patient and health provider rarely overlap. An encounter perceived by both sides as satisfactory demands reciprocal efforts in integrating the two agendas. Exploring the patient's agenda by giving voice to the patient increases diagnostic accuracy and therapeutic efficacy via personalised treatment programmes but is also considered a prerequisite for therapeutic alliance.

The criteria of efficacy

The three functions of a clinical encounter can be said to be fulfilled by the health provider, if the patient (a) offers in reasonable time, in a precise and reliable way, the maximum of relevant information necessary to understand his/her current health and life problems; (b) feels understood and sustained by the health provider and free to express emotions, fears, worries and doubts, including discontent; (c) obtains and understands all information that is relevant to him/her [3], is involved in the encounter, participates in decisions and collaborates with the treatment programme.

Pendleton et al. [4] suggest that health providers answer a short list of questions to regularly check their efficacy after each clinical encounter, such as: 'Do I know more about the patient than I knew before the encounter?' 'Did I listen?' 'Did I explore the patient's worries, expectations and ideas (patient agenda)?' 'Did I recognise and acknowledge the patient's view?' 'Was I facilitating?' 'Did I involve the patient in the information and decision process?' 'Did the patient feel understood and sustained?' Phrased as third-person questions, we found these questions to be also useful for peer assessment.

Cue

There is evidence that patients, including psychiatric patients, rarely express their views and their informative and emotional needs spontaneously [24, 45]. Instead, they offer 'cues', hinting that there is still something not explored or not dealt with enough in the encounter. Cues may refer to a variety of patient's agenda items – symptoms, expectations, ideas, worries and feelings such as sadness, anxiety, anger, discontent and disappointment – and can be expressed in many ways, by tone of voice, body language, emphasis, exclamations, unusual words or repetitions [11]. Recognition and acknowledgement of cues is difficult to put into practice because of their elusive and vague nature, but once identified and explored, they offer access to otherwise 'hidden' but important items of the patient's agenda. Cues signalling negative emotions alert the health provider to relationship problems. If such cues are ignored, strains in the relationship may exacerbate and increase the risk of dropout of care and poor treatment adherence, a familiar and well-documented phenomenon in psychiatric patients [46, 47]. In contrast, alliance ruptures can be repaired if such cues are picked up, explored and the emerging underlying negative emotion is handled empathically.

Empathic communication and active listening

The identification of and the response to the patient's cues are the essentials of 'empathic communication'. It is defined as the cognitive ability to identify and understand the patient's emotions and the behavioural ability to convey understanding of those emotions back to the patient, to check its accuracy and to act on that understanding with the patient in a helpful way [12, 48–50]. This definition refers to the learnable, professional communication skill of empathy. Empathic communication needs 'active listening', defined as intense concentration on the patient's verbal and nonverbal expressions [10]. This is facilitated by the use of patient-centred communication tools such as summarising, open-ended emotion-focusing questions and emotion handling expressions which legitimate the patient's emotions and convey understanding. Empathic communication has been shown to have positive effects on immediate and long-term patient outcomes in medical settings, such as satisfaction and treatment adherence [48]. Similar findings are now also emerging for psychiatric patients [51].

Implications for training

The aforementioned key concepts create the framework that ensures a proper use of communication skills by improving trainees' understanding of the issues behind a constructive use of these skills. They regard different, although interrelated, training aspects which may be approached in a variety of ways, ranging from time-expensive methods such as observation and peer feedback on trainees' videotaped encounters to time-economic group exercises in analysing consultation transcripts or critical incident reports of communication failures, elaborating solutions and practising them in role playing. In the following paragraphs, we show how the different key concepts are integrated in trainees' learning process, as shown also by Rimondini et al. [9, 52] for psychiatric residents. As a first step, we prefer to propose to trainees some anonymous transcripts of audiotaped routine interviews of professionals with real psychiatric patients. In our case, we may use transcripts from the pool of psychiatric interviews examined in detail in the observational studies by Goss et al. [22] and Del Piccolo et al. [24] or transcripts of audiotaped patient encounters provided by senior colleagues of other mental health professions of the South Verona Community Mental Health Service. Trainees critically assess these provider–patient interactions under the lens of the acquired key concepts and receive trainer feedback on their conclusions. Only subsequently do trainees analyse their own videotaped or transcribed interview performance and start with interviewing exercises.

The following paragraphs provide some practical examples of how the clinical relevance of the proposed key concepts may give structure to the training and exercise tasks.

Information gathering and patient agenda

In small groups, trainees identify the information gathering expressions used by anonymous mental health professionals (nurse, psychiatrist, social worker or psychologist) and study the transcripts and the type and quality of information obtained. They look for the use of information gathering skills comprising patient facilitating and other space providing expressions, active listening skills, and check which items of the patient agenda were collected or were missing. A similar procedure may then be applied later on to trainees' own audiotaped or transcribed encounters with patients.

The next step in improving information gathering at a higher activity level consists in each trainee conducting an interview with a peer trainee who simulates a patient according to a precise role script. The information obtained can then be compared with the information on the 'patient's' role script about symptoms, worries, life problems, values, expectations and preferences. The reasons for missing agenda items can be discussed within the group, and constructive peer and trainer feedback keeps the trainee on track. Videotapes of such simulated patient interviews, observed and commented within the group, are a powerful educational method to promote the desired communication changes.

Establishing a collaborative relationship

This function is often poorly performed in routine psychiatric practice despite its diagnostic and therapeutic implications for psychiatry and certainly deserves greater attention in training programmes. For this function to be met, the concepts of cue and that of empathic communication as guiding principle are of particular importance, as shown in the following description of some training exercises.

Trainees' first task consists in identifying on the provided transcripts patient cues which signal emotions and the professionals' responses to these cues. In performing this task, they use the consensus-based cue definitions of the Verona

Coding Definitions of Emotional Sequences (VR-CoDES) [11], a system which also defines the different provider responses to cues that can be observed in clinical practice [53], for example, replies that allow or reduce the space given to the exploration of the cues or replies that refer either to the emotional or the factual component of the cue or the expressed concern.

The recognition of such distinct types of cues is particularly important when they signal relationship problems such as disagreement, resistance or hostility of the patient, frequently reported by mental health staff members. For this purpose, we propose brief vignettes of critical communication incidents, asking trainees to apply empathic communication strategies which open patient's emotional agenda and can repair the relationship. Following are two examples, with cues underscored.

The mother of a son with an early onset psychosis has an appointment with the case manager nurse of her son.

MOTHER: *Marco does not feel well. After a month I see no improvements with your medicines. I thought of looking for a private specialist.*

NURSE: *You should wait a bit to see the effects of the treatment. You will see that we will obtain results.*

MOTHER: *I would like to see another doctor.*

NURSE: *If you agree, I will fix an appointment with your son's psychiatrist to discuss the therapy.*

MOTHER: *If you think so …*

Mother does not turn up at the appointment and Marco is admitted to a private psychiatric hospital.

Mr. Dossi had to be compulsorily admitted to the psychiatric ward.

RESIDENT: *Hi, Mr. Dossi, how are you today?*

PATIENT: *I will not tell you.*

RESIDENT: *Ok, I see. However, it is important that I get to know how you feel today, given that you are in the hospital to improve and to be helped.*

PATIENT: *I have been admitted illegally. I will sue you. I feel fine. Why don't you bother someone else. I will leave the hospital!*

RESIDENT: *I think that you need to stay here for some days, just to undergo some exams so that we can fix the right medicine for you.*

PATIENT: *I do not believe in medicines and pills, I do not want any therapy.*

RESIDENT: *Mr. Dossi, why do you not understand that we are here to help you?*

Patient turns away and does not talk any more, leaving the resident helpless.

These two examples of critical communication incidents illustrate the general pattern that characterises communication failures: providers stick to their own agenda by informing, convincing or too quickly reassuring the patient; they overlook the relationship-building function of the medical interview, often reacting defensively. As in the aforementioned examples, the cues are not acknowledged and not used to open patients' emotional agenda.

The task of trainees is first to identify the patient cue of the vignettes, then to use the cue or the situation which has led to the cue and to propose different empathic communication options:

Reflections (e.g. *you saw no improvement.... You want to look for a private specialist; you don't want to talk...*)

Summary (e.g. *You perceived no improvement in your son despite a month of therapy and you thought of looking for a private specialist, right? You consider your admission illegal; you don't want to talk and do not want to have any medicine. You just want to go home, right?*)

Open-ended emotion-focusing questions (e.g. *I wonder, how are your feelings after a month's therapy without any apparent improvement? To be admitted against your will, how does this make you feel?*)

Empathic statement (e.g. *You must feel quite disappointed not having perceived any improvement after a month's therapy. To be admitted to a psychiatric ward without your consent must be an upsetting experience*)

Legitimating statement (e.g. *A therapy which doesn't seem to work indeed makes people want to change doctors. If you consider your admission illegal, and don't feel ill, I fully understand that you don't want any medicine and wish to go home*)

Trainees are invited to contribute with own critical incidents, to report the precise phrasing and words of the critical interaction to be subjected to group analysis for repair solutions, which may then be tried and tested by role play. They are also encouraged to experiment with empathic communication and active listening skills in their routine clinical work and to report back in subsequent training sessions, presenting own audio- or videotapes. Compared to consultation transcripts, audio- and videotapes offer the opportunity to focus trainees' attention on nonverbal cues which may convey a whole range of different emotions.

Informing and educating patients about their problem and patient agenda

Central to this function is the final information exchange which, if successful, incorporates the previously obtained information on the patient's agenda, in particular the core values, life aims, the views of the patient on the presented problem and his/her social context, all factors which may be obstacles to a patient's adherence to the treatment programme and require negotiating skills. Patients should feel that their contributions are essential for the therapeutic process and that they are not passive recipients of a therapy decided by the health provider.

Trainees approach this function first by returning to the supplied transcript of the patient–provider encounter. They check how the provider engages and involves the patient by applying the operational definitions given in the OPTION scale [54]. For example: Does the health professional try to find out what the patient wants to know by encouraging question asking? Is he/she interested to hear what the patient already knows? Does the professional provide the patient with the desired amount and type of information without being too restrictive or overloading? Does he/she ensure the patient's understanding and check the emotional impact of the given information? Does he/she assess the patient's desired level of involvement in decisions?

Subsequent to this exercise, the application of such information-providing and patient-involving skills can be practised in simulated information-giving dialogue. A peer acts as the patient who has to be informed about diagnosis (depression, panic attack, psychosis, etc.) or treatment options (medication, group psychotherapy, hospital admission, attendance to the mental health centre, etc.). Group and trainer feedback and repeated rehearsal strengthen the learning process.

Implications for assessment and evaluation

Trainees are invited to apply the efficacy questions of Pendleton et al. [4] not only to the transcripts and the vignette material but also to their own interviewing performance and to that of their peers. The accuracy of self-assessment is important for health provider professions from whom self-regulation is expected. Self-assessment is known to tend to overestimate one's own performance competence compared to peer ratings and objective evaluations [55]. To improve the accuracy of self-assessments, they were corroborated in our training sessions by corresponding peer assessment. In routine clinical work, regular confrontation with peers becomes crucial since health providers who suffer from inaccurate self-assessments are unlikely in future to pursue or seek out continuing education and professional development experiences from which to benefit. Similarly, the discussion within the mental health team of stressful critical communication incidents represents an important occasion not only for feedback but also for reciprocal support in the handling of difficult provider–patient relationships.

Research instruments, such as the OPTION scale [54] and the VR-CoDES [45, 53], were developed as objective measures for the analysis of interaction sequences of the medical encounter and for the evaluation of educational interventions. In the training context, they guided trainees' learning process and helped critically evaluate the quality of patient–provider interactions. The same instruments may be used to follow up how trainees implement what they learned into their routine clinical practice. The findings of Rimondini et al. [52] who evaluated the efficacy of a training course on patient-centred communication skills for psychiatric residents showed that residents, despite improving their skills, had difficulties in putting the learned skills into daily practice. Post-training exercise and supervised practice are needed in order to establish a regular performance at a higher skill level, which, in order to become observable, would require a prolonged follow-up period for evaluation. Therefore, special thought should be dedicated to the organisational and content-related aspects of the follow-up period.

Despite the value of self, peer and expert assessments, for communication to be effective, it must be perceived by the patient. The most reliable assessments of the quality of patient–provider communication remain the subjective reports of patients themselves. Patient satisfaction with communication appears to have the greatest impact on treatment outcome in terms of treatment adherence, as was shown for patients of medical specialties [48, 56]. How this important voice of our patients may be integrated into communication skills training as feedback to trainees or as criteria for the evaluation of efficacy of the training itself presents one of the challenges for future training and research agenda on communication issues in mental health care.

Conclusions

To conclude this chapter, the main messages we would like mental health providers to take home after a training course are as follows. Attending a training course in communication is not enough to become a good communicator in clinical practice. It merely provides trainees with a toolbox and some basic instructions to take along to their patient encounters. A comfortable command of these tools develops over time and improves by trial and error and patient feedback. It requires motivation and commitment not to be discouraged by occasional lapses in communication and to resist adverse professional contexts. This challenging and in many cases self-directed apprenticeship stage will be greatly compensated by the satisfaction that the mental health provider would derive from rewarding and collaborative relationships with psychiatric patients.

References

[1] Cohen-Cole SA. (1991) *The Medical Interview: The Three-Function Approach*. St. Louis: Mosby-Year Inc.
[2] Lazare A, Putnam S, Lipkin M. (1995) Three functions of the medical interview. In: Lipkin M, Putnam SM, Lazare A (eds.), *The Medical Interview*. New York: Springer, pp. 3–9.
[3] Priebe S, Dimic S, Wildgrube C et al. (2011) Good communication in psychiatry – a conceptual review. *European Psychiatry* **26**: 403–407.
[4] Pendleton D, Schofield T, Tate P et al. (2002) *The New Consultation: Developing Doctor-Patient Communication*. Oxford/New York: Oxford University Press.

[5] Tate P. (1994) *The Doctor's Communication Handbook*. Oxford/New York: Radcliff Medical Press.

[6] Goldberg D, Hobson RF, Maguire P et al. (1984) The clarification and assessment of a method of psychotherapy. *British Journal of Psychiatry* **144**: 567–580.

[7] Del Piccolo L, Saltini A, Zimmermann C et al. (2000) Differences in verbal behaviours of patients with and without emotional distress during primary care consultations. *Psychological Medicine* **30**: 629–643.

[8] Heaven C, Green C, Schofield N et al. (2004) *Medical Interview Aural Rating Scale. CRC Psychological Medicine Group*. Unpublished Manuscript, University of Manchester.

[9] Rimondini M, Del Piccolo L, Goss C et al. (2006) Communication skills in psychiatry residents. How do they handle patient concerns? An application of sequence analysis to interviews with simulated patients. *Psychotherapy and Psychosomatics* **75**: 161–169.

[10] Ford S, Hall A, Ratcliffe D et al. (2000) The Medical Interaction Process System (MIPS): an instrument for analysing interviews of oncologists and patients with cancer. *Social Science & Medicine* **50**: 553–566.

[11] Zimmermann C, Del Piccolo L, Bensing J et al. (2011) Coding patient emotional cues and concerns in medical consultations: the Verona Coding Definitions of Emotional Sequences (VR-CoDES). *Patient Education and Counseling* **82**: 141–148.

[12] Mercer SW, Reynolds WJ. (2002) Empathy and quality of care. *British Journal of General Practice* **52**: 9–13.

[13] Cox K, Stevenson F, Britten N et al. (2003) *A Systematic Review of Communication Between Patients and Health Providers About Medicine Taking and Prescribing*. London: GKT Concordance Unit, Kings College.

[14] Swanson KA, Bastani R, Rubenstein LV et al. (2007) Effect of mental health care and shared decision making on patient satisfaction in a community sample of patients with depression. *Medical Care Research and Review* **64**: 416–430.

[15] Patel SR, Bakken S, Ruland C. (2008) Recent advances in shared decision making for mental health. *Current Opinion in Psychiatry* **21**: 606–612.

[16] Maguire P. (1982) Psychiatrists also need interview training. *British Journal of Psychiatry* **141**: 423–424.

[17] Maguire P, Goldberg D, Hobson RF et al. (1984) Evaluating the teaching of a method of psychotherapy. *British Journal of Psychiatry* **144**: 575–580.

[18] McCabe R, Heath C, Burns T et al. (2002) Engagement of patients with psychosis in the consultation: conversation analytic study. *BMJ* **325**: 1148–1151.

[19] Cruz M, Pincus HA. (2002) Research on the influence that communication in psychiatric encounters has on treatment. *Psychiatric Services* **53**: 1253–1265.

[20] Mitchell AJ. (2007) Reluctance to disclose difficult diagnoses: a narrative review comparing communication by psychiatrists and oncologists. *Support Care Cancer* **15**: 819–828.

[21] Goosensen A, Zijlstra P, Koopmanschap M. (2007) Measuring shared decision making process in psychiatry: skills versus patient satisfaction. *Patient Education and Counseling* **67**: 50–56.

[22] Goss C, Moretti F, Mazzi M et al. (2009) Involving patients in decisions during psychiatric consultations. *British Journal of Psychiatry* **193**: 416–421.

[23] Adams JR, Drake RE, Wolford GL. (2007) Shared decision making preferences of people with severe mental illness. *Psychiatric Services* **38**: 1219–1221.

[24] Del Piccolo L, Mazzi MA, Goss C et al. (2012) How emotions emerge and are dealt with in first diagnostic consultations in psychiatry. *Patient Education and Counseling* **88**: 29–35.

[25] Committee on Quality of Health Care in America. (2006) *Improving the Quality of Health Care for Mental and Substance Abuse Conditions*. Quality Chasm Series. Washington, DC: Institute of Medicine, National Academy Press.

[26] National Collaborating Centre for Mental Health. (2009) *Schizophrenia: Core Interventions in the Treatment and Management of Schizophrenia in Adults in Primary and Secondary Care*. NICE Clinical Guidelines No. 82. London: National Institute for Health and Clinical Excellence.

[27] Goodwin GM. (2003) Evidence-based guidelines for treating bipolar disorder, recommendations from the British Association for Psychopharmacology. *Journal of Psychopharmacology* **17**: 149–173.

[28] Walton H, Gelder M. (1999) Core curriculum in psychiatry for medical students. *Medical Education* **33**: 204–211.

[29] Swick S, Hall S, Beresin E. (2006) Assessing the ACGME competencies in psychiatry training programs. *Academic Psychiatry* **30**: 330–351.

[30] Smith RC, Lyles JS, Mettler J et al. (1998) The effectiveness of intensive training for residents in interviewing. A randomized, controlled study. *Annals of Internal Medicine* **15**: 118–126.

[31] Mead N, Bower P. (2002) Patient-centred consultations and outcomes in primary care: a review of the literature. *Patient Education and Counseling* **48**: 51–61.

[32] Stewart M, Brown JB, Donner A et al. (2000) The impact of patient-centered care on outcomes. *Journal of Family Practice* **49**: 796–804.

[33] Gask L, McGrath G, Goldberg et al. (1987) Improving the psychiatric skills of established general practitioners: evaluation of group teaching. *Medical Education* **21**: 362–368.

[34] Gask, L, Goldberg D, Lesser A et al. (1988) Improving the psychiatric skills of the general practice trainee: an evaluation of a group training course. *Medical Education* **22**: 132–138.

[35] Gask L. (1992) Training general practitioners to detect and manage emotional disorders. *International Review of Psychiatry* **4**: 293–300.

[36] Maguire P, Booth K, Elliot C et al. (1996) Helping health professionals involved in cancer care acquire interviewing skills-the impact of workshops. *European Journal of Cancer* **32**: 1457–1459.

[37] Jenkins V, Fallowfield L. (2002) Can communication skills training alter physicians' beliefs and behaviour in clinics? *Journal of Clinical Oncology* **20**: 765–769.

[38] Fallowfield L, Jenkins V, Farewell F et al. (2003) Enduring impact of communication skills training: results of a 12-month follow-up. *British Journal of Cancer* **89**: 1445–1449.

[39] Quirk A, Chaplin R, Lelliott P et al. (2012) How pressure is applied in shared decisions about antipsychotic medication: a conversation analytic study of psychiatric outpatient consultations. *Sociology of Health and Illness* **34**: 95–113.

[40] Paccaloni M, Pozzan T, Zimmermann C. (2004) Being informed and involved in treatment: what do psychiatric patients think? A review. *Epidemiologia e Psichiatria Sociale* **13**: 270–283.

[41] Hamann J, Cohen R, Leucht S et al. (2005) Do patients with schizophrenia wish to be involved in decision about their medical treatment? *American Journal of Psychiatry* **162**: 2382–2384.

[42] Simon D, Wills CE, Härter M. (2009) Shared decision-making in mental health. In: Edwards A, Elwyn G (eds.), *Shared Decision Making in Health Care: Achieving Evidence Based Patient Choice*, 2nd edn. Oxford: Oxford University Press, pp. 269–276.

[43] Clafferty RA, McCabe W, Brown KW. (2001) Conspiracy of silence. Telling patients with schizophrenia their diagnosis. *Psychiatric Bulletin* **25**: 336–339.

[44] Hamann J, Cohen R, Leucht S et al. (2007) Shared decision making and long-term outcomes in schizophrenia. *Journal of Clinical Psychology* **68**: 962–997.

[45] Zimmermann C, Del Piccolo L, Finset A. (2007) Cues and concerns by patients in medical consultations. A literature review. *Psychological Bulletin* **133**: 438–463.

[46] Rossi A, Amaddeo F, Ruggeri M et al. (2002) Dropping out of care. Inappropriate terminations of contact with community based psychiatric services. *British Journal of Psychiatry* **181**: 331–338.

[47] Nosé M, Barbui C, Tansella M. (2003) How often do patients with psychosis fail to adhere with treatment programs? A systematic review. *Psychological Medicine* **33**: 1149–1160.

[48] Kim SS, Kaplowitz S, Johnston MV. (2004) The effect of physician empathy on patient satisfaction and compliance. *Evaluation & the Health Professions* **27**: 237–251.

[49] Stepien KA, Baernstein A. (2006) Educating for empathy. a review. *Journal of General and Internal Medicine* **21**: 524–530.

[50] Neumann M, Scheffer C, Tauschel D et al. (2012) Empathy: definition, outcome-relevance and its measurement in patient care and medical education. *GMS Zeitschrift für Medizinische Ausbildung* **21**: Doc 11.

[51] Priebe S, Richardson M, Cooney M et al. (2011) Does the therapeutic relationship predict outcomes of psychiatric treatment in patients with psychosis? A systematic review. *Psychotherapy and Psychosomatics* **80**: 70–77.

[52] Rimondini M, Del Piccolo L, Goss C et al. (2010) The evaluation of a training in patient-centred interviewing skills for psychiatric residents. *Psychological Medicine* **40**: 467–476.

[53] Del Piccolo L, de Haes H, Heaven C et al. (2011) Coding provider responses to cues and concerns. Development of the Verona-CoDES-P framework. *Patient Education and Counseling* **82**: 149–155.

[54] Elwyn G, Hutchings H, Edwards A et al. (2005) The OPTION scale: measuring the extent that clinicians involve patients in decision-making tasks. *Health Expectations* **8**: 34–42.

[55] Violato C, Lockyer J. (2006) Self and peer assessment of paediatricians, psychiatrists and medicine specialists. Implications for self directed learning. *Advances in Health Sciences Education* **11**: 235–244.

[56] Zachariae R, Pedersen CG, Jensen AB et al. (2003) Association of perceived physician communication style with patient satisfaction, distress, cancer-related self-efficacy, and perceived control over the disease. *British Journal of Cancer* **88**: 658–665.

CHAPTER 13

Making an economic case for better mental health services

Martin Knapp[1,2]

[1] Personal Social Services Research Unit, London School of Economics and Political Science, London, UK
[2] Centre for the Economics of Mental and Physical Health, Institute of Psychiatry, King's College London, London, UK

Introduction: The relevance of economics

The primary aims of a health system are to improve the health and health-related well-being of individuals, both immediately and over the longer term. Preventing health needs from emerging in the first place is obviously an important related aim. But every health system in the world is constrained in the pursuit of such aims by the availability of resources. Staff numbers and skill levels are fixed in the short term, and usually cannot easily be increased in the medium term; buildings and other physical capital take a long time to alter; and consumables such as medications can only be purchased if there is a budget of sufficient size. Even the unpaid resources of family carers, volunteers and communities are not limitless.

The scarcity of resources is probably more apparent today than for some time, given the state of the world economy and the austerity measures being introduced by some national governments. Until recently, and for a few decades, health budgets in most high-income and many low- and middle-income countries tended to grow year on year, albeit quite modestly. But in a period of global economic downturn, those health budgets will remain unchanged or – as is the case in some countries today – they will shrink. Health-care funders of all types have fewer resources today than in the recent past to devote to health care. This applies whether they are collective ('risk-pooling') funders like governments, social insurance agencies and private health insurance companies, or individual funders paying out-of-pocket for their own or a family member's care. At the same time as health budgets are tightening, the funders of services and activities in adjacent systems with potentially sizeable impacts on health (such as housing, employment, education and criminal justice) are also increasingly constrained, which will potentially put even more pressure on health systems.

Improving Mental Health Care: The Global Challenge, First Edition.
Edited by Graham Thornicroft, Mirella Ruggeri and David Goldberg.
© 2013 John Wiley & Sons, Ltd. Published 2013 by John Wiley & Sons, Ltd.

Careful choices therefore have to be made by budget holders and decision-makers wherever they sit within health and related systems about how they should use the resources at their disposal. This means that health systems are now pursuing aims related not only to health improvement and illness prevention, but also to the 'appropriate' or 'better' use of resources. In this chapter, I will focus on these latter aims and how choices might be and have been informed by economic evaluation. I will first introduce a simple conceptual framework in order to show how needs, resources and outcomes are connected and to highlight two key criteria that are often invoked in resource allocation decisions: efficiency and equity. Next, I will look at economic evaluation and the tools commonly employed to examine efficiency (and to some extent also equity). The most familiar of those tools is cost-effectiveness analysis, and I briefly discuss what is meant by each of its main ingredients, providing some illustrations along the way. In the final section of the chapter, I then discuss some of the ways in which decision-making processes in mental health systems can be and have been supported by evidence from economic evaluations.

Efficiency and equity

Economics is the study of how choices are made in the face of scarcity. Although a lot of attention in a lot of countries is today focused on how to respond to – indeed, how to survive – the challenges of economic recession, the need for careful choices in the face of scarcity, and so the need for economic analysis, has clearly always been there. There have never been and there never will be enough resources to meet all mental health needs. Tough choices therefore need to be made between competing uses of those scarce resources. These include decisions about how to allocate resources across service providers and between medical specialties or diagnostic groups, about which needs to target and which individuals to prioritise for support, about the most appropriate treatments or care arrangements for meeting those needs and about the best ways to train staff so that they can deliver those treatments or services. Broader strategic choices need to be made about what proportion of available resources should be devoted to addressing today's needs rather than trying to prevent the emergence of new needs. Broader still, choices have to be made about what proportion of public or private expenditure should be devoted to health rather than, say, to education, nutrition or defence.

Although none of these choices is solely or even primarily an economic issue, decision-makers can benefit from evidence generated by economic analysis. This is because behind each of the choices listed in the previous paragraph are various possible relationships between resources expended, services or support arrangements delivered and outcomes achieved for individuals, families and the wider society. It is therefore helpful to be explicit about those relationships between needs, resources, outputs and outcomes.

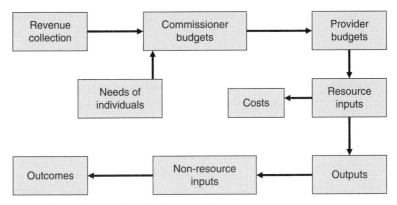

Figure 13.1 The production of welfare framework.

A simple conceptual framework

A straightforward way to represent these potential relationships between the resources that are available in a mental health system and the outcomes they might achieve is with 'the production of welfare framework' illustrated in Figure 13.1. This is adapted from work I undertook with Bleddyn Davies many years ago in the context of long-term care [1, 2]. This conceptual framework is a considerable simplification of the myriad links between budgets, the staff and other 'inputs' employed (and the costs of employing them), the services that are thereby produced and the health, behavioural and quality of life outcomes that (potentially) will result for the people who use these services, their families and relevant others. The framework helps to explain and (conceptually speaking) to locate economic analysis, how to interpret the evidence thus generated, and to highlight the issues faced by strategic and clinical decision-makers.

The framework in Figure 13.1 shows the connections between:

- The *needs* of individuals for care, treatment and support, defined by reference to national and local policies, agreed service objectives and the views of service users and relevant others.
- *Resource inputs* used in an attempt to alleviate symptoms, promote better health, improve quality of life and so on. Important resource inputs include staff, physical capital, medications and other consumables, but the *most* important input in the lives of many people with mental health needs is unpaid care and support from family members and friends.
- The *costs* of these resource inputs expressed in monetary terms. Aggregations of some of these costs are of course the budgets available to decision-makers.
- Service volumes and qualities that are achieved ('produced') by combining the resource inputs; these are commonly called *outputs*, sometimes 'intermediate outputs'. They are not the ultimate objectives of a mental health system but they are obviously achievements.

- The *outcomes* achieved by these services, that is, from treatment, care and rehabilitation (and also from prevention). Outcomes are achieved principally for
the individuals who are treated or who use the services, and will be gauged in
terms of symptom alleviation, changes in behavioural patterns, better personal
and social functioning, improved quality of life (including for families) and
perhaps some wider social consequences. Other terms for these achievements
are 'final outcomes' and 'effectiveness'.
- *Non-resource inputs*, which do not have a readily identified cost (since they
are not directly marketed and do not have a 'price') but which exert potentially sizeable influences on outcomes and also mediate the influences of
the resource inputs. Examples of non-resource inputs would be the social
milieu of a congregate care setting, the inpatient ward 'environment', the
personal histories and experiences of service users (especially previous
treatment/care experiences), their resilience and their preferences and the
attitudes of staff.
- *Commissioning* or funding links between costs (or budgets) and the (service)
outputs: the channels along which funds flow from the agencies seeking to
encourage the delivery of outputs to the agencies that actually do the
delivery.
- *Revenue collection*, which is the process by which funds reach a health system
from households, organisations, companies and donors [3].

The 'production of welfare' framework has various resonances with the approach
outlined by Michele Tansella and Graham Thornicroft in their own conceptual
work [4].

This framework emphasises that the success of a mental health system in
assessing and meeting needs by improving health and quality of life outcomes
depends on the mix, volume and deployment of resource inputs and the services
they deliver, mediated through or by the non-resource inputs, and dependent
on the finances made available through various funding or commissioning channels, and raised through revenue collection. It also makes it relatively straightforward to identify the criteria that mental health decision-makers might employ
to choose how to use their available resources. Contingent on the resources
available, they will want to achieve the greatest benefit for service users and
their families, as well as (depending on their span of responsibility) perhaps the
greatest benefit for the broader community, contingent on the resources available. They might also or alternatively want to allocate resources and services in
ways that are deemed to be fair by some criterion, or that are empowering for
individuals with mental health needs, or that offer sufficient protection to individuals with mental health needs from discrimination or ridicule, or that improve
their social inclusion, or that are 'socially solidaristic'. Although there are actually many criteria that might be deployed to decide what is and what is not a
'good' use of available resources, the two that have been discussed more than
most are efficiency and equity.

Efficiency

Efficiency means achieving the maximum effect in terms of outcomes achieved, defined in terms of needs met, symptoms alleviated or quality of life improved, from a specified volume of resources (such as an available budget). Efficiency may also be expressed in terms of the services delivered for a given level of resources – the 'outputs' – but this is less helpful than focusing on outcomes, given that health and quality of life improvements are the core purposes of the health system.

At a strategic level, many factors can prevent a mental health system from being efficient [5]. It is not infrequent for resources to be used in inappropriate combinations, for example, because there is too much emphasis on hospital compared to community treatment or too heavy a presence of managerial staff over those who deliver treatment at the front line. Support from professions outside the clinical fields, such as social work or employment support expertise, can in some cases improve efficiency, as can a good administrative structure that allocates routine administrative tasks to lower-salaried staff. Inefficiencies can also arise because resources are poorly targeted, for instance, because they are not provided to the people who need them most (perhaps due to inappropriate systems of access, or due to discrimination on grounds of age or race or gender) or because ineffective interventions are used when more effective alternatives are available. The fragmented nature of many mental health systems, with multiple sources of funding and multiple service delivery mechanisms, both within health care and across other sectors such as social care, can also contribute to inefficiencies, especially where insufficient attention is paid to coordination and cooperation. Inter- and intra-agency rivalries, administrative bureaucracy and a desire to protect existing budgets may mean that resources are not always efficiently used, especially where treatments are increasingly based in the community.

Of course, inefficiencies may also arise because of a lack of understanding by decision-makers of the relative costs and effectiveness of treatment options, both narrowly and broadly. Cost-effectiveness analyses can prove particularly helpful, and this is the aspect of efficiency on which I will concentrate later.

Equity

Equity relates to the extent to which outcomes, access to outputs and payments for them are distributed fairly across individuals, regions or parts of a society. Most mental health systems are inequitable in that their benefits are not distributed in ways that might widely be seen as fair, due to the influence of social, economic, political or underlying demographic factors. Access to treatments (and, hence, their impact) may be unfairly distributed by gender, ethnicity, age, language, religion, income, socioeconomic group or place of residence.

But this begs the question of what is meant by 'fair'. Equity is clearly not the same as *equality* in the provision of services, as people do not have identical needs, so that an equitable allocation of resources would likely mean giving more resources to people with greater needs. Similarly, it might be seen to be more equitable to ensure that individuals with the least ability to pay for care or treatment are asked to pay lower amounts than those with greater ability to pay (higher incomes). The most commonly discussed aspects of equity are (a) whether incidence and prevalence are linked to socioeconomic status, ethnicity or other personal characteristics, (b) whether access to (evidence-based) treatment and support is linked to type and level of need, as well as to these personal characteristics, and (c) whether individual financial contributions are linked to ability to pay. There is certainly plenty of evidence of inequalities that appear not to be fair. In work by my own research group, for example, we found that income-related inequality in relation to mental health is actually worse than in relation to general health in the United Kingdom [6] and that it varies by ethnicity [7]. Worryingly, there is evidence from South Korea that income-related inequalities in relation to depression and suicide worsen considerably during periods of macroeconomic difficulty, such as during a sustained recession [8].

Among the reasons for low use of mental health services are poor identification of need, low or slow availability of treatment and care, financial barriers to access (particularly a problem in low-income countries) [9] and stigma and discrimination [10]. Stigma is also a key factor in the widespread social exclusion of people with mental disorders.

Economic evaluation

There are two key questions that must be addressed when considering whether to license, recommend, prescribe, purchase or use a particular mental health intervention. (I use the term 'intervention' quite broadly here to include preventive strategies, treatments, service configurations, local policies and so on.) The first question is 'Does it work?' – that is, is the intervention effective in reducing or removing symptoms, or improving health-related quality of life, without unacceptable side effects? If the answer to the first question is likely to be yes – that is, if the intervention appears to be effective (on the basis of experience with use, backed up by robust research) – then the second question must be 'Is it worth it?' – that is, is the cost of the intervention worth incurring in order to achieve that level of effectiveness? The second of the two questions – 'Is it worth it?' – is what a cost-effectiveness analysis seeks to answer. Neither of these two questions can be answered without reference to some comparator, even if that comparator is the option of 'doing nothing'.

Thus the three principal components of cost-effectiveness are (a) two or more interventions that are being compared, including perhaps the option of doing nothing; (b) the outcomes of each intervention, measured in terms of changes in symptoms and quality of life over time; and (c) the associated costs of each intervention, measured in terms of health system resources used to deliver the interventions, plus perhaps some measure of the wider resource implications (to other agencies, service users, families and others). An evaluation that has each of these core ingredients can provide decision-makers with potentially very helpful insights into the efficiency with which resources are deployed and, in some respects, some of the equity implications too. An analysis that misses one or more of these ingredients – for example, one that looks only at comparative outcomes and ignores costs or adds up the costs of different interventions without assessing the outcome implications – could still be useful, but it cannot provide evidence on efficiency, and only a partial perspective on equity.

Economic evaluations come in different forms, as I shall describe later, but they have a lot in common. For instance, they share a common approach to the conceptualisation, definition and measurement of costs. The main differences between them are how they define and assess outcomes, and these differences arise primarily because they seek to answer slightly different questions. It is helpful to describe these different evaluative approaches by discussing, first, the questions that an economic evaluation might address, and, second, the measurement of costs and outcomes, and how trade-offs are made between them. It is also instructive to introduce utility and benefit measurement, both of which can be relevant when addressing certain policy or practice questions through economic evaluation.

The evaluative question to be answered

If the question that is addressed by an economic evaluation is solely concerned with improving the mental health and associated well-being of (say) patients with severe depression, then information will be needed on the comparative costs of the available treatments, and also on the comparative outcomes of those treatments (measured in terms of symptom alleviation, improved functioning, quality of life and so on). This is what health economists would call a *cost-effectiveness analysis*, and it is the most prevalent form of economic evaluation to be found in the health field, with hundreds of new studies published each year, quite a few of them in the mental health area. It tells decision-makers what course of action most efficiently meets a specific set of clinical needs.

However, many decision-makers face broader questions. They may need to choose whether to treat more people with depression rather than spending their available funds elsewhere in the health system, say on coronary heart disease. If that is the case, they not only need to know the costs of the different options but also some common measure of outcome that would allow them to compare the impact of treatment for depression with the impact of treatment of coronary heart disease. Given that the diagnosis-specific symptoms are rather different between depression and coronary heart disease, it is clearly necessary to find a sufficiently generic outcome measure that has relevance in both clinical areas. A commonly used metric is 'utility', often operationalised in terms of quality-adjusted life year (QALY), which I define and discuss later; another is the disability-adjusted life year (DALY), more commonly used in low-income countries but a poorer measure in most circumstances. Using such a generic outcome measure, the health economist would conduct a *cost-utility analysis*. This form of evaluation tells the strategic decision-maker whether there is a better impact in terms of health-related quality of life from allocating resources in one clinical area compared to another.

It is possible to broaden the evaluative aperture even further, particularly useful if decision-makers face the challenge of deciding between expenditure on health care, broadly defined, and expenditure in another arena, such as education or transport or defence. In this case, an economic evaluation would again need to ask about the comparative costs and impacts of these very different options, but would also need to ensure that the definition of 'impact' has relevance across each policy area. This is where a *cost-benefit analysis* can be helpful.

The policy or practice question to be addressed influences the type of economic evaluation needed, but a single study can usually support more than one approach if the right measures are employed.

Costs

Some costs are directly associated with a disorder or its treatment, such as the money spent on medications and other health services. Other costs are indirect, such as lost productivity because of ill-health, which can be very high [11], or the family cost of unpaid care and support, which can be even higher, for example, in the case of dementia [12]. Productivity losses stem from short- and long-term absenteeism, reduced performance while people are actually at work ('presenteeism'), early retirement, reduced opportunities for career development, days 'out of role' for people not in paid work, and reduced lifetime productivity due to premature mortality. Costs for unpaid carers stem from similar productivity losses, as well as out-of-pocket expenses (payments for treatment or to transport the person with mental health needs to services) and psychological strain.

An economic evaluation needs data on what services individuals use and how frequently. Such information might come from organisational billing systems, which record amounts transferred between purchasers and providers for services used, or from routine computerised information systems that record service contacts such as a case register [13, 14]. Alternatively, data might be collected specifically for the purposes of the research, for instance, through interviews with service users, caregivers or service professionals. One instrument that has been widely used is the Client Service Receipt Inventory [15], which has literally hundreds of adaptations, including for cross-country studies [16] and in Italian translation [17].

The next task is to calculate and attach unit cost estimates to these service use data. These are the average costs per unit of output for different services, such as the cost per session of psychological therapy or the cost per day for inpatient hospital stay. Such information is now quite readily available for England [18], but is not routinely available for most countries. Economics researchers must therefore calculate unit costs themselves, as was done some years ago by Michele Tansella's team in Verona [19]. When carrying out cost-effectiveness evaluations in the mental health field, the main cost categories that would need to be included in calculating a unit cost are salaries of staff employed in prevention; treatment and care services; facility operating costs, for example, cleaning and catering; overhead costs, for example, personnel, finance; and capital costs for buildings and durable equipment. A range of data sources can be used to build up these cost measures, including government statistics, health system expenditure figures and specific facility or organisation accounts.

Even without conducting a full economic evaluation, cost calculations and comparisons can be informative, perhaps comparing between diagnostic groups [13], or examining the influence of psychiatric history [20] or making comparisons between different mental health systems [21]. However, cost evidence is most powerful and helpful when combined with effectiveness evidence.

Effectiveness

The most appealing and intuitively familiar type of economic evaluation – and the most common – is cost-effectiveness analysis (CEA), which measures costs as set out earlier, and measures outcomes along dimensions that would be recognised by clinicians and other service professionals, such as changes in symptoms, behaviour and functioning. A CEA can then help decision-makers choose between interventions aimed at specific health needs, such as two different treatments for mild/moderate depression.

Strictly speaking, CEA looks at a single outcome dimension, such as, for instance, a change in depressive symptoms using the Hamilton rating scale [22], and then compares the difference in costs between two interventions and the difference in the primary outcome. If one intervention is both more effective in terms of improvement on the Hamilton scale and also less costly than the other, then it would clearly be seen as the more cost-effective. But if one intervention is both more effective and more costly than the other, then a trade-off has to be made (see following text).

There are different forms of CEAs, including cost-consequences analysis, where the cost differences and a *range* of effectiveness differences – one for each relevant outcome dimension – are computed. This approach has the advantage of breadth, but poses a challenge if one intervention is found to be comparatively better on one outcome measure, but comparatively worse on another. The preferred option in this case is not clear and decision-makers must weigh up the strength of evidence, perhaps on the basis of value judgements about the relative importance of the respective outcome dimensions. For this reason, attempts have been made to find summary outcome measures that cover all dimensions.

Making trade-offs

The most intriguing and difficult challenge in an economic evaluation – and of course in the very real world of decision-making – is when one intervention is more effective than another but also has higher costs. In these circumstances, which of the two represents the best use of resources? The answer hinges on the extent to which the decision-maker is prepared to trade off better outcomes for lower costs. In other words, since it is not possible to achieve them without incurring additional cost, what is the decision-maker's willingness to pay for the better outcomes? Not surprisingly, there is no single or simple answer: it is a matter of value judgement.

The classical way of presenting the evidence from an economic evaluation to illustrate the nature of this trade-off is to calculate the incremental cost-effectiveness ratio (ICER). This ratio divides the extra cost associated with a new intervention by its additional effect. For example, in a study of computerised cognitive behavioural therapy (CCBT) compared to treatment as usual for people with depression or anxiety, it was found that CCBT was better in terms of alleviating symptoms and improving work and social functioning over an eight-month follow-up period [23], but that it was also more expensive to the health service [24]. The cost of achieving an incremental improvement in symptoms as measured by the Beck Depression Inventory was calculated to be £21, equivalent to a cost of £2.50 per depression-free day over the follow-up period. Is that additional cost worth paying?

In recent years, health economists have begun to use cost-effectiveness accept-ability curves (CEACs) to show the trade-off that a decision-maker will need to make in order to decide whether the higher costs are justified by the better out-comes [25]. In the case of the evaluation of CCBT, the plotted cost-effectiveness acceptability curves showed that, even if the value placed by the decision-maker in the health system (perhaps on behalf of society or of taxpayers) on a unit reduction in the Beck Depression Inventory was as little as £40, there was an 81% probability that CCBT would be viewed as cost-effective. Similarly, assign-ing a societal value of just £5 to each additional depression-free day would result in an 80% probability that CCBT would be cost-effective.

Utility measurement

As I noted earlier, some resource allocation decisions require comparisons to be made that are beyond a specific diagnostic context, such as when setting depart-mental budgets within a hospital, or taking decisions at a locality level. In these circumstances it helps to have a single, overarching measure. Most health economists today favour a preference-weighted, health-related quality of life measure, gauged in units of utility, and usually expressed by a combined index of mortality and quality of life. The QALY is the best known and most widely used in high- and medium-income countries [25]. Values are elicited from the general public on the quality of life associated with different states of health (through a series of robust field studies), with a value of 1 being assigned to a state of perfect health and a value of 0 assigned to death. The extra years of life that flow from an intervention can then be weighted by the quality of each of those years.

The study of computerised cognitive behavioural therapy described earlier included an assessment of QALYs approximated from the Beck Depression Inventory. The cost per QALY was £2190, which compares very favourably with suggested cost-effectiveness thresholds used in England and Wales to guide some health service decisions (see the section 'Evidence appraisal and guideline development'). Although this particular study was able to approximate a measure of QALYs from a clinical tool, this is quite a crude approach. It is more common to use a tool that can *directly* (and therefore generally more robustly) measure QALYs. There are tools now very widely used in health services research (and indeed in health-care systems themselves) to generate such measures. Probably the best known, certainly in Europe, is the EuroQol or EQ-5D [26]. The EQ-5D does not always perform as sensitively as needed in research on treatments for some severe mental health problems [27]. This difficulty has encouraged the development of disease-specific tools to measure QALYs, such as the DEMQOL-U for studies of people with dementia [28].

Monetary benefits

If it is possible to convert the outcomes of an intervention into a monetary value, then another form of economic evaluation is possible: a cost–benefit analysis. Because costs and outcomes (benefits) are now measured in the same monetary units it is possible to see whether the benefits exceed costs, that is, whether the evaluation provides support for the intervention to go ahead. With two or more interventions to be compared, the one with the greatest difference between costs and benefits would be seen as the most efficient.

Cost–benefit analyses are intrinsically attractive, as they can help decision-makers to allocate resources across different sectors, for example, comparing investments in health care with those in housing, education or transport. But they are also intrinsically difficult to do, and there have been only a few cost–benefit analyses of mental health interventions. One that was completed recently looked at Individual Placement and Support (IPS) for people with severe mental health problems who are unemployed but would like to work. IPS has been shown to be a promising approach to establishing people in paid employment [29]. Our randomised controlled trial was conducted across six European countries [30], and included an investigation into the economic case for IPS compared to standard vocational rehabilitation [31]. The two primary outcomes were additional days worked in competitive settings, and additional percentage of individuals who worked at least one day. The former could be converted to a monetary measure by attaching a value equal to average gross wage (assumed to be equal to the value of productivity added to the economy). The analysis revealed a large difference in net cost–benefit in favour of IPS, which thus represented the more efficient use of resources than standard vocational rehabilitation.

Links to policy and practice

Decision-makers and other stakeholders in mental health systems across the world are increasingly turning to economics for evidence to help inform and support their actions, no doubt prompted by the parlous state of many national economies and the gloomy forecasts for global economic growth. Some brief examples can be offered to illustrate how information on costs and cost-effectiveness can be used to inform their decisions.

Comparison

Every region of the world comprises a highly heterogeneous collection of countries, and that variety is reflected in the needs of people with mental health problems, their material and social circumstances, their access to treatment and support and their quality of life. Logically, it should also lead to heterogeneity in policy responses to these heterogeneous needs (and individual preferences). Similarly, there are wide variations *within* countries in terms of needs, capabilities and resources; and similarly again, one would expect these to be reflected in variations in the level and nature of response from health-care and other systems. These differences, whether between or within countries, and indeed *between individuals* in those settings, will have economic implications. It can be instructive to present descriptive information on patterns of service use, employment difficulties, costs and other economic dimensions as a basis for the discussion of policy frameworks and practice-level implementation. A study mentioned earlier, which collected data from approximately 100 people with schizophrenia in each of six European countries, generated some interesting descriptive data on costs and their patterns of association with the characteristics of individuals and localities [21].

Lobbying

Studies that identify, measure and sum the various economic impacts of a condition or disability – so-called cost-of-illness calculations – are quite common. They seek to aggregate all of the direct costs associated with treatment and support of a particular condition, as well as all of the indirect costs of (say) reduced productivity because of interrupted employment and the unpaid support provided by family members. These cost-of-illness studies are popular with patient organisations and advocacy groups as they usually find that the disorder or illness generates high costs, and these figures can then be quoted in making arguments for more resources. In turn, it is expected that more resources will mean better health and quality of life for people with the condition and their families.

An example would be the way Alzheimer's Disease International calculated and used estimates of the global cost of dementia to support its case for earlier diagnosis, better care and treatment, more research on causes and so on [32].

Marketing

While their underlying motivations are different, pharmaceutical companies and other manufacturers also find cost-of-illness studies useful, because they help to draw attention to what might be considered a neglected set of needs, and thus the aggregate cost information might encourage health-care funding bodies to invest more in treatments that can meet unmet needs. More helpful than such cost descriptions are analyses of cost-effectiveness, and in some countries there are now formal requirements for manufacturers (particularly of new pharmaceuticals) to submit evidence of cost-effectiveness to regulatory bodies. Even where there are no such regulations, pharmaceutical companies may commission economics studies to demonstrate how their product is more cost-effective than other available treatments. Of course, there are no 'product champions' for interventions such as psychological therapies or service configurations, and so evidence about their effectiveness or cost-effectiveness will need to be generated from elsewhere, perhaps a professional body or the government or some independent research-funding body.

Policy development and monitoring

Evidence on economic impacts can also be used to inform the development of mental health services and then subsequently monitor the consequences of policy change. An early example of the role of economics in informing policy development was in relation to plans to close psychiatric hospitals in England. Research was commissioned by both central government and some local health and other bodies to examine the financial and economic impacts of closing long-stay institutions and investing in alternative community-based services. A later systematic review of the evidence on the economic consequences of hospital closure concluded that community-based models of care are *not* inherently more costly than institutions, once account is taken of individuals' needs and the quality of care. And even if new community-based care arrangements are more expensive than long-stay hospital care, they may still be seen as more cost-effective because, when properly set up and managed, they deliver better outcomes. Understanding the economic consequences of deinstitutionalisation, including the budgetary impacts for the various public and non-public sector bodies involved, was fundamental to the planning of this major policy strategy [33]. Today there is wide acknowledgement that a 'balanced care' approach is required, with front-line services based in the community but hospitals and other congregate care settings playing important roles as specialist providers [34].

A more recent example of how economics evidence can feed into policy development is work by researchers at the London School of Economics and

King's College London that investigated 25 evidence-based mental health interventions and modelled 15 of them. For each intervention, there was already well-established evidence of effectiveness [35]. The aim was to examine whether there were economic pay-offs from these interventions in terms of direct (immediate or longer term) cash savings to the public sector or to employers or to the wider society (e.g. through crimes averted). Investigating the wider impacts was important, given the extensive impact of many mental health problems. The research was able to feed directly into policy because it gave national and local decision-makers the confidence of knowing that interventions they were keen to promote on the grounds of health improvement and quality of life gains were also at least affordable and in many cases would generate significant economic gains.

Evidence appraisal and guideline development

Many countries have now established mechanisms to consider formally the cost-effectiveness of new technologies (such as new medications and medical devices) as part of reimbursement and coverage decision-making processes [36]. The work of the National Institute of Health and Clinical Excellence (NICE) in England and Wales is quite widely known for its technology appraisals and its development of clinical guidelines. Through literature review, meta-analysis and expert appraisal, NICE synthesises information on both clinical effectiveness and potential cost-effectiveness, using the cost per QALY gained compared with current treatment as a major element in its decision-making. Effective interventions that are found to have a cost per QALY gained of less than £30 000 are likely to be recommended for use within the National Health Service [37].

Commissioning

Economic information and associated 'levers' can also be used to help direct resources in the health system. For instance, the implementation of clinical guidelines might be helped by offering specific bonus payments or other financial incentives to practitioners seen to be adhering to clinical guidelines, or reaching out to specific vulnerable population groups such as people from some ethnic minorities with low levels of contact with services. More generally, commissioners and purchasers of services will clearly find it helpful to know the economic impacts of decisions they might be contemplating.

Conclusions

Decision-makers within health systems across the world need to balance their budgets. They need to do so while pursuing their primary objective, which is to maximise the impact that services and treatments can have on the health and quality of life of patients and families. This is a tough task. Resources are scarce relative to the demands for them, and also scarce relative to the needs of the population, and therefore, careful choices have to be made about to utilise them. Economic analysis certainly does not have a magic solution to resolve once and for all the challenge of scarcity, but what it can offer is a coherent framework and a set of empirical techniques that can provide decision-makers with evidence to inform their responses to that challenge.

References

[1] Davies B, Knapp M. (1981) *Old People's Homes and the Production of Welfare*. London: Routledge and Kegan Paul.

[2] Knapp M. (1984) *The Economics of Social Care*. Basingstoke: Macmillan.

[3] World Health Organization. (2000) *The World Health Report 2000. Health Systems: Improving Performance*. Geneva: World Health Organization.

[4] Thornicroft G, Tansella M. (1999) *The Mental Health Matrix: A Manual to Improve Services*. Cambridge: Cambridge University Press.

[5] Knapp M, Funk M, Curran C et al. (2006) Mental health in low- and middle-income countries: economic barriers to better practice and policy. *Health Policy and Planning* **21**: 157–170.

[6] Mangalore R, Knapp M, Jenkins R. (2007) Income-related inequality in mental health in Britain: the concentration index approach. *Psychological Medicine* **37**: 1037–1045.

[7] Mangalore R, Knapp M. (2011) Income-related inequalities in common mental disorders among ethnic minorities in England. *Social Psychiatry and Psychiatric Epidemiology* **47**: 351–359.

[8] Hong J, Knapp M, McGuire AJ. (2011) Income-related inequalities in depression prevalence: a 10-year trend following economic crisis. *World Psychiatry* **10**: 40–44.

[9] Lund C, de Silva M, Plagerson S et al. (2011) Poverty and mental disorders: breaking the cycle in low-income and middle-income countries. *Lancet* **378**: 1502–1514.

[10] Thornicroft G. (2006) *Shunned: Discrimination Against People with Mental Illness*. Oxford: Oxford University Press.

[11] Organization for Economic Cooperation and Development. (2012) *Sick on the Job? Myths and Realities About Mental Health and Work*. Paris: OECD.

[12] Alzheimer's Disease International. (2010) *World Alzheimer's Report 2010: The Global Economic Impact of Dementia*. London: Alzheimer's Disease International.

[13] Amaddeo F, Beecham J, Bonizzato P et al. (1997) The use of a case register for evaluating the costs of psychiatric care. *Acta Psychiatrica Scandinavica* **95**: 189–198.

[14] Amaddeo F, Beecham J, Bonizzato P et al. (1998) The costs of community-based psychiatric care for first-ever patients: a case register study. *Psychological Medicine* **28**: 173–183.

[15] Beecham J, Knapp M. (2001) Costing psychiatric interventions. In: Thornicroft G (ed.), *Measuring Mental Health Needs*, 2nd edn. London: Gaskell, pp. 93–108.

[16] Chisholm D, Knapp M, Knudsen HC et al. (2000) Client socio-demographic and service receipt inventory – EU version: development of an instrument for international research. *British Journal of Psychiatry* **177**: 28–33.

[17] Amaddeo F, Bonizzato P, Beecham J et al. (1996) ICAP: Un'intervista per la raccolta dei dati necessari per la valuataziane dei costi dell'assistenza psichiatria. *Epidemiologia e Psichiatria Sociale* **5**: 201–213.

[18] Curtis L. (2011) *Unit Costs of Health and Social Care 2011*. Personal Social Services Research Unit, University of Kent, Canterbury.

[19] Ammadeo F, Bonnizato P, Rossi F et al. (1995) La valutazione dei costi delle malattie mentali in Italia. Sviluppo di una metodologie e possibili applicazioni. (Evaluating costs of mental illness in Italy. The development of a methodology and possible applications). *Epidemiologia e Psichiatria Sociale* **4**: 145–162.

[20] Mirandola M, Amaddeo F, Dunn G et al. (2004) The effect of previous psychiatric history on the cost of care: a comparison of various regression models. *Acta Psychiatrica Scandinavica* **109**: 132–139.

[21] Knapp M, Chisholm D, Leese M et al. (2002) Comparing patterns and costs of schizophrenia care in five European countries: the EPSILON study. *Acta Psychiatrica Scandinavica* **105**: 42–54.

[22] Hamilton M. (1960) A rating scale for depression. *Journal of Neurology, Neurosurgery and Psychiatry* **23**: 56–62.

[23] Proudfoot J, Ryden C, Everitt B et al. (2004) Clinical efficacy of computerised cognitive-behavioural therapy for anxiety and depression in primary care: randomised controlled trail. *British Journal of Psychiatry* **185**: 46–54.

[24] McCrone P, Knapp M, Proudfoot J et al. (2004) Cost-effectiveness of computerised cognitive behavioural therapy for anxiety and depression in primary care: randomised controlled trial. *British Journal of Psychiatry* **185**: 55–62.

[25] Petrou S, Gray A. (2011) Economic evaluation alongside randomised controlled trials: design, conduct, analysis, and reporting. *BMJ* **342**. Available from: http://www.bmj.com/content/342/bmj.d1548. Accessed on 20 February 2013.

[26] EuroQol Group. (1990) EuroQoL: a new facility for the measurement of health-related quality of life. *Health Policy* **16**: 199–208.

[27] Brazier J. (2010) Is the EQ-5D fit for purpose in mental health? *British Journal of Psychiatry* **197**: 348–349.

[28] Mulhern B, Rowen D, Brazier J et al. (2013) Development of DEMQOL-U and DEMQOL-Proxy-U: Generation of preference-based indices from DEMQOL and DEMQOL-proxy for use in economic evaluation. *Health Technology Assessment* **17** (5): 1–140.

[29] Bond GR, Drake RE, Becker DR. (2012) Generalizability of the Individual Placement and Support (IPS) model of supported employment outside the US. *World Psychiatry* **11**: 32–39.

[30] Burns T, Catty J, Becker T et al. (2007) The effectiveness of supported employment for people with severe mental illness: a randomised controlled trial in six European countries. *Lancet* **370**: 1146–1152.

[31] Knapp M, Patel A, Curran C et al. (2013) Supported employment: cost-effectiveness across six European sites. *World Psychiatry* **12** (1): 60–68.

[32] Knapp M, McDaid D. (2004) Financing and funding mental health care services. In: Knapp M, McDaid D, Mossialos E et al. (eds.), *Mental Health Policy and Practice Across Europe*. Maidenhead: McGraw Hill.

[33] Knapp M, Beecham J, McDaid D et al. (2011) The economic consequences of deinstitutionalisation of mental health services: lessons from European experience. *Health and Social Care in the Community* **19**: 113–125.

[34] Thornicroft G, Tansella M. (2004) Components of a modern mental health service: a pragmatic balance of community and hospital care. *British Journal of Psychiatry* **185**: 283–290.

[35] Knapp M, McDaid D, Parsonage M (eds.). (2011) *Mental Health Promotion and Mental Illness Prevention: The Economic Case*. London: Department of Health.

[36] McDaid D, Cookson R. (2003) Evaluating health care interventions in the European Union. *Health Policy* **63**: 133–139.

[37] Appleby J, Devlin N, Parkin D. (2007) NICE's cost-effectiveness threshold. *BMJ* **335**: 358–359.

SECTION 3
New research methods

CHAPTER 14

Incorporating local information and prior expert knowledge to evidence-informed mental health system research

Luis Salvador-Carulla[1,2], Carlos Garcia-Alonso[3], Karina Gibert[4] and Javier Vázquez-Bourgon[5]

[1] Centre for Disability Research and Policy, Faculty of Health Sciences, University of Sydney, Australia
[2] Spanish Research Network on Mental Health Prevention an Promotion (Spanish IAPP Network)
[3] Department of Management and Quantitative Methods, Loyola University Andalusia, Cordoba, Spain
[4] Knowledge Engineering and Machine Learning Group, Department of Statistics and Operations Research, Universitat Politècnica de Catalunya, Barcelona, Spain
[5] Department of Psychiatry, Psychiatric Research Unit of Cantabria, University Hospital "Marqués de Valdecilla", IFIMAV, CIBERSAM, Santander, Spain

Introduction

Health care has been recognised as a highly complex, dynamic and adaptive system [1, 2]. Within this context, and as was foreseen by Leon Eisenberg in the 1970s [3], mental health has moved from the marginal areas of health to play a central role in the general care system [4], being a prototype of dynamic, community-based and integrated long-term care in upper-income countries. Mental health systems entail very complex structures and high-dimensional interactions among multiple factors, where the meaning of the measurements becomes central for proper interpretation and where phenomena are very difficult to model under classical approaches. Mental health systems are non-linear, self-organised and fragmented but highly interconnected, history-dependent and non-stationary (i.e. characterised by constant change over time). Furthermore, data on mental health systems are intrinsically heterogeneous, highly imprecise and depend on multiple factors which act at many different spatial and temporal scales (dimensional and multi-scaled) in the context of highly complex multifaceted care [5].

Seventeen years ago, E.R. Epstein envisioned the major challenges derived from the shift from a model based on acute care of infectious diseases to a model of highly complex integrated care of chronic diseases. He sensibly titled his paper

Improving Mental Health Care: The Global Challenge, First Edition.
Edited by Graham Thornicroft, Mirella Ruggeri and David Goldberg.
© 2013 John Wiley & Sons, Ltd. Published 2013 by John Wiley & Sons, Ltd.

'A guide for the perplexed', linking his analysis to the long history of paradigm shifts in scientific knowledge since Averroes in the eleventh century [6]. While this shift to complexity is progressively accepted in several areas of clinical practice such as mental health, primary care, rehabilitation and long-term care, there has not been a parallel change in health policy, where research methods for generating evidence and supporting decision-making are mainly based on the 'classical' approach of Evidence-Based Medicine (EBM) [7] and the related Evidence-Based Care (EBC) [8]. Instead of vanishing, the perplexity derived from this paradigm change has substantially increased during the last decade, posing constant challenges to data management and usability of information in Health System Research, which is increasingly regarded as a separate specialty within the health policy and services field.

The four axioms of this 'aversion to complexity' in health system research based on EBC may be identified as follows: (a) Experimental method is the only gold standard of EBC. (b) Observational data are part of the same dimension of evidence as experimental data, and therefore they should be rated lower than evidence derived from Randomised Controlled Trials (RCTs). (c) Classical statistics based on algebraic formalism are the reference standard techniques for data analysis. (d) Expert knowledge is regarded as a source of bias, and therefore it is excluded from data processing.

In this chapter, we review these axioms and provide alternatives to improve the assessment of highly complex phenomena in health service research, mainly local information and prior expert knowledge (PEK), using a novel approach called Expert-based Cooperative Analysis (EbCA). A case study of the applicability to mental health system research is also provided.

Evidence-based care in health system research

During recent years, an increasingly heated debate has taken place with regard to the usability of the EBM approach in clinical practice [9–12]. Surprisingly enough, this debate has been mainly focused on EBM and not on EBC, where problems and challenges are more prominent and require urgent solutions [13].

The medical advance due to the development of RCTs during the 1950s is uncontested. This method followed a strict experimental approach and relied on the analysis of homogeneous and comparable samples of patients. In order to reach experimental conditions, restrictive inclusion criteria and extensive exclusion criteria were applied to identify 'prototypical' samples of patients and controls. As far as medicine could focus on acute diseases and rely on the advance of health-care technology, this formulation proved extremely successful, but as health shifted to long-term care of complex cases and integrative care approaches appeared, the advantages of 'complexity aversion' and its related axioms were nullified. As an example, the experimental approach was very successful for the analysis of antibiotics and other medical drugs, but disparities emerged between results obtained under experimental conditions and in routine clinical practice. In order to describe the usability of tested interventions in actual medical practice, the concept of *effectiveness* was added to the traditional concepts of efficacy and safety [14], and EBM was introduced to fill the gap between RCT-related efficacy and practical effectiveness [15].

EBM introduced meta-analyses and systematic reviews of available 'evidence' as well as quality guidelines, which graded RCT efficacy studies at the highest level of quality whilst rating observational/ecological/local data at the lower level of quality in the so-called levels of evidence. However, this rating of available evidence constituted in itself an oversimplification of the original EBM approach, as the EBM model incorporated training in 'rational thinking' and patients' values and preferences as key components in the decision-making process [7]. Although mentioned in its theoretical framework, expert opinion and narrative reviews were not even taken into consideration in the EBM/EBC evidence set.

The gap between RCT and practice widened when comparing care interventions, particularly in the mental health field and when the local context was considered. A classical example was provided by the comparison of the effectiveness of Assertive Community Treatment in the United States and the United Kingdom [16]. However, problems in results were attributed to difficulties in getting a proper rating. A more detailed analysis of the grading of RCT was suggested [17], and a series of extended guidelines were developed such as QUOROM (Quality of Reporting of Meta-analyses) [18] or CONSORT recommendations [19, 20].

The main problems identified were related to the design of RCT, such as lack of allocation concealment, lack of blinding, incomplete accounting of patients and outcome events, selective outcome reporting and other factors (e.g. stopping early for benefit; use of non-validated patient-reported outcomes; carry-over effects in cross-over trials; recruitment bias in cluster randomised trials). On the other hand, critics of EBM were focused on the need for practical interpretation of results, other relevant sources of evidence for clinical decision and lack of recognition of clinically sound, practical tools [9].

More recently, the 'Grades of Recommendation, Assessment, Development, and Evaluation' (GRADE) approach [21] has recognised that early systems of grading which focused almost exclusively on randomised trials were inadequate, as a series of factors may decrease its quality while increasing the value of observational studies. These factors include lower quality of evidence, uncertainties about the balance of benefits versus harms and uncertainties in values or in opportunity costs. However, these factors are all related to problems in RCT and insufficient information, and they do not recognise the value of observational data and expert knowledge. GRADE and similar rankings of evidence have been adopted by the Scottish Intercollegiate Guidelines Network (SIGN), the British National Institute for Health and Clinical Excellence (NICE), the US Preventive Services Task Force, the New Zealand Guideline Group and the Australian NHRMC, and also suggested for WHO recommendations [22].

Hence, the consensus raised on the capacities of EBM to provide ample response to Epstein's challenge were not hastened by critics to this approach, and EBM/EBC is still regarded as the fundamental research response to the paradigm shift in health care [10]. At least in theory, EBM provides a sound combination of new information-processing techniques such as meta-analysis, with health economics and modelling tools (i.e. Markov analysis) to guide evidence-based decision-making, mainly via clinical practice guidelines. However, the overall value of the restrictive experimental approach which is based on RCT may decrease as the levels of complexity of the analysed phenomenon increases; it may even become irrelevant in highly complex situations as those occurring in health system research, where organisations behave as a complex adaptive system [12]. This is also a problem when applying the EBM paradigm to effectiveness analysis in social and psychological domains [23].

There are also relevant conceptual and terminological problems in the use of terms such as evidence-based medicine, health technology assessment, comparative effectiveness research and other related terms which lack clarity and so could lead to confusion and miscommunication in health system research, often leading to poor decision-making [13].

'Consilience' approach to health service research

The quality ratings used in EBM/EBC are based on an implicit assumption: the hypothetical–deductive approach and its related experimental method is the *only* system able to generate scientific evidence, and therefore, observational 'evidence' should be graded as 'second level' in a unidimensional rating scale of quality of evidence.

This implicit statement is against the history and the progress of scientific knowledge since the mid 1800s when William Whewell coined the term 'consilience' to name one of the tests of the inductive inference process of empirical science. Before it can be confirmed as an 'empirical truth', induction should accomplish three criteria: prediction ('our hypotheses ought to *fortel* [sic] phenomena which have not yet been observed'), consilience ('explain and determine cases of a *kind different* from those which were contemplated in the formation') and coherence, which is in itself an iterative process where hypotheses must 'become more coherent' over time. The consilience approach underlies the theory of evolution [24], and Charles Darwin combined experiments with natural observations followed by inductive reasoning and was fully aware of Whewell's approach [25].

The consilience approach based on the systematic collection of multiple sources of observational data and modelling was applied to economics and policy by John Stuart Mill, although with a different perspective [26]. This approach was restated as a valid system to generate scientific evidence in complex domains by E.O. Wilson in the late 1990s [27]. Wilsonian consilience [28] provides a different kind of value to observational data from heterogeneous sources as basic information for modelling phenomena that can generate predictions and incorporate PEK to interpret the information and increase coherence in an iterative process to improve hypotheses and to generate a theory. In summary, consilience and experimental approaches are complementary and use observational information in different ways.

The consilience approach has recently been suggested as a relevant source of evidence in health care [29]. In complex dynamic systems, the RCT/experimental approach should be complemented by the consilience/modelling approach, where observational data (local, national or global), expert opinion and pragmatic approaches play a significant role. As a matter of fact, observational data may provide critical information to understand non-linear phenomena and successfully complement evidence obtained from experimental designs. Clinical guidelines based on meta-analysis from RCT do not provide enough information on effectiveness in the real setting, and they may largely underestimate the real value of a treatment alternative. In order to be of practical use, evidence from RCT should be contrasted with observational data, if possible, from high-quality large databases.

Incorporating observational/local information to the evidence base

The WHO Advisory Committee on Health Research has recently recognised that all evidence is context sensitive – and therefore indirect to some extent – and both global and local evidence should be combined to develop usable recommendations. Local evidence (from the specific setting or territory in which decisions and actions will be taken) is needed for most other judgements, including the presence of modifying factors in specific settings, need (prevalence, baseline risk or status), values, costs and the availability of resources [30]. The relevance of local (meso-level) and global/national/regional information (macro-level) has been reviewed in the context of the SUPPORT programme for improving decision-making about health policies and programmes in the new evidence-informed paradigm [31]. The combination of bottom-up and top-down local information to generate evidence-based health-care management has also been promoted in the United Kingdom [32].

This combined approach is essential to generate knowledge. Criticisms were previously made on the use of an exclusive pragmatic approach instead of a theory-based approach [33] and on the quality of information resulting from non-randomised studies. A systematic review indicated that 'non-randomised studies may give seriously misleading results when treated and control groups appear similar in key prognostic factors. Standard methods of case-mix adjustment do not guarantee removal of bias. Residual confounding may be high even when good prognostic data are available, and in some situations adjusted results may appear more biased than unadjusted results' [34]. A problem identified in this review was the lack of adequate quality guidelines of observational studies. This problem may be at least partly surmounted by the development of guidelines such as STROBE [35]. On the other hand, to be useful for EBC, observational studies of highly complex phenomena should use new data analysis methods and incorporate PEK alongside all the data management.

Incorporating prior expert knowledge to data analysis

As discussed earlier, exclusion and inclusion criteria are defined in RCTs to reduce the complexity of the phenomena observed, while expert knowledge is disregarded as it is considered a source of bias which should be excluded from the analysis. Recently, the importance of incorporating a qualitative approach both prior to RCT and in the post-processing phase has been recognised in the context of the evidence-informed approach to policy planning when evaluating 'complex' interventions – that is, those 'made up of various interconnecting parts' that act both 'independently and inter-dependently' [36]. Pooling available knowledge and taking into account historical perspectives are important elements. As Hanney and Gonzalez-Block have pointed out, 'the importance of this historical perspective is that it helps to underline the difficulties, and complexities, of making progress in the field of greater exploitation of research or evidence in health policy making' [37].

However, taking the PEK into account is not necessarily related to a loss of scientific rigour, since, from the beginnings of the Artificial Intelligence in the mid 1950s, there have been strict procedures, based on the logical paradigm, to handle expert knowledge in a formal and automatic way [38]. Hence, methods for generalising classical data analysis guided by PEK may permit better modelling of very complex phenomena and improve the quality of the results.

The suppression of expert knowledge in data processing may also be related to the lack of formal tools to analyse the health-related expert knowledge in its declarative form. To be formalised, explicit knowledge and implicit knowledge (IK) require different approaches. Explicit knowledge can be defined as the knowledge which is more or less directly available and can be explained by experts through standard tools like books, standard *If–Then* rules and so on [39]. On the other hand, IK, sometimes called *expertise*, comes from people, places, ideas, experiences, habits or culture and 'cannot be found in books' [40]. It is derived from the experience of the learner and it is not easily accessible while, at the same time, it is constantly used in reasoning processes and unconsciously activated for decision-making. Therefore, IK is extremely difficult to formalise. It can be transferred to a system by using interactive approaches of knowledge engineering to help the expert make his/her IK explicit; machine learning techniques (from artificial intelligence) can be used to automatically induce it from data; or the Knowledge Discovery from Data (KDD) approach [41] can be used for extracting valuable knowledge from databases. As domain complexity increases, so too does the quantity of IK *implicitly* used in reasoning and decision-making, and more powerful tools are required for elicitation.

The evidence-based cooperative analysis approach

Recently, some new approaches have defended the advantages of incorporating PEK into the analysis itself. As an example, the EbCA has been proposed as a general framework suitable for research in very complex medical problems where classical approaches provide poor results (e.g. in the analysis of 'integrated care' regarded as a holistic system). EbCA is based on formally including expert knowledge in the analysis. This proposal is, in fact, a methodology for generalising any classical analysis method to incorporate well-established knowledge as an essential part of the analysis [36]. The EbCA is based on the KDD approach and it is structured by the following steps (Figure 14.1):

1 Data collection and Data preparation: includes selection of relevant variables to be considered and inclusion and exclusion criteria, data representation, missing data analysis, outlier detection and treatment, etc.

2 PEK: acquisition and design of the Prior Knowledge Base (PKB) using qualitative approaches for knowledge exchange (e.g. nominal groups).

3 PKB-guided analysis: PKB is used to guide the analysis in different ways depending on the underlying method selected (e.g. cluster based on rules (ClBR), Data Envelopment Analysis (DEA), etc.).

4 Support interpretation: including tools to evaluate results and detect inconsistencies. In this step, new IK is elicited. Visualisation techniques play a critical role to facilitate IK. These representation techniques include dendograms, semaphores, class panel graphs, spider-web graphs and spatial analysis mapping, among others.

5 Incorporation of IK in PKB and repetition from step 3 until a satisfactory solution is found after an iterative process.

6 Post-processing results for decision support.

The evidence-based cooperative analysis approach could be applied to any technique currently available for health service research. For example, two separate ways of proceeding are ClBR, which has been used in a case-mix study functional dependency in schizophrenia, in the analysis of integrated home care support system and to define the characteristics of deficit and response to neuro-rehabilitation treatment [36, 42, 43]; and DEA, which has been used in benchmarking analysis of small mental health areas [36, 44].

As an example, EbCA-ClBR has been used in a case-mix study of functional dependency in schizophrenia [36, 42]; and EbCA-DEA has been used for benchmarking analysis of small mental health areas [36, 43].

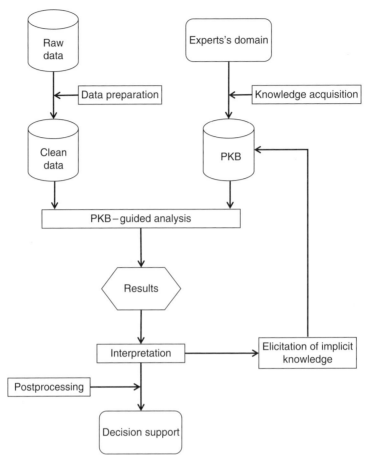

Figure 14.1 Steps in data analysis and knowledge management in expert-based cooperative analysis.

Findings from PKB allowed a refinement of the models in all these cases. For example, the functional dependency case-mix study in Catalonia (Spain) [42] allowed for the identification of a class of functional dependent patients with schizophrenia not previously identified by the panel expert group. This group included patients living alone, with low adherence to treatment and who did not use intermediate services whilst over-utilising emergency and acute hospital care. The use of PEK in the second study (benchmarking of small catchment areas in Spain) allowed for designing a model of basic mental health community care that has been used for assessing small catchment areas in Spain and in Chile [45]. It also allowed for a better understanding of the differences between adequacy/ appropriateness and technical efficiency for ranking small mental health areas. The combination of this technique with systematic data collection and representation of regional mental health atlases in Spain such as in Cantabria [46] and Catalonia [47] allows for evidence-informed planning and policy decision-making.

Case Study: Use of EbCA and combined DEA and Bayesian networks to model technical efficiency of small health areas in Andalusia (Spain)

We have used Bayesian network-DEA combined with EbCA for analysing technical efficiency of small mental health areas in Andalusia. This is a new approach to improve the former DEA method used for the analysis of technical efficiency of small health areas. 'Technical efficiency' uses proxy measures to assess the proportion of outputs produced (i.e. hospital bed utilisation) related to the resources available (i.e. hospital bed availability), when actual efficiency based on population outcome indicators cannot be estimated due to incomplete information, complex units of analysis (e.g. general hospitals, health areas) and use of ordinal outcomes [44].

Our former DEA model assumed that there were no dependence relationships between inputs and outputs (I/O) [44]. However, this assumption does not hold – or is difficult to assess – when the random variables are not identically distributed, especially in uncertain environments as occurs in health-care systems. Although dependence relationships between I/O in DEA models are evident in many contexts, formalising them in a way which may be understandable to both experts and computer systems is a major unsolved problem.

One practical approach to this is to consider a knowledge representation framework expressive enough to catch causal relationships among variables. Causal phenomena and the behaviour of complex systems in uncertain environments can be formalised and represented in probabilistic terms to produce a Bayesian network [48] used as framework F to formalise the PEK. $K_0 = F(D)$ is a Bayesian network expressing the a priori known dependences among variables in D. The Bayesian network can be rewritten as a fuzzy rules base interpreting these causal relationships. In this particular case, the fuzzy rules contain composite and conjunctive antecedents (*AND*'s in K_0). The consequents of these rules can also have mixed effects (usually expressed in a conjunctive way) on dependent variables in D.

$$K_0 : \underset{j=1}{\overset{c}{\text{ALSO}}} \left[\text{IF} \left(x_{ik} \in X_k \text{ isr } A_{jk} \right) \text{THEN } x'_{ik} = f \left(x_{ik} \right) \right]$$

In this example, K_0 can be obtained directly from the experts or by inducing the Bayesian network from some previous data, when available. In order to design the algebraic DEA model, I/O should be transformed mathematically using linear, exponential and other functions. Hence, the interpretation of the I/O which 'feed' the DEA models using causal dependence relationships is richer but more computer demanding than previous alternatives.

In this case study, we analyse the relative technical efficiency of 71 small mental health areas in Andalusia (Spain). To make comparisons across areas, all services identified were coded using the ESMS/DESDE-LTC classification system [49]. Basic expert-driven assumptions based on the previous model [44] included types and places of residential and day care (inputs) and its utilisation (outputs) (Table 14.1).

The new Bayesian model incorporated characteristics of staff and outpatient care. These characteristics are summarised in Figure 14.2.

The arrows represent expert-based relations of causality. The variable new patients_t (treated incidence: patients who contact the mental health community centre of a small health area in a given year t) depends in this model on two other variables – *accessibility* and *psychiatric morbidity* – with the value of the former depending on the values of the latter. The boxes represent variables that can be numeric (new patients_t) or constructs (*risk factors for mental health*). The efficiency of the small health areas depends directly on two main global variables: 'professional workers' (that can be obviously disaggregated in psychiatrists, psychologists, etc.) and the 'activities with patients', the second depending on the first (Figure 14.2). There is an additional dependence relationship between the 'public health budget' variable and 'professional workers'. This Bayesian

Table 14.1 Inputs and outputs of residential and day care at the Basic Model of Mental Health Community Care for the EbCA-DEA model.

Grouping of services	ESMS/DESDE-LTC Coding[a]	Description of ESMS 'Main Types Care'	Variables: Types (T)1, Utilisation (U)2, Places (P)3	Technical characteristics of the Expert-driven model of community care (B-MHCC) (Types: T: units available per small health area (SHA); P & U: rates per 100000 population)
Acute care	R2	Residential/hospital/acute	Types TR2 Places (beds) PR2 Utilisation UR2	High availability and utilisation by users from the area BUT avoiding over-use 1. TR2 within a [1, 1.5] range 2. PR2 within a [9, 20] range 3. UR2 medium-high to high avoiding over-use. Within a [10, 19] range. T9 [0, 6], T1 [6, 19], T9 [19, 100]. Uw [0.10, 0.15]
Non-acute hospital care	R4, R5, R6 and R7	Residential/hospital/non-acute	Types TR4R7 Places (beds) PR4R7 Utilisation UR4R7	Low availability and utilisation BUT not '0' 4. TR4-R7 Low, within [1, 3.1]. T9 [0, 1.9], T1 [1.9, 3.1], T11 [3.1, 15]. Uw [0.20, 0.25] 5. PR4-R7 Low, within [3, 13]. T9 [0, 3], T1 [3, 13], T7 [13, 200]. Uw [0.10, 0.15] 6. UR4-R7: Low use, within [3, 12]. T9 [0, 3], T1 [3, 13], T9 [13, 100]. Uw [0.13, 0.17]
Residential community care	R8, R9, R10, R11, R12 and R13	Residential/non-hospital	Types TR8R13 Places (beds) PR8R13 Utilisation UR8R13	High availability and utilisation 7. TR8-R13: High [>3]. T9 [0, 3], T2 [3, 20]. Uw [0.18, 0.23] 8. PR8-R13: High [>10]. T9 [0, 3], T1 [3, 13], T8 [13, 20]. Uw [0.10, 0.15] 9. UR8-R13 High avoiding over-use, within [10, 40]
Day care	D1+D45	D1: Day care/acute (day hospitals) D4: Day care/non-acute/other structured activities	Types TD1+D4 Places PD1+D4 Utilisation UD1+D4	High availability and utilisation 10. TD1+D4 High [>3]. T9 [0, 3], T2 [3, 20]. Uw [0.25, 0.3] 11. PD1+D4 High [>34]. T12 [0, 28], T11 [28, 100]. Uw [0.025.0.05] 12. UD1+D4 High [>33]. T9 [0, 15], T1 [15, 37], T2 [37, 100]. Uw [0.13, 0.17]

[a]For an explanation of ESMS/DESDE-LTC service coding system see [51]. (a) T: Number of 'main types of care' (R2, R4–R7, R8–R13 and D1+D4) available within a small health area; (b) U: Utilisation per 100000 inhabitants of the codes or 'main type of care' by patients from the small health area; (c) P: Places or beds available per 100000 inhabitants at the small health area; (d) Selected variables, T1, T2, …, T12: Selected variables in a specific range; (e) Uw: Uniform statistical distribution of the I/O weight; (f) work (D2), work-related (D3) and non-structured care (D5) have not been included in this model.

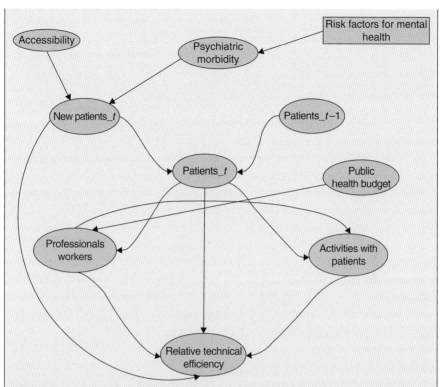

Figure 14.2 Case study of expert-based cooperative analysis (EbCA): Bayesian network for the EbCA-BNW-DEA model evaluating the relative technical efficiency of 71 small health areas in Andalusia (Spain). *T*, time (year); Patients_*t*, annual treated prevalence; New patients_*t*, annual treated incidence; Patients *t–1*, patients already in contact with the system at the beginning of the reference year.

network model helps us design the DEA models and to understand the treated prevalence in a small health area in a specific year *t* ('patients_*t*') as a result of a combination of patients already in contact with the mental health community service in the year *t* – 1 (patients_*t*–1) and the new patients that can contact the specialised community services in this year *t* (new patients_*t*).

Causal dependence relationships described in Bayesian networks were used to define a new and more complex model of Basic Mental Health Community Care (K_0) than the one used in previous analysis [44]. The Bayesian network can be rewritten in the form of rules with more than one variable in the antecedent.

For example, the experts found that the first version of the model did not identify the relevance of a high rate of staff per 100 000 population in relation to the relative activity of the community mental health centres in certain rural areas of Andalusia. Thus, a formal rule was included, which was related to the proportion of the rate of different professionals providing care in every small health area:

IF 'number of psychiatrists' IS high_psych AND

    'number of psychologists' IS high_psycho AND

    'number of other staff' IS high_ostaff AND

    'their sum'* IS high_sum

THEN
  'number of psychiatrists' = 'number of psychiatrists' + 20
(*) 'number of psychiatrists' + 'number of psychologists' + 'number of other staff'
(the number of psychiatrists – input – is penalised when the DEA model is solved).

Here *high_psych* is a linguistic or semantic label used in fuzzy logic, which, in this case, is associated to the variable *number of psychiatrists* that can be considered 'high' (*high_psych*) when its value is greater than or equal to 3. Similarly, *number of psychologists* is 'high' (*high_psycho*) when its value is greater than or equal to 2; *number of other staff* becomes 'high' (*high_ostaff*) for values greater than or equal to 2; and, finally, *their sum* can be considered 'high' (*high_sum*) when its value is greater than or equal to 10.

This rule was used in this particular technical efficiency exercise to penalise the community mental health centres with higher *number of psychiatrists* at the same level of population coverage (in comparison to the *number of psychologists*, the *number of other staff* and *their sum*). When the formal rule is activated by the values of the variables (a rate of psychiatrists per 100 000 population over 3), the model sums a number (in this case 20) to the real value of the variable *number of psychiatrists*. When this happens, the DEA interprets that the real local system – small health area – cannot be considered efficient with respect to *number of psychiatrists*. In this particular case, the experts identified that the original allocation of staff resources to the different community mental health centres by the planning agency was not adjusted to population size and urbanicity and followed fixed standards by centre. The formal rules introduced in the model during the EbCA process are explicit and available so they can be removed or modified when there is a significant change in the system (e.g. a reduction of intermediate services due to the financial crisis or a quick increase in the immigration rates that changes the demographics of the area).

Some results from the EbCA-BNW-DEA model are shown in Figure 14.3.

DEA models evaluate the relative technical efficiency of the small health areas by comparing their I/O values once they are appropriately interpreted by the rules (a DEA score equal to 1 means that the small health area is efficient; values of the DEA score lower than 1 mean that the small health area is inefficient – the lower the score, the lower the efficiency). There is only one sector that can be considered efficient and can be used as a reference for the rest (benchmark). Obviously, it is efficient because it has the best relationship between inputs consumed (resources) and outputs produced (outcomes). In this case, the model identified 6 other 'nearly efficient' areas, and 64 'inefficient' sectors, that is, sectors with a technical efficiency which could be improved over their current performance level in comparison with the benchmark. The model also identified

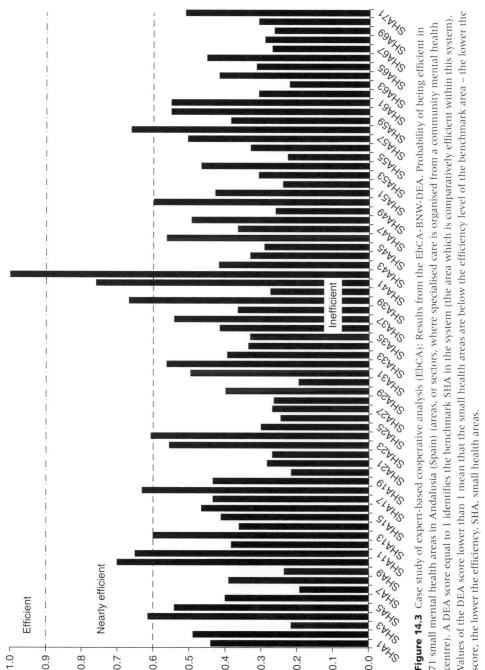

Figure 14.3 Case study of expert-based cooperative analysis (EbCA): Results from the EbCA-BNW-DEA. Probability of being efficient in 71 small mental health areas in Andalusia (Spain) (areas, or sectors, where specialised care is organised from a community mental health centre). A DEA score equal to 1 identifies the benchmark SHA in the system (the area which is comparatively efficient within this system). Values of the DEA score lower than 1 mean that the small health areas are below the efficiency level of the benchmark area – the lower the score, the lower the efficiency. SHA, small health areas.

16 small health areas with a very low technical efficiency performance in comparison to the benchmark area (values below 0.3).

Apart from providing a better technique for benchmarking, this DEA model allows for identification of the optimal values of indicators within the system by comparing the values found in the benchmark with other decision units (in our case, the 71 sectors). Nearly efficient or inefficient areas can be improved if decision-makers are able to modify their I/O values to approximate them to the values of the benchmark (efficient sector). Therefore, it is possible to model the technical efficiency of the small health areas in Andalusia and rank them at least in three levels (efficient, nearly efficient and inefficient) by combining hybrid modelling techniques with local information and experts' opinion. It is important to take into account that this case study is just an example that has not been cross-validated with local experts and health policy officers yet.

As a mater of fact, second-level expert knowledge from local managers and health officers is essential to further refine the available model for its use in actual policy planning. Once the model – including its formal rules – is finally agreed upon by local experts and planners, it can be used for targeting objectives and priority setting. Health planners can design incentives and disincentives aimed at improving the efficiency of target areas as well as the overall efficiency of the health system. For example, the 16 very low-efficiency sectors identified in the preliminary model may deserve special attention by the regional planners who now can use locally driven indicators and perform comparisons within the territory. From a practical point of view, the adequate use of infographics and visualisation is also very important for policy planning.

This Bayesian network and the derived PK base are now being applied to the analysis of technical efficiency in Catalonia and the Basque Country, where the second-level expert knowledge has been incorporated into the EbCA process. In both regions, we have carried out a systematic analysis and mapping of local information. These regional atlases of mental health include social and demographic indicators relevant for mental health in Spain [50, 51], availability of services for mental disorders using a standard and comparable coding system (DESDE-LTC) [49] and its geographical representation. The systematic local information also includes the utilisation of hospital and outpatient care at macro-level (health districts in Catalonia and provinces in the Basque Country) and at meso-level (small mental health catchment areas, or sectors, where care is organised from a community mental health centre), as well as spatial analysis of the use of services [47]. Hence, it will be possible to explore the general applicability of EbCA for mental health policy decision-making in Spain in the future.

Conclusion

Science is all about combining systematic observation, experiments and shared expert knowledge. Polanyi [40] and others highlighted the role of tacit knowledge in this process, and observation-driven models have guided relevant research since William Whewell's time to our day [27]. Charles Darwin combined observations and experiments in Down House garden and the surrounding area to advance his Theory of Evolution [25].

In the generation of scientific knowledge, observational data are not at the same dimension as experimental data nor should they be downrated and written off in systematic reviews. Comprehensive, reliable and comparable local information registries are essential for the analysis of complex health systems and do constitute a second source of information absolutely necessary to interpret and to apply the evidence derived from RCTs. Our understanding of the observational and local data in mental health research was improved greatly by the development of the standard assessment framework provided by the Mental Health-Care Matrix and its later developments [52]. Within this context, the new balance-of-care-model in mental health [53] cannot be properly understood and analysed without taking into account a system dynamics approach [2], a common and well-accepted method in the public and private sector for policy analysis and design, probably with the exception of health care [54].

Due to its non-linearity and dynamics, uncertainty may be regarded as an unavoidable component of mental health systems. The aim of any study in health service research is to – temporarily – reduce uncertainty so as to increase the strength of the decision-making. In order to accomplish this aim and to develop knowledge usable for policy decision-making and priority setting in mental health, it may be necessary to move away from the traditional EBC paradigm to the new evidence-informed one [55], taking into account observational and local information as well as PEK to guide the decision-making process. This information cannot be analysed using only the techniques designed for experimental data. As an example, imputation of missing data, sensitivity analysis and modelling should be used in health system research as these techniques are routinely used in health economics. In this process, expert knowledge has to be applied not only at the pre-processing of data and at the post-processing interpretation of results, but throughout the whole data analysis, as it has been shown in the EbCA approach.

In this approach, prior knowledge is an information base as relevant as data itself, and both information sources need to be integrated instead of being managed in separate ways. The PEK base does not need to be complete. A partial description of the domain elicits IK, which is transformed in formal rules that are incorporated into the model to obtain a practical and usable knowledge model at the end of the process. In real applications of EbCA methods, experts can incorporate their explicit prior knowledge into the analysis and use the provided interpretation-support tools to learn from the results of the analysis in a virtuous cycle to create new knowledge. After iteration, the relevant knowledge for the decisional problem to be solved is elicited, and complex decisions can be taken based on extracted knowledge. Hence, EbCA may integrate standard strategies already available to improve information transfer from experts and decision-makers to knowledge engineers and vice versa. As formal rules are available, they can be tested by external observers and changed if found inadequate or questioned by new evidence.

EbCA can potentially produce a new family of data analysis methods placed in a novel paradigm where expert knowledge is used together with data to obtain results that may have a better practical use in health decision-making and may fill the existing gap between academic health service research and policy decision-making [56, 57]. This does not replace EBC but complements it by combining knowledge-driven and data-driven systems within the general framework of KDD, where analysts and experts work together in a formal iterative process throughout the whole data analysis (from the pre-processing to the post-processing of results).

References

[1] Edgren L. (2008) The meaning of integrated care: a systems approach. *International Journal of Integrated Care* **8**: e68.

[2] Savigny D, Adams T. (2009) *Systems Thinking for Health Systems Strengthening*. Geneva: World Health Organization.

[3] Eisenberg L. (1973) The future of psychiatry. *Lancet* **ii**: 1371–1375.

[4] Goldman HH, Glied SH, Alegria M. (2009) Conclusion: mental health in the mainstream on public policy. *American Journal of Psychiatry* **166** (11): 1215.

[5] Salvador-Carulla L, Haro JM, Ayuso-Mateos JL. (2006) A framework for evidence-based mental health care and policy. *Acta Psychiatrica Scandinavica* **111** (Suppl. 432): 5–11.

[6] Epstein RS, Sherwood LM. (1996) From outcomes research to disease management: a guide for the perplexed. *Annals of Internal Medicine* **124** (9): 832–837.

[7] Sackett DL, Rosenberg WMC, Gray JAM et al. (1996) Evidence based medicine: what it is and what it isn't. *BMJ* **312** (7023): 71–72.

[8] Gray JAM. (1997) *Evidence-Based Healthcare. How to Make Health Policy and Management Decisions*. Edinburgh: Churchill Livingstone.

[9] Casali PG, LicitraL, Bruzzi P. (2000) Editorial: QUOROM and the search for an updated 'clinical method' in the era of evidence-based medicine. *Annals of Oncology* **11**: 923–925.

[10] Montori VM, Guyatt GH. (2008) Progress in evidence-based medicine. *Journal of American Medical Association* **300** (15): 1814–1816.

[11] Djulbegovic B, Guyatt GH, Ashcroft RE. (2009) Epistemologic inquiries in evidence-based medicine. *Cancer Control* **16**: 158–168.

[12] Sturmberg JP. (2009) EBM: a narrow and obsessive methodology that fails to meet the knowledge needs of a complex adaptive clinical world: a commentary on Djulbegovic, B., Guyatt, G. H. & Ashcroft, R. E. (2009). *Cancer Control* **16**, 158–168; *Journal of Evaluation in Clinical Practice* **15** (6): 917–923.

[13] Luce BR, Drummond M, Jönsson B et al. (2010) EBM, HTA, and CER: clearing the confusion. *Milbank Quarterly* **88** (2): 256–276.

[14] Schwartz JS, Ball JR, Moser RH. (1982) Safety, efficacy, and effectiveness of clinical practices: a new initiative. *Annals of Internal Medicine* **96** (2): 246–247.

[15] Guyatt G. (1991) Evidence-based medicine. *ACP Journal Club* **114** (Suppl. 2): A16.

[16] Burns T. (2010) The rise and fall of assertive community treatment? *International Review of Psychiatry* **22** (2): 130–137.

[17] Moher D, Cook DJ, Jadad AR et al. (1999) Assessing the quality of reports of randomised trials: implications for the conduct of meta-analyses. *Health Technology Assessment* **3** (12): i–iv, 1–98.

[18] Moher D, Cook DJ, Eastwood S et al. (1999) Improving the quality of reports of meta-analyses of randomised controlled trials: the QUOROM statement. *Lancet* **354**: 1896–1900.

[19] Begg C, Cho M, Eastwood S et al. (1996) Improving the quality of reporting of randomized clinical trials. The CONSORT statement. *Journal of American Medical Association* **276**: 637–639.

[20] Schulz KF, Altman DG, Moher D et al. (2010) CONSORT Statement: updated guidelines for reporting parallel group randomised trials. *Journal of Clinical Epidemiology* **63** (8): 834–840.

[21] Guyatt G, Oxman AD, Akl EA et al. (2011) GRADE guidelines: 1. Introduction-GRADE evidence profiles and summary of findings tables. *Journal of Clinical Epidemiology* **64** (4): 383–394.

[22] Schünemann HJ, Fretheim A, Oxman AD. (2006) WHO Advisory Committee on Health Research. Improving the use of research evidence in guideline development: 1. Guidelines for guidelines. *Health Research Policy and Systems* **4**: 13.

[23] Kelly M, Morgan A, Ellis S et al. (2010) Evidence based public health: a review of the experience of the National Institute of Health and Clinical Excellence (NICE) of developing public health guidance in England. *Social Science & Medicine* **71** (6): 1056–1062.

[24] Ruse M. (2008) *Charles Darwin*. Oxford: Wiley-Blackwell, p. 65.

[25] Boulter M. (2008) *Darwin's Garden. Down House and the Origin of Species*. London: Constable & Robinson, p. 8.

[26] Snyder LJ. (2006) *Reforming Philosophy: A Victorian Debate on Science and Society*. Chicago/London: University of Chicago Press.

[27] Wilson EO. (1998) *Consilience: The Unity of Knowledge*. New York: Knopf.

[28] Emery R. (2003) Could a "philosophical fitness landscape" foster Wilsonian consilience in biosystems debates? *Biosystems* **72** (3): 217–227.

[29] Kellermann AL. (2010) Consilience. *Annals Emergency Medicine* **56** (5): 568–570.

[30] Oxman AD, Schünemann HJ, Fretheim A. (2006) Improving the use of research evidence in guideline development: 7. Deciding what evidence to include. *Health Research Policy and Systems* **4**: 19.

[31] Lewin S, Oxman AD, Lavis JN et al. (2009) SUPPORT tools for evidence-informed policy-making in health 11: finding and using evidence about local conditions. *Health Research Policy and Systems* **16** (7 Suppl. 1): S11.

[32] Hamlin R. (2001) *Support of Evidence-Based Healthcare Management: an empirical study of managerial effectiveness within an NHS trust hospital*. Working Paper Series 2001, WP 004/01. Telford: University of Wolverhampton.

[33] Oxman AD, Fretheim A, Flottorp S. (2005) The OFF theory of research utilization. *Journal of Clinical Epidemiology* **58**: 113–116.

[34] Deeks J, Dinnes J, D'Amico R et al. (2003) Evaluating non-randomised intervention studies. *Health Technology Assessment* **7** (27): 1–173.

[35] Vandenbroucke JP, Von Elm E, Altman DG et al. (2009) Iniciativa STROBE. [STrengthening the Reporting of OBservational studies in Epidemiology (STROBE): explanation and elaboration]. *Gaceta Sanitaria* **23** (2): 158.

[36] Gibert K, García-Alonso C, Salvador-Carulla L. (2010) Integrating clinicians, knowledge and data: expert-based cooperative analysis in healthcare decision support. *Health Research Policy and Systems* **8**: 28.

[37] Hanney SR, González-Block MA. (2009) Evidence-informed health policy: are we beginning to get there at last? *Health Research Policy and Systems* **7**: 30.

[38] Russell SJ, Norvig P. (2003) *Artificial Intelligence: A Modern Approach*. Upper Saddle River: Prentice Hall.

[39] Gupta JND, Sharma SK. (2004) *Creating Knowledge Based Organizations*. Hershey: Idea Group Publishing.

[40] Polanyi M. (1967) *The Tacit Dimension*. New York: Anchor Books.

[41] Fayyad U, Piatetsky-Shapiro G, Smyth P et al. (eds) (1996) Advances in knowledge discovery and data mining. In *From Data Mining to KDD: An Overview*. Columbia: AAAI/MIT Press.

[42] PRODEP (Catalan Agency of Dependency). (2006) Estudi DEFDEP: Definició operative de dependència en persones amb discapacitat psíquica (vol. 2). Generalitat de Catalunya. Available from: http://www.dincat.cat/definici%C3%B3-operativa-de-depend%C3%A8ncia-en-persones-amb-discapacitat-ps%C3%ADquica-2-_21311. Accessed on 3 January 2013.

[43] Gibert K, García-Rudolph A, García-Molina A et al. (2008) Response to TBI-neuro-rehabilitation through an AI & Stats hybrid KDD methodology. *Medical Archives* **62** (3): 132–135.

[44] Salvador-Carulla L, García-Alonso C, Gonzalez-Caballero JL et al. (2007) Use of an operational model of community care to assess technical efficiency and benchmarking of small mental health areas in Spain. *Journal of Mental Health Policy and Economics* **10** (2): 87–100.

[45] Salvador-Carulla L, Saldivia S, Martinez-Leal R et al. (2008) Meso-level comparison of mental health service availability and use in Chile and Spain. *Psychiatric Services* **59** (4): 421–428.

[46] Vázquez-Barquero JL, Gaite Pindado L, Salvador Carulla L et al. (2010) *Atlas de Salud Mental de Cantabria*. Santander: Consejería de Sanidad.

[47] Salinas-Perez JA, Garcia-Alonso C, Molina-Parrilla C et al. (2012) Identification and location of hot and cold spots of treated prevalence of depression in Catalonia (Spain). *International Journal of Health Geographics* **11**: 36.

[48] Pearl J. (2000) *Causality: Models, Reasoning, and Inference*. Cambridge: University Press.

[49] Garrido-Cumbrera M, Almenara-Barrios J, López-Lara E et al. (2008) Development and spatial representation of synthetic indexes of outpatient mental health care in Andalusia (Spain). *Epidemiologia e Psichiatria Sociale* **17** (3): 192–200.

[50] Salvador-Carulla L, Salinas-Pérez JA, Martín M et al. (2010) A preliminary taxonomy and a standard knowledge base for mental-health system indicators in Spain. *International Journal of Mental Health Systems* **4**: 29.

[51] Salvador-Carulla L, Dimitrov H, Weber G et al. (eds.). (2011) *DESDE-LTC: Evaluation and Classification of Services for Long-Term Care in Europe*. Barcelona: PSICOST and CatalunyaCaixa. Available from: http://www.edesdeproject.eu/images/documents/eDESDE-LTC_Book.pdf. Accessed on 27 December 2012.

[52] Thornicroft G, Tansella M. (2009) *Better Mental Health Care*. Cambridge: Cambridge University Press.

[53] Thornicroft G, Tansella M. (2012) The balanced care model for global mental health. *Psychological Medicine* :1–15. July 11 [Epub ahead of print].

[54] Radzicki MJ, Taylor RA. (1997) Introduction to system dynamics. A systems approach to understanding complex policy issues. U.S. Department of Energy's. Available from: http://www.systemdynamics.org/DL-IntroSysDyn/intro.htm. Accessed on 3 January 2013.

[55] Lavis JN, Røttingen JA, Bosch-Capblanch X et al. (2012) Guidance for evidence-informed policies about health systems: linking guidance development to policy development. *PLoS Medicine* **9** (3): e1001186.

[56] Hanney SR, González-Block MA. (2011) Yes, research can inform health policy; but can we bridge the 'Do-Knowing It's Been Done' gap? *Health Research Policy and Systems* **9**: 23.

[57] Lewin S, Bosch-Capblanch X, Oliver S et al. (2012) Guidance for evidence-informed policies about health systems: assessing how much confidence to place in the research evidence. *PLoS Medicine* **9** (3): e1001187.

CHAPTER 15

Innovative epidemiological methods

Francesco Amaddeo, Valeria Donisi, Laura Grigoletti and Alberto Rossi

Department of Public Health and Community Medicine, Section of Psychiatry, University of Verona, Verona, Italy

Introduction

Epidemiology in the field of mental health is facing new challenges and is now tracing new perspectives. A wide literature is available to explain how psychiatric illnesses are distributed, and scientific articles have contributed to hypotheses about which factors influence the distribution of these conditions [1, 2], though the role played by single social determinants still remains not sufficiently clear. Furthermore, we remain unable to predict mental health service utilisation and their costs. After a person is diagnosed with a mental disorder, the consequent access and utilisation of services are influenced by a complex variety of interacting factors. Some of these factors have been explored using innovative epidemiological approaches; in particular, researchers are interested in the interaction between individual and environmental characteristics. The components of the environment where patients live are, for example, the social milieu, the availability and accessibility of health services and the organisation of social and health services that are mainly based on political choices. To investigate these complex models, studies have to be conducted comparing different places, linking together data from different settings of care, and using health geographic techniques such as Geographic Information Systems (GIS). For example, they can be conducted at the international level or by comparing large regions within one same country, and by using data from social, general health (including primary care), mental health and other specialty sectors.

A greater understanding of which patient characteristics influence service utilisation and costs in psychiatry as well as economic evaluation of services is crucial in helping decision-makers to achieve a more cost-efficient use of resources. An increasing number of research studies have attempted to identify

Improving Mental Health Care: The Global Challenge, First Edition.
Edited by Graham Thornicroft, Mirella Ruggeri and David Goldberg.
© 2013 John Wiley & Sons, Ltd. Published 2013 by John Wiley & Sons, Ltd.

factors related to psychiatric service utilisation and costs using data on individual people; however, the studies included different numbers and types of variables and used different approaches. A recent study conducted on a large representative sample of patients receiving psychiatric care in a Spanish hospital confirms that mental health costs were not evenly distributed throughout the patient population [3]. In a cross-national study conducted in five European countries, investigating patterns and costs of care for patients with schizophrenia, higher needs, greater symptom severity and longer psychiatric history were associated with higher costs [4]. With regard to the previous psychiatric history, patients with a long history of care present higher costs [5–7], and in previous studies conducted in South Verona, the best predictor of future costs was previous psychiatric history: first-time patients and patients with a new episode of care after three years were less costly than patients with an ongoing episode and patients having a new episode after less than three years [8].

A recent review [9], which examined the prediction of service utilisation and costs in psychiatry, confirmed that no single variable alone is able to predict costs, and that clinical factors, as diagnosis, alongside other individual personal characteristics, as gender and age, and previous use of psychiatric services, as the most consistent predictor of higher psychiatric cost, could explain the variations in costs between patients. However, most studies have explained only 25–50% of the total variations in costs, and the authors concluded that it seems plausible that the inclusion of ecological measures in predictive models, such as socio-economic status (SES), the geographical characteristics and social cohesion of areas where patients live, could improve the explanation of the variation in psychiatric costs. Urbanisation, gender, age and number of immigrants are reasons for differences in direct psychiatric costs aggregated and analysed at the county level per capita in Sweden [10].

Analyses of costs in mental health

The growing movement in many European countries towards new prospective systems for financing mental health care has generated increasing interest in developing appropriate models to predict mental health costs.

A study was conducted on all patients in contact with the South Verona community-based psychiatric service (CPS) during the last quarter of 1996 [11]. Clinical and service-related variables were collected at first index contact; three months later, patients were interviewed using the Client Services Recipient Interview. For those who completed both the clinical assessments and the services receipt schedule ($N=339$), one-year psychiatric and non-psychiatric direct care costs were calculated. Weighted backward regression analyses were performed. The most significant variables associated with psychiatric costs were admission to hospital in the previous year, intensity and duration of previous contacts with South Verona CPS, being unemployed, having a diagnosis of affective disorder and the Global Assessment of Functioning (GAF) score. The final model explained 66% of the variation in costs of psychiatric care and 13% of variation in non-psychiatric medical costs. The model explains a higher degree of cost variance than previously published studies. In community-based services, more resources are targeted towards the most disabled patients. Previous psychiatric history (number of admissions in the previous year and intensity of psychiatric contacts lifetime) is strongly associated with psychiatric costs.

Following these results, a further study was carried out to obtain a new, well-balanced mental health funding system, through the creation of (a) a list of psychiatric interventions provided by Italian CPSs and associated costs and (b) a new prospective funding system for patients with a high use of resources, based on packages of care. Five Italian CPSs collected data from 1250 patients during October 2002. Socio-demographical and clinical characteristics and GAF scores were collected at baseline. All psychiatric contacts during the following six months were registered and categorised into 24 service contact types. Using elasticity equation and contact characteristics, the costs of care were estimated. Cluster analysis techniques allow to identify packages of care, and logistic regression defined predictive variables of high-use patients. Multinomial Logistic Model assigned each patient to a package of care. The sample's socio-demographic characteristics are similar, but variations exist between the different CPSs. Patients were then divided into two groups, and the group with the highest use of resources was divided into three smaller groups, based on number and type of services provided. Our findings show how it is possible to develop a cost predictive model to assign patients with a high use of resources to a group that can provide the right level of care. For these patients, it might be possible to apply a prospective per-capita funding system based on packages of care [12].

Social conditions and mental health

The study of the relationship between social conditions and health services utilisation is of crucial importance for all those interested in mental health services evaluation at different spatial levels. As the Nobel Prize winner Amartya Sen [13] has demonstrated, the incidence of deprivation, in terms of *capability*,[1] can be surprisingly high even in the most developed countries of the world. For this reason, interest in this topic has grown among mental health researchers, aware that relative deprivation in their own countries has an impact upon the utilisation of mental health services. The results of research studies in this field will enable us to develop the principal tools required to develop and maintain modern, effective and safe mental health services that can be accessed and used by all those who need them.

SES is a complex concept with no universal definition [14]. When one looks at the international research literature on SES, it is evident that it is related to social class, social position, occupational status, educational attainment, income, wealth and standard of living [15]. It also appears that there are different ways of measuring SES, something that is often country-specific and related to the different questions asked in national population censuses. For example, a number of well-known census-based SES indices in the United Kingdom, such as those developed by Jarman [16] and Townsend [17], include the census variable 'car ownership' as an indicator of SES. However, in other countries, such as in Italy, this question is not asked in a national census. Accordingly, many SES indices are country- or even place-specific, for example, the Carstairs indices developed in Scotland [18]; a community-based index created in Turin, Italy [19]; the Rome SES index [20]; the deprivation index of Tuscany Region in Italy [21]; and the Barcelona index from Spain [22].

Regarding the relationship between SES and mental health, existing studies demonstrate that people from a more deprived social background, with a lower SES, are more likely to have a higher psychiatric morbidity [15, 23, 24]. We also know that socio-economic deprivation is particularly associated with rates of depression and anxiety disorders [14, 25, 26].

As discussed by various authors, the culmination of research findings over the years suggest two possible classical explanations for the concentration of mentally ill people in particular localities: social causation and social selection. Social causation suggests that a lower individual SES, or lower SES in the community where people live (i.e. ecological), may produce or contribute to mental illness because of deprivation, poor living and housing standards and a lack of social cohesion. The second explanation supports the hypothesis that the relationship between SES and mental disorders results from a drift of mentally ill people to lower SES conditions, with people's SES worsening as their mental health declines. More deprived areas also offer more affordable accommodation, and frequently there will already be specialist mental health-care services being provided in the neighbourhood, which may provide a 'pull' factor for mentally ill people. Recently, studies have been published that argued the importance of urbanicity as a risk factor for schizophrenia [27–30], and the correlation between urbanicity and socio-economic conditions remains ambiguous. For example, it is possible that some influential factors, such as population density or concentration of ethnic minority groups, may be hidden beneath the concept of urbanicity, and a high incidence of infective diseases could also be related with poorer living conditions found in some parts of urban areas.

Mental health services utilisation and socio-economic status

The association between socio-economic characteristics and rates of psychiatric service utilisation is also well established, with a number of studies demonstrating that psychiatric service use is more prevalent in geographical areas characterised by social deprivation, particularly in urban environments [31–33], although studies from the United Kingdom, the United States and Italy show that the strength of association varies according to psychiatric diagnosis [34–37]. A study, conducted in South Verona, Northern Italy, has highlighted the fact that ecological characteristics, derived from district-level census data, can be good *predictors* of psychiatric service used by patients with a diagnosis of psychosis, but not by people suffering from a neurotic and somatoform disorder [34, 38]. Using 1981 Census data, this study identified four socio-demographic variables that were associated with psychiatric service utilisation: living alone, unemployment, the percentage of the total population who are dependent (dependent ratio) and the percentage of people who are separated, divorced or widowed [39].

Lower SES groups are more likely to be compulsorily admitted and have longer average length of stay when admitted to hospital [40]. Low SES is also associated with an increased risk of suicide [41, 42] and depression persistence [43]. New epidemiological approaches have studied the interaction between individual and socio-economic environmental characteristics. For example, poverty and socio-economic deprivation, social fragmentation, high concentration of minority ethnic groups and close spatial proximity to services are positively associated with higher levels of psychiatric hospital use [44]. Evidence for an association between neighbourhood SES and objective and subjective mental health status has also been found, especially for young children [45].

In Sweden, neighbourhood socio-economic deprivation was found to be positively associated with psychopharmacological prescription for antipsychotic and anxiolytic drugs [46]. Although psychiatric costs showed a relationship with socio-demographic and clinical patient's characteristics [47], Donisi and colleagues [48] indicated that they are not significantly influenced by SES.

Overall, such research has revealed that a wide range of environmental factors may be associated with psychiatric service use. Resources such as leisure and park facilities, day-care centres, parking places, social activities, opportunities and other institutional resources are usually more scarce in poor neighbourhoods [49], and it seems plausible that the effect of neighbourhood characteristics increases in particular groups, such as the elderly and people in psychiatric treatment, whose activity space and mobility is limited [50, 51].

Peen and collaborators [52], considering the literature, suggested marginally higher overall prevalence rates of psychiatric disorders, with higher rates of depression in urban areas. A higher incidence rate of schizophrenia in urban areas is now well recognised [28], and a range of socio-environmental markers, measured across the life course, are associated with increased rates of psychotic illness [53].

The introduction in the 1990s of multilevel analyses added predictive power and precision in explaining the causal effects at the ecological level. Nevertheless, to date little research has simultaneously considered the influence of both individual- and ecological-level socio-economic factors upon the utilisation of the full range of hospital and community psychiatric services.

A study conducted in South Verona allowed to assess the effect of SES on psychiatric service use in an Italian area with a well-developed community-based psychiatric service [54, 55]. An index of SES was calculated from nine census variables and grouped into four categories, ranging from SES-I-affluent to SES-IV-deprived, for each of 328 census blocks (CB) of our catchment area. Fifteen indicators of psychiatric service use were collected using the psychiatric case register. All patients resident in the catchment area, who had at least one psychiatric contact in 1996 ($N=989$), were included in the study. Indicators of inpatient, daypatient, outpatient and community service use showed an inverse association with SES. Only first-time and long-term psychotic patients were equally distributed in the four SES groups. The inverse association between SES and most indicators of psychiatric service use suggests that the planning of community-based services and resource allocation should take into account the SES of residents.

The results highlighted that, in an area with a community-based system of care, socio-economic characteristics of the place of residence are associated with psychiatric service use by patients. SES and distance from hospital or other community-based services should not prevent the access to the care, but for some type of care (e.g. day care) there is a relation between services utilisation and nearness between place of residence and services. Accessibility is a surprisingly complex concept, since it includes many factors, like the cost of the travel, the availability of public transports, psychological and physical barriers, social and cultural factors and environment characteristics as well as social capital and social cohesion.

These findings seem to suggest that SES has a potential to worsen among those suffering from psychiatric illnesses (social selection), whilst the equal distribution of incidence rates by SES seems to exclude the possibility that SES is a contributory casual factor to becoming mentally unwell. However, important theoretical questions regarding the effects of social conditions on mental illness and vice versa cannot be answered by case register studies; rather, they require population studies. Nevertheless, it is important to reflect upon the findings that two service use variables, length of stay in hospital and number of day contacts, were not significantly associated with SES group. This finding could be because of the relatively small capacity of hospital beds (which determines, in most cases, a relatively short length of stay and a relatively high turnover of patients) and also the small number of day-care places available. Only when mental health care is easily accessible to all and free of charge can the quantity and type of service consumption be regarded as an indicator of the level of severity of the mental illness.

Further studies whose main aim was to analyse the effect of urbanicity, SES and distance from services on the incidence and prevalence of treated patients and on mental health services utilisation have been conducted in the same catchment area.

Low SES was also found to be associated with more community service contacts. When controlling for other individual and ecological variables, SES was negatively associated only with the number of home visits, which was about half the rate in deprived areas. An association between service utilisation and the resources of the catchment area was also detected.

Accessibility to mental health services

Equal access to health care is a guiding principle in countries where health care is mainly provided within public health-care systems; an important objective of such systems is to meet the population needs as close as possible to where people live.

Access to health-care services varies according to both non-spatial and spatial factors. Non-spatial factors encompass economic, cultural and social issues, as well as factors related to health-care organisation and network [56], whilst spatial factors concern the environmental context, the availability of facilities, the public transport and the road network structure. Their respective importance depends on the type of health-care framework (e.g. general practitioners, general hospitals, etc.) and on the type of health problem considered.

Concerning spatial factors, Jarvis in the late 1850s postulated the 'distance decay effect' – an inverse association between home to hospital distance and the rates of admission – subsequently confirmed for utilisation of emergency services, of psychiatric hospitals [57–60] and of community-based psychiatric services [61]. However, the association between geographical distance and service utilisation is complex, being an interaction between geographical proximity to services, socio-economic conditions in local communities, service provision and pathways of care [56, 62, 63].

For dealing with such complex issues, it appears crucial to implement reasonably simple methods to assess access, when both spatial and non-spatial factors are involved [64]. Moreover, it is important to build models for assessing access to specific health-care services, such as mental health services, for which continuity and regularity in attending the services are a fundamental part of treatments. In fact, for the most part, research on access to health services has focused on general practitioners and primary care services [65, 66], general health services as neighbourhood opportunities [67] and emergencies [68]. As an example, Haynes and co-workers [59] used distance as a convenient, although crude, summary measure of relative differences in geographical accessibility. They were interested in the effect of distance on hospital inpatient episodes, and they pointed out that measures of need, provision and distance were all significant predictors of small area variations in inpatient admissions for GP surgery, accounting for a high proportion of the variations between census wards. This trend was confirmed by other authors [69–71]. Other studies pointed out that the extent of the relationship between distance and mental health service utilisation decreases for severe clinical conditions, but it is strong for the less critical clinical conditions [72, 73].

Previous research on mental health service utilisation suggests a universal pattern of 'distance decay effect'. Nevertheless, the relationship is not a simple or consistent one, with a complex interaction between geographical proximity to services, socio-economic conditions in local communities and the organisation of care [63]. Whetten and co-workers [74] examined whether distance (calculated from an individual's zip code of residence to treatment provision site) predicts the utilisation of a mental health service when transportation is provided as a part of the programme. Bürgy and Häfner-Ranabauer [57, 58] explored the relationship between the utilisation of a psychiatric emergency service and distance in Mannheim, Germany. In a first study [57], they analysed contacts with the psychiatric emergency service between 1982 and 1993. As a proxy of accessibility, they used the straight line distance and the time-related distance estimated for the public transport available as aggregated data for the 23 districts of Mannheim. They found an association between ecological variables and distance on utilisation rates. In the second study [58], the authors investigated the association between need and demand of psychiatric emergency provision and ecological, socio-demographic and distance factors. They demonstrate that, in Mannheim, demand correlates with ecological, socio-demographic and distance-related factors and need correlates only with age.

Still using aggregate data, Curtis and colleagues analysed small area variations of acute psychiatric hospital admission in New York City [75] and then compared admissions in New York and London [43]. Both studies focused on the variation in the use of inpatient psychiatric care due to the proximity of facilities and the SES of the population. The question of proximity was addressed in two ways: by observing whether there is a hospital in the geographic unit of analysis and by using a gravity model of access opportunity to psychiatric beds in the city. Findings showed that the use of psychiatric beds is significantly and positively associated with immediate proximity and potential access to opportunities. Tseng and colleagues [60] examined the variations in hospitalisations among patients affected by schizophrenia in Taiwan. They found that travel distance did not significantly account for lower readmission rates after an index admission, but explained the longer length of stay of an index admission between remote and non-remote regions. Other studies focused on hospitalisation in psychiatric wards using potential accessibility models, commonly used for evaluating the potential delivery of care [76].

Determinants of different pathways of care

It is reasonable to assume that an episode of care should usually end when an episode of illness finishes. When these two end-points do not coincide, we need to understand why there has been an end to a period of treatment, although the illness has not yet been resolved. To clarify this, it is necessary first to define both types of episode and then to operationalise such definitions.

An 'episode of care' can be simply defined as the time interval between a first service contact for a mental health problem and a 'last' contact with the services. The most useful definition of last contact in the field of mental health care, which has been tested using case register data, is 'a contact, after which there is a gap of 90 days or more without any further contact' [77]. This has been applied to the end of a single episode of care, but may not be a sufficiently long period of time without contact to establish that treatment has truly been terminated.

Few studies have investigated thus far factors that predict inappropriate terminations (dropout) of clinical contact with mental health services. A three-month cohort study conducted in South Verona [78], with a two-year follow up, showed that 26.8% of all patients treated in one year terminated their contact with the services; of these, 62.9% were rated as having inappropriate terminations (the 'dropout' group) and 37.1% had appropriate terminations of contact. Dropouts were younger, less likely to be married and their previous length of contact with services was shorter. No dropouts had a diagnosis of schizophrenia. Multivariate analysis revealed that those who drop out of care were younger patients without psychoses who were generally satisfied with their treatment.

Another study examined variables associated with having a once-only contact with the outpatient department of two community mental health services in Italy and Australia [79]. Two eight-year cohorts of patients, who had a new episode of care with outpatient psychiatric departments in South Verona and in Western Australia, were followed up for three months after the first contact, to identify those patients who had no further contact with services. Thirty percent of new episodes of care for persons who met the inclusion criteria of the study were once-only contacts with the service in South Verona. In Western Australia, the figure was 24%. Moreover, the proportion of once-only contact patients has increased over time in South Verona, whereas in Western Australia it has remained stable. In Western Australia, once-only contact patients were younger, whereas in South Verona they tended to be older. At both research sites, patients who had a once-only contact were more likely to be male and to have a less severe mental illness. It seems that only clinical characteristics were significant determinants of this pattern of contact with services consistently at both sites: the less severe the patient's diagnosis, the more likely the patient is to have a once-only contact. This may well indicate good screening at the initial point of contact by both sets of mental health service providers.

Mortality studies in mental health

Research on the causes of death of psychiatric patients is a worthwhile endeavour as it has long been recognised that death rates among patients with chronic mental illnesses are higher than among the general population [80, 81].

In a meta-analysis of 152 reports about the mortality of patients with mental disorders, Harris and Barraclough [81] found that although people with mental disorders have an increased risk of premature death, the highest risks from both natural and unnatural causes are from substance abuse and eating disorders. They also found that the risk of death from unnatural causes is especially high among people with schizophrenia and major depression, whilst the risks of death from natural causes are markedly increased for organic mental disorders, mental retardation and epilepsy.

Regarding organic mental disorders, some studies have identified a high association between mortality and antipsychotic drugs in patients with dementia, although it is not clear whether this is due to a direct medication effect or to the pathophysiology underlying neuropsychiatric symptoms that prompt antipsychotic use [82–84].

Most previous mortality studies have been conducted in areas where hospital-based systems of mental care are the norm. For example, a study by Craig and Lin [85] suggested that, in the United States, deinstitutionalisation, through a variety of mechanisms, may have had a beneficial effect on the mortality of elderly patients who remain hospitalised. Other studies showed a decrease in the excess mortality of psychiatric patients after the reduction in the provision of long-stay psychiatric hospital care [86–88]. Deinstitutionalisation, however, seems also to be associated to increased rates in deaths for causes considered 'behaviourally avoidable' (i.e. preventable with adequate health promotion policies) such as cardiovascular and unnatural causes for both genders [89] and for suicide [90, 91].

Vreeland [92] stated that the problem of increased morbidity and premature death in people with serious mental illness must be addressed with a transformation of the current mental health system and the integration of physical and mental health care, towards a system that utilises a coordinated, multidisciplinary holistic approach. This should be done to overcome some of the multiple barriers that make it difficult for individuals with serious mental illness to access quality health care.

Research and intervention studies for improving medical care for people with serious mental illness have spanned a continuum of inter-professional involvement, ranging from staff and patient training to on-site consultation by medical staff, multidisciplinary collaborative care approaches and facilitated linkages between community and mental health and medical providers. On the other hand, great attention should be paid to those patients who develop psychiatric symptoms as comorbidity of cardiovascular accident and stroke [93]. This would contribute to diminish the mortality of people with a secondary psychiatric diagnosis.

However, there is still a need to explore mortality in different service settings, such as community services, because mortality is a useful indicator of the quality of a health-care system over time.

A study conducted in South Verona explored the effect of those causes of death considered avoidable [94]. All patients with an ICD-10 psychiatric diagnosis, living in the catchment area of about 100 000 inhabitants, seeking care in 1982–2005 (23 years), were included in this study. Standardised Mortality Ratios (SMRs) were calculated for each cause including those considered avoidable, using the mortality of the general population in the Veneto Region to estimate the expected number of deaths. For avoidable causes, a list derived from the Rutstein's list and from an EC version set up in the 1980s was used, and then causes were divided into two groups: indicators of quality of (a) health care and (b) health policies. The observed number of deaths for avoidable causes was four times greater than the expected ($P<0.01$). SMR was higher for deaths preventable with adequate health promotion policies than for those preventable with appropriate health care. Males, alcohol/drug addicts and young patients had the highest avoidable SMRs. Another study [95] evaluated not only avoidable mortality but the relation among mortality, causes of death and associated risk factors among psychiatric patients. Patients were followed up over a 20-year period in an area where psychiatric care is entirely provided by community-based psychiatric services. Many of the mortality studies published so far were conducted in areas where a hospital-based system of care is available for the mentally ill. All subjects who had at least one contact with the South Verona CPS during a 20-year period and who at the first contact or later received an ICD-10 psychiatric diagnosis were included in this study (59 139 person years). Total SMR of our psychiatric population was 1.88, mortality in outpatients was significantly high (SMR = 1.70, 95% CI 1.6–1.8), and, as expected, it becomes higher after the first admission (SMR = 2.61, 95% CI 2.4–2.9). SMRs for infectious diseases are higher among younger patients and extremely high in patients with drug addiction (216.40, 95% CI 142.5–328.6) and personality disorders (20.87 CI 5.2–83.4). Our data show that, also in a community-based mental health service, psychiatric patients are at almost twofold higher risk of death than the general population, and this becomes extremely high for those diagnosed with drug addiction or personality disorders.

Conclusions

Very few epidemiological studies have been carried out until now using innovative approaches, and all of them have recognised methodological difficulties and biases that affect their results. These studies have highlighted that, in areas where care is provided by community-based systems, social and economic characteristics of the place of residence are associated with psychiatric service use by patients. However, SES and distance from hospital or other community-based services should not prevent access to care, but for some types of care (e.g. day care) there is a relation between service utilisation and proximity between place of residence and services [61]. Moreover, accessibility is a many-sided concept that regards many factors, like the cost of travel, the availability of public transport, psychological and physical barriers, social and cultural factors and environment characteristics as well as social capital and social cohesion.

The economic crisis in Europe is increasing the inequality of wealth distribution, and so paying attention to these socio-economic characteristics at both the individual and the ecological levels is likely to become increasingly important in understanding patterns of psychiatric service utilisation and planning care accordingly.

Another important issue for psychiatric epidemiology is to find strong and widely agreed indicators of the quality of care provided by mental health services. One of these, even if open to criticism and not exhaustive, is the excess of mortality, and of avoidable mortality, among users of mental health services. In the mortality studies conducted in South Verona described in this chapter, the observed number of deaths from avoidable causes among users of community-based mental health services was shown to be four times greater than expected. The SMR is higher for deaths preventable with adequate health promotion policies than for those preventable with appropriate health care. From these results it seems important that the implementation, by specialist psychiatric services, of health promotion and preventive programmes specifically targets psychiatric patients [94–96].

If, on the one hand, it is complex to conduct studies at the international level, on the other hand, this is the only way to obtain answers to the research questions that will allow in the future greater understanding and, as consequence, improved quality of mental health services.

Note

1 A. Sen proposed to replace the concept of utility with the concept of capability in assessing inequalities. Capability is defined by Sen as 'the capability of a person reflects the alternative combination of functionings the person can achieve, and from which he or she can choose one collection. The approach is based on a view of living as a combination of various "doings and beings", with quality of life to be assessed in terms of the capability to achieve valuable functionings'.

References

[1] Alonso J, Codony M, Kovess V et al. (2007) Population level of unmet need for mental healthcare in Europe. *British Journal of Psychiatry* **190**: 299–306.

[2] Lund C, Breen A, Flisher AJ et al. (2010) Poverty and common mental disorders in low and middle income countries: a systematic review. *Social Science & Medicine* **71**: 517–528.

[3] Baca-Garcia E, Perez-Rodrigues MM, Basurte-Villamor I et al. (2008) Patterns of mental health service utilization in a general hospital and outpatient mental health facilities: analysis of 365,262 psychiatric consultations. *European Archives of Psychiatry and Clinical Neuroscience* **258**: 117–123.

[4] Knapp M, Chisholm D, Leese M et al. (2002). Comparing patterns and costs of schizophrenia care in five European countries: the EPSILON study. European Psychiatric Services: Inputs Linked to Outcome Domains and Needs. *Acta Psychiatrica Scandinavica* **105**: 42–54.

[5] Beecham J, Hallam A, Knapp M et al. (1997) Costing care in the hospital and the community. In: Leff J (ed.), *Care in the Community; Illusion or Reality?* Chichester: John Wiley & Sons, Ltd, pp. 93–108.

[6] Amaddeo F, Beecham J, Bonizzato P et al. (1997) The use of a case register to evaluate the costs of psychiatric care. *Acta Psychiatrica Scandinavica* **95**: 189–198.

[7] McCrone P, Thornicroft G, Parkman S et al. (1998) Predictors of mental health service costs for representative cases of psychosis in south London. *Psychological Medicine* **28**: 159–164.

[8] Mirandola M, Amaddeo F, Dunn G et al. (2004) The effect of previous psychiatric history on the cost of care: a comparison of various regression models. *Acta Psychiatrica Scandinavica* **109**: 132–139.

[9] Jones J, Amaddeo F, Barbui C et al. (2007) Predicting costs of mental health care: a critical literature review. *Psychological Medicine* **37**: 467–477.

[10] Tiainen A, Edman G, Flyckt L et al. (2008) Regional variations and determinants of direct psychiatric costs in Sweden. *Scandinavian Journal of Public Health* **36**: 483–492.

[11] Bonizzato P, Bisoffi G, Amaddeo F et al. (2000) Community-based mental health care: to what extent are services costs associated with clinical, social and service history variables? *Psychological Medicine* **30**: 1205–1215.

[12] Grigoletti L, Amaddeo F, Grassi A et al. (2006) Proposal for a new funding system for mental health departments. Results from an evaluative multicentre Italian study (I-psycost). *Epidemiololia e Psichiatria Sociale* **15**: 295–306.

[13] Sen A. (1992) *Inequality Reexamined*. Oxford: Oxford University Press.

[14] Dohrenwend BP. (1990) Socioeconomic status (SES) and psychiatric disorders. Are the issues still compelling? *Social Psychiatry and Psychiatric Epidemiology* **25**: 41–47.

[15] Bonizzato P, Tello JE. (2003) Socio-economic inequalities and mental health. I. Concepts, theories, and interpretations. *Epidemiologia e Psichiatria Sociale* **12**: 205–218.

[16] Jarman B. (1983) Identification of underprivileged areas. *British Medical Journal* **286**: 1705–1709.

[17] Townsend P. (1987) Deprivation. *Journal of Social Policy* **16**: 125–146.

[18] Carstairs V, Morris R. (1991) *Deprivation and Health in Scotland*. Aberdeen: Aberdeen University Press.

[19] Cadum E, Costa G, Biggeri A et al. (1999) Deprivation and mortality: a deprivation index suitable for geographical analysis of inequalities. *Epidemiologia e Prevenzione* **23**: 175–187.

[20] Michelozzi P, Perucci CA, Forastiere F et al. (1999). Inequality in health: socioeconomic differentials in mortality in Rome, 1990–95. *Journal of Epidemiology and Community Health* **53**: 687–693.

[21] Regione Toscana (2001) *SLTo (Studio Longitudinale Toscano). Condizione socio-economica e mortalità in Toscana. Informazioni Statistiche.* Firenze: Edizioni Regione Toscana.

[22] Benach J, Yasui Y, Borrell C et al. (2001) Material deprivation and leading causes of death by gender: evidence from a nationwide small area study. *Journal of Epidemiology and Community Health* **55**: 239–245.

[23] Bijl RV, Ravelli A, van ZG. (1998) Prevalence of psychiatric disorder in the general population: results of The Netherlands Mental Health Survey and Incidence Study (NEMESIS). *Social Psychiatry and Psychiatric Epidemiology* **33**: 587–595.

[24] Glover GR, Leese M, McCrone P. (1999) More severe mental illness is more concentrated in deprived areas. *British Journal of Psychiatry* **175**: 544–548.

[25] Ostler K, Thompson C, Kinmonth AL et al. (2001) Influence of socio-economic deprivation on the prevalence and outcome of depression in primary care: the Hampshire Depression Project. *British Journal of Psychiatry* **178**: 12–17.

[26] World Health Organisation. (2001) *The World Health Report 2001. Mental Health: New Understanding, New Hope.* Geneva: World Health Organisation.

[27] Amaddeo F, Tansella M. (2006) Urbanicity and schizophrenia. From statistical association to causality? *Epidemiologia e Psichiatria Sociale* **15**: 239–241.

[28] McGrath J, Scott J. (2006) Urban birth and risk of schizophrenia: a worrying example of epidemiology where the data are stronger than the hypotheses. *Epidemiologia e Psichiatria Sociale* **15**: 243–246.

[29] Pedersen CB, Mortensen PB (2006) Why factors rooted in the family may solely explain the urban-rural differences in schizophrenia risk estimates. *Epidemiologia e Psichiatria Sociale* **15**: 247–251.

[30] Spauwen J, van Os J. (2006) The psychosis proneness: psychosis persistence model as an explanation for the association between urbanicity and psychosis. *Epidemiologia e Psichiatria Sociale* **15**: 252–257.

[31] Faris REL, Dunham HW. (1939) *Mental Disorders in Urban Areas: An Ecological Study of Schizophrenia and Other Psychoses.* Chicago: University of Chicago Press.

[32] Jarman B, Hirsch S, White P et al. (1992) Predicting psychiatric admission rates. *BMJ* **304**: 1146–1151.

[33] Thornicroft G. (1991) Social deprivation and rates of treated mental disorder. Developing statistical models to predict psychiatric service utilisation. *British Journal of Psychiatry* **158**: 475–484.

[34] Tansella M, Bisoffi G, Thornicroft G. (1993) Are social deprivation and psychiatric service utilisation associated in neurotic disorders? A case register study in south Verona. *Social Psychiatry and Psychiatric Epidemiology* **28**: 225–230.

[35] Harrison J, Barrow S, Creed F. (1995) Social deprivation and psychiatric admission rates among different diagnostic groups. *British Journal of Psychiatry* **167**: 456–462.

[36] Boardman AP, Hodgson RE, Lewis M et al. (1997) Social indicators and the prediction of psychiatric admission in different diagnostic groups. *British Journal of Psychiatry* **171**: 457–462.

[37] Koppel S, McGuffin P. (1999) Socio-economic factors that predict psychiatric admissions at a local level. *Psychological Medicine* **29**: 1235–1241.

[38] Thornicroft G, Bisoffi G, De Salvia D et al. (1993) Urban-rural differences in the associations between social deprivation and psychiatric service utilization in schizophrenia and all diagnoses: a case-register study in Northern Italy. *Psychological Medicine* **23**: 487–496.

[39] Amaddeo F, Jones J. (2007) What is the impact of socio-economic inequalities on the use of mental health services? *Epidemiologia e Psichiatria Sociale* **16**: 16–19.

[40] Lorant V, Kampfl D, Seghers A et al. (2003) Socioeconomic differences in psychiatric in-patient care. *Acta Psychiatrica Scandinavica* **107**: 170–177.

[41] Lorant V, Deliège D, Eaton W et al. (2003) Socioeconomic inequalities in depression: a meta-analysis. *American Journal of Epidemiology* **157**: 98–112.

[42] Li Z, Page A, Martin G et al. (2011) Attributable risk of psychiatric and socio-economic factors for suicide from individual-level, population-based studies: a systematic review. *Social Science & Medicine* **72**: 608–616.

[43] Melchior M, Chastang JF, Leclerc A et al. (2010) Low socioeconomic position and depression persistence: longitudinal results from the GAZEL cohort study. *Psychiatry Research* **177**: 92–96.

[44] Curtis S, Copeland A, Fagg J et al. (2006) The ecological relationship between deprivation, social isolation and rates of hospital admission for acute psychiatric care: a comparison of London and New York City. *Health Place* **12**: 19–37.

[45] Drukker M, Gunther N, Van Os J. (2007) Disentangling associations between poverty at various levels of aggregation and mental health. *Epidemiologia e Psichiatria Sociale* **16**: 3–9.

[46] Crump C, Sundquist K, Sundquist J et al. (2011) Neighborhood deprivation and psychiatric medication prescription: a Swedish National Multilevel Study. *Annals of Epidemiology* **21**: 231–237.

[47] Grigoletti L, Amaddeo F, Grassi A et al. (2010) A predictive model to allocate frequent service users of community-based mental health services to different packages of care. *Epidemiologia e Psichiatria Sociale* **19**: 168–177.

[48] Donisi V, Jones J, Pertile R et al. (2011) The difficult task of predicting the costs of community-based mental health care. A comprehensive case register study. *Epidemiology and Psychiatric Sciences* **20**: 245–256.

[49] Leventhal T, Brooks-Gunn J. (2000) The neighborhoods they live in: the effects of neighborhood residence on child and adolescent outcomes. *Psychological Bulletin* **126**: 309–337.

[50] Gale CR, Dennison EM, Cooper C et al. (2011) Neighbourhood environment and positive mental health in older people: the Hertfordshire Cohort Study. *Health & Place* **17**: 867–874.

[51] Vallée J, Cadot E, Roustita C et al. (2011) The role of daily mobility in mental health inequalities: the interactive influence of activity space and neighbourhood of residence on depression. *Social Science & Medicine* **73**: 1133–1144.

[52] Peen J, Schoevers RA, Beekman AT et al. (2010) The current status of urban-rural differences in psychiatric disorders. *Acta Psychiatrica Scandinavica* **121**: 84–93.

[53] Kirkbride JB, Lunn DJ, Morgan C et al. (2010) Examining evidence for neighbourhood variation in the duration of untreated psychosis. *Health & Place* **16**: 219–225.

[54] Tello JE, Mazzi M, Tansella M et al. (2005) Does socioeconomic status affect the use of community-based psychiatric services? A South Verona case register study. *Acta Psychiatrica Scandinavica* **112**: 215–223.

[55] Tello JE, Jones J, Bonizzato P et al. (2005) A census-based Socio-Economic Status (SES) index as a tool to examine the relationship between mental health services use and deprivation. *Social Science & Medicine* **61**: 2096–2105.

[56] Amaddeo F, Zambello F, Tansella M et al. (2001) Accessibility and pathways to psychiatric care in a community-based mental health system. *Social Psychiatry and Psychiatric Epidemiology* **36**: 500–506.

[57] Bürgy R, Häfner-Ranabauer W. (1998) Utilization of the psychiatric emergency service in Mannheim: ecological and distance related aspects. *Social Psychiatry and Psychiatric Epidemiology* **33**: 558–567.

[58] Bürgy R, Häfner-Ranabauer W. (2000) Need and demand in psychiatric emergency service utilization: explaining topographic differences of a utilization sample in Mannheim. *European Archives of Psychiatry and Clinical Neuroscience* **250**: 226–233.

[59] Haynes R, Bentham G, Lovett A et al. (1999) Effects of distances to hospital and GP surgery on hospital inpatient episodes, controlling for needs and provision. *Social Science & Medicine* **49**: 425–433.

[60] Tseng KC, Hemenway D, Kawachi I et al. (2008) Travel distance and the use of inpatient care among patients with schizophrenia. *Administration and Policy in Mental Health* **35**: 346–356.

[61] Zulian G, Donisi V, Secco G et al. (2011) How are caseload and service utilisation of psychiatric services influenced by distance? A geographical approach to the study of community-based mental health services. *Social Psychiatry and Psychiatric Epidemiology* **46**: 881–891.

[62] Hansson L. (2003) Inequality and inequity in use of mental health services. *Acta Psychiatrica Scandinavica* **107**: 161–162.

[63] Curtis S. (2007) Socio-economic status and geographies of psychiatric inpatient service use; places, provision, power and wellbeing. *Epidemiologia e Psichiatria Sociale* **16**: 10–15.

[64] Wang FH, Luo W (2005) Assessing spatial and nonspatial factors for healthcare access: towards an integrated approach to defining health professional shortage areas. *Health & Place* **11**: 131–146.

[65] Lovett A, Haynes R, Sunnenberg G et al. (2002) Car travel time and accessibility by bus to general practitioner services: a study using patient registers and GIS. *Social Science & Medicine* **55**: 97–111.

[66] Luo W. (2003) Measures of spatial accessibility to health care in a GIS environment: synthesis and a case study in the Chicago region. *Environment and Planning B: Planning and Design* **30**: 865–884.

[67] Pearce J, Witten K, Bartie P. (2006) Neighbourhoods and health: a GIS approach to measuring community resource accessibility. *Journal of Epidemiology and Community Health* **60**: 389–395.

[68] Nicholl J, West J, Goodacre S et al. (2007) The relationship between distance to hospital and patient mortality in emergencies: an observational study. *Emergency Medicine Journal* **24**: 665–668.

[69] Bille M. (1963) The influence of distance to mental hospital; first admission. *Acta Psychiatrica Scandinavica* **39** (Suppl. 169): 226–233.

[70] Cohen J. (1972) The effect of distance on use of outpatient services in a rural mental health center. *Hospital and Community Psychiatry* **23**: 79–80.

[71] Shannon GW, Bashur LR, Lovett JE. (1986) Distance and the use of mental services. *Milbank Quarterly* **64**: 302–320.

[72] Joseph A, Boeckh J. (1981) Location variation in the mental health care utilization departments upon diagnosis: a Canadian example. *Social Science & Medicine* **15**: 395–404.

[73] Stampfer H, Reymond J, Burvill PW et al. (1984) The relationship between distance from inpatient facilities and the rate of psychiatric admissions in western Australia. *Social Science & Medicine* **19**: 879–884.

[74] Whetten R, Whetten K, Pence BW et al. (2006) Does distance affect utilization of substance abuse and mental health services in the presence of transportation services? *AIDS Care* **18** (Suppl. 1): 27–34.

[75] Curtis SE, Southall H, Congdon P et al. (2004) Area effects on health variation over the life-course: analysis of the longitudinal study sample in England using new data on area of residence in childhood. *Social Science & Medicine* **58**: 57–74.

[76] Luo W. (2004) Using a GIS-based floating catchment method to assess areas with shortage of physicians. *Health & Place* **10**: 1–11.

[77] Tansella M, Micciolo R, Biggeri A et al. (1995) Episodes of care for first-ever psychiatric patients. A long-termcase-register evaluation in a mainly urban area. *British Journal of Psychiatry* **167**: 220–227.

[78] Rossi A, Amaddeo F, Bisoffi G et al. (2002) Dropping out of care: inappropriate terminations of contact with community-based psychiatric services. *British Journal of Psychiatry* **181**: 331–338.

[79] Rossi A, Morgan V, Amaddeo F et al. (2005) Psychiatric out-patients seen once only in South Verona and Western Australia. A comparative case-register study. *Australian and New Zealand Journal of Psychiatry* **39**: 414–422.

[80] Goff DC, Cather C, Evins AE et al. (2005) Medical morbidity and mortality in schizophrenia: guidelines for psychiatrists. *Journal of Clinical Psychiatry* **66**: 183–194.

[81] Harris EC, Barraclough B. (1998) Excess mortality of mental disorder. *British Journal of Psychiatry* **173**: 11–53.

[82] Wang PS, Schneeweiss S, Avorn J et al. (2005) Risk of death in elderly users of conventional vs. atypical antipsychotic medications. *New England Journal of Medicine* **353**: 2335–2341.

[83] Schneider LS, Dagerman KS, Insel P. (2005) Risk of death with atypical antipsychotic drug treatment for dementia: meta-analysis of randomized placebo-controlled trials. *Journal of American Medical Association* **294**: 1934–1943.

[84] Kales HC, Valenstein M, Kim HM et al. (2007) Mortality risk in patients with dementia treated with antipsychotics versus other psychiatric medications. *American Journal of Psychiatry* **164**: 1568–1576.

[85] Craig TJ, Lin SP. (1981) Death and deinstitutionalization. *American Journal of Psychiatry* **138**: 224–227.

[86] Allebeck P, Wistedt B. (1986) Mortality in schizophrenia. A ten-year follow-up based on the Stockholm County inpatient register. *Archive of General Psychiatry* **43**: 650–653.

[87] Casadebaig F, Quemada N. (1991) Changes in mortality among psychiatric inpatients, 1968–1982. *Social Psychiatry and Psychiatric Epidemiology* **26**: 78–82.

[88] Tsuang MT, Simpson JC. (1985) Mortality studies in psychiatry. Should they stop or proceed? *Archive of General Psychiatry* **42**: 98–103.

[89] Hansen V, Jacobsen BK, Arnesen E. (2001) Cause-specific mortality in psychiatric patients after deinstitutionalisation. *British Journal of Psychiatry* **179**: 438–443.

[90] Mortensen PB, Juel K. (1993) Mortality and causes of death in first admitted schizophrenic patients. *British Journal of Psychiatry* **163**: 183–189.

[91] Martiello MA, Cipriani F, Voller F et al. (2006) The descriptive epidemiology of suicide in Tuscany, 1988–2002. *Epidemiologia e Psichiatria Sociale* **15**: 202–210.

[92] Vreeland B. (2007) Bridging the gap between mental and physical health: a multidisciplinary approach. *Journal of Clinical Psychiatry* **68** (Suppl. 4): 26–33.

[93] Politi P, Sciarini P, Lusignani GS et al. (2006) Depression and stroke: an up-to-date review. *Epidemiologia e Psichiatria Sociale* **15**: 284–294.

[94] Amaddeo F, Barbui C, Perini G et al. (2007) Avoidable mortality of psychiatric patients in an area with a community-based system of mental health care. *Acta Psychiatrica Scandinavica* **115**: 320–325.

[95] Grigoletti L, Perini G, Rossi A et al. (2009) Mortality and cause of death among psychiatric patients. A twenty year case-register study in an area with a community-based system of care. *Psychological Medicine* **39**: 1875–1884.

[96] Amaddeo F, Tansella M. (2010) Mortality among people with mental disorders. *Epidemiologia e Psichiatria Sociale* **19**: 1–3.

CHAPTER 16

Routine outcome monitoring: A tool to improve the quality of mental health care?

Sjoerd Sytema and Lian van der Krieke

University Center for Psychiatry, University Medical Center Groningen, University of Groningen, Groningen, The Netherlands

Introduction

In this chapter, we will explore whether routine outcome monitoring (ROM), integrated in daily practice, can improve the quality of mental health care. As there is no uniform definition of ROM [1], we will use outcome assessment, outcome measurement and outcome interchangeably.

Principally, there are two different ways of using ROM data. The first is direct feedback of individual outcome data to clinicians and patients to evaluate treatment progress at patient level. The second way is at different aggregated levels. These can serve the purpose of (a) monitoring, in order to evaluate and improve treatments within teams or services; (b) research, in order to publish outcome in mental health care in a region or country; and (c) benchmarking, in order to make comparisons between teams or services. Ultimately, benchmark outcomes may be used by various stakeholders to choose between service providers (patients or insurance companies) or to monitor the quality of services (government).

The South Verona Community Mental Health Service, for decades developed and directed by Michelle Tansella, is the best and most well-known example of a mental health-care service in which ROM has been fully implemented. It is renowned mainly due to the high level of research it conducts with the ROM data, resulting in a continuous stream of publications. The key elements of the South Verona Outcome Project (SVOP) present an outline of what ROM should ideally look like [2]. The basic elements are as follows:

1 Data are collected in the daily routine of a clinical practice setting, and these data are collected from all patients contacting the mental health-care service.

Improving Mental Health Care: The Global Challenge, First Edition.
Edited by Graham Thornicroft, Mirella Ruggeri and David Goldberg.

2 All primary clinicians are involved in the assessment process and properly trained in the use of the instruments.

3 The assessment includes both clinician- and patient-rated outcomes.

4 Reliability and quality of the data are closely monitored.

In the SVOP, the ROM data are mainly used at an aggregated level for research purposes and not for direct feedback of individual patient data to the clinician. The latter is the key aim of a different ROM project, namely, the Groningen ROM project, which will be discussed later in this chapter.

In the daily practice of mental health services, the first and principal aim of ROM is to support clinical decision-making at the patient level. Decisions might be related to, for instance, as to whether to continue treatment because symptom reduction has not yet progressed to normal levels or when to reconsider treatment because no change in symptom severity was established. This surely is the basic level of ROM, where it all starts. But aggregated ROM data provide outcome data at various other levels that support clinical decision-making. This aggregated data can be used, for instance, to evaluate the effectiveness of a treatment, by taking the percentage of patients recovered after treatment as an indicator.

The matrix model of Tansella and Thornicroft is an excellent model to describe the interconnectedness between the different levels of ROM data [3]. In this model, a distinction is made between two dimensions: (a) the geographical dimension, which is subdivided into patient level, local level and regional/country level; and (b) the temporal dimension, which is subdivided into input phase, process phase and outcome phase. The input phase includes national or regional budgets available for mental health, mental health laws and government directives. The process phase includes mental health performance indicators, such as admission rates, contact rates and pathways to care.

A cross-tabulation of both the geographical and the temporal dimension gives six cells, which are all interconnected (see Table 16.1). This implies that 'outcome' at the patient level (e.g. symptom reduction) is to some degree dependent on 'input' at the country level (e.g. how many psychotherapy contacts are covered by national insurance regulations) and on 'process' at the local level (e.g. caseloads and waiting lists). It is important to consider this interconnectedness between various levels and phases when we want to compare outcome results between services, regions or countries. Such comparisons can only be interpreted properly when the content of all six cells are taken into account. We will explore this point further when we discuss one of the central aims of the national Dutch ROM project, which is benchmarking of aggregated outcome results between mental health services at a national level.

In the remainder of this chapter, we will first describe the similarities and the differences between the Australian and the Dutch national ROM models. Australia was the first country where ROM was implemented, whereas in the Netherlands ROM has only been introduced recently. Second, we will outline the application of the Routine Outcome and Quality Assessment (RoQua) tool,

Table 16.1 Overview of the matrix model, with examples of key issues in each cell of the matrix.

Geographical dimension	Temporal dimension		
	Input phase (A)	Process phase (B)	Outcome phase (C)
Country/region level	1A Expenditure on services Role of the media Mental health law Government directives Special interest groups	1B Performance/activity indicators (e.g. admission rates, bed occupancy rates, compulsory treatment rates)	1C Suicide rates SMRs Homelessness Special enquiries
Local level (catchment area)	2A Population needs assessment Population characteristics Budget Staff Fixed expenditure Consumer participation	2B Operational policies Pathways to care Patterns of service use Caseloads Contact rates Targeting of special groups	2C Outcome studies at group level Secondary and tertiary prevention Decrease of local stigma Better access to services
Patient level	3A Individual needs assessment Demands made by patients Demands made by family	3B Quality of treatments Frequency and duration of treatment Continuity of care Income support Vocational services	3C Symptom reduction Satisfaction Quality of life/accommodation Disability/work rehabilitation Burden on care-givers

Derived from Tansella and Thornicroft [3].

developed by the University Medical Center Groningen, which is used in the northern and central parts of the Netherlands. This is a catchment area covering a total population of three million people, comprising 150000 mental health service users. Furthermore, we will briefly consider ROM instruments and discuss ROM implementation. The final sections of this chapter deal with outcomes for and feedback to clinicians and patients.

The Australian and Dutch national ROM models

Australian model

Australia was the first country where ROM was implemented at a national level [4–6]. A consortium known as the Australian Mental Health Outcomes and

Classification Network (AMHOCN; http://amhocn.org/) is responsible for data management and reporting. This consortium also offers online training in the instruments selected for ROM, collected in the National Outcomes and Casemix Collection (NOCC). At present, all public-sector inpatient and community mental health services collect data according to the NOCC protocol. The NOCC protocol includes subprotocols for children and adolescents, adults and the elderly. Two clinician-rated instruments, the Health of the Nation Outcome Scales (HoNOS [7]) and the Life Skills Profile 16 (LSP-16 [8]), are the core instruments. But the protocol also includes a self-report instrument (see [5] for details). The NOCC protocol is administered at admission, at reviews during treatment and at discharge of an 'episode of care', which is defined as a continuous period of contact in one mental health setting (inpatient or community).

All Australian ROM data are submitted to AMHOCN. The data in this national database is freely available through http://amhocn.org. By means of a Web Decision Support Tool, selections in the data can be made. For instance, it is possible to compare an individual score (e.g. a female patient aged 26 who scored 20 on the HoNOS with a diagnosis of schizophrenia, who was voluntarily admitted to acute ambulatory care) with the HoNOS scores of other patients with similar characteristics (e.g. female patients in the age range between 25 and 34 with psychotic disorders, who were admitted to ambulatory care). The outcome is a distribution chart and a comparison statistic (percentile score=91, meaning that 91% of patients within this selection of characteristics have lower HoNOS total scores; this female patient also belongs to the 10% of patients with the highest HoNOS scores).

The Australian ROM model might be the most elaborate in the world. However, there is room for improvement as far as the completion rates are concerned. As the AMHOCN website shows, the overall tendency is that the clinician-rated HoNOS family of measures have the highest completion rates, while patient-rated measures have much lower rates. For instance, if we take a look at adults in outpatient care, the HoNOS completion rate is about 80% at admission, but only about 25% for the patient-rated questionnaires at the same point in time. At discharge, the HoNOS completion rate dropped to about 60% and rates of patient-rated instruments dropped to about 10%. These percentages are stable throughout the years (2006–2011). Comparable completion rates were reported for the young and the elderly patients.

From this, we may conclude that the implementation of ROM in Australia has been passed off favourably among clinicians. However, it has been less successful at the patient level, as response rates of self-report instruments are low. In the future, this drawback might be obviated by directing more efforts to engage patients in ROM and enabling them to benefit from ROM results. Computerised ROM systems, offering patients the opportunity to complete self-report questionnaires at home, as the one we will describe later in this chapter, might increase completion rates.

Dutch model

The Dutch ROM model has had a recent onset and was started only in 2011 as result of an agreement between insurance companies and mental health-care organisations. Consequently, the ROM system relies heavily on the Dutch financial system. Health care in the Netherlands, including mental health care, is financed by a dual system. Long-stay living arrangements (e.g. sheltered homes, permanent hospitalisation) are covered by state-controlled mandatory insurance. For all other treatments, there is a system of obligatory health insurance with private health insurance companies. The latter must offer a core universal insurance package. (More information about the dual system can be found at http://en.m.wikipedia.org/wiki/Healthcare_in_the_Netherlands.)

The financing system, introduced in 2005, is based on so-called diagnosis treatment combinations (DTCs). A DTC includes all registered activities carried out by the mental health-care service during the complete treatment process of an individual patient. A DTC is opened when a patient has received a diagnosis, and it is closed when the treatment has ended or after 365 days. Each DTC must be validated (using information technology (IT)-based validation modules) before it can be sent for billing to the insurance company. The payment for each DTC varies according to the diagnosis and the type of treatment. As the name 'diagnosis treatment combination' indicates, each diagnosis is linked to specific treatment options with a pre-specified price. These prices are fixed at the national level.

Budgets for mental health services largely depend on the DTC system. Insurance companies have additional tools to force services into desired directions. For instance, they are entitled to punish health-care services by withholding all DTC reimbursements when the health-care services do not stick to the rules that had been agreed upon. In addition, insurance companies negotiate with services about their total production of care delivery in a financial year. A certain growth percentage in total production may be allowed for the next year, provided that a number of goals in the present year, directed by the insurance company, have been realised. If not, the service is punished by not being allowed to realise growth.

At present, insurance companies make an all-out effort to introduce ROM in mental health care, as they consider ROM a valuable instrument to keep track of the quality of delivered care. Mental health services are now forced to introduce ROM into their clinical practice. The incentive for compliance is high, since mental health-care services face penalties if they do not reach the desired response rates.

In order to construct a national database of ROM data, a trusted third party (TTP) has been appointed, paid by the insurance companies, to collect ROM data from all mental health services (see www.sbggz.nl for more information). The

TTP has developed a model in which ROM data are connected to DTCs. According to this model, each DTC should include a ROM measurement at the start and one at the end of a treatment episode with the same instrument, allowing the calculation of effect (the change in scores between first and last measurement). Services are free to choose instruments from a core set of instruments selected for each category of service users by a scientific board of researchers. Moreover, a timeline for implementation of ROM was agreed upon by national representative bodies of both insurance companies and mental health-care institutions. In 2012, 30% of all DTCs delivered for billing had ROM assessments. This percentage will increase to 50% by 2014.

The aim of insurance companies is to use the database for benchmarking between mental health services, as they believe that ROM will increase the quality of treatment and that it will create transparency in the effectiveness of mental health treatments. Ultimately, insurance companies want to use the database to be able to contract those mental health-care services that are most cost-effective. At present, there is a heated debate between insurance companies and researchers about the value of this benchmarking model. Researchers criticise the model, arguing that it is unreliable because differences in effectiveness might be due to confounders not being taken into account [9]. This includes, for example, case mix differences (two groups of patients within the same diagnostic category might be different in severity of the illness) and regional differences (deprived areas in cities vs countryside areas). Another major point of criticism is that the DTC financial-based system is not congruent to the treatment process. The ROM assessment instances specified in the DTCs do not reflect relevant evaluation points during treatment. To evaluate a treatment process, one usually needs more information than a ROM assessment at the beginning and the end of a DTC trajectory.

Finally, the obligatory core set of instruments that mental health-care services must choose from, usually constituted by instruments which measure global aspects of mental health, might not be the right choice for many teams.

Advantages and drawbacks of the Australian versus the Dutch model

The Australian ROM model has some advantages compared with the Dutch model:

- First, in the Australian model, one small set of ROM instruments was selected based on a series of field trials. In the Dutch model, each mental health service can choose instruments according to their own preferences, from a large set of global instruments. Comparisons between services using different instruments may be possible after some statistical transformations, but results will remain questionable.
- Second, the Australian model includes assessments at admission, discharge and in between these two ends of a treatment episode, whereas the Dutch

model only includes assessments at admission and discharge. Therefore, the Australian model provides more information about the course of progress during treatment.

- Third, the Dutch ROM model is linked to a financial declaration system, which may not reflect the dynamics of the treatment process. The Australian model is much more linked to daily practice.

On the other hand, the Dutch model, which is in an early stage of development, might have the following advantages over the Australian model:

- The Dutch model relies more strongly on patient-rated instruments, particularly for patients with non-psychotic disorders. This might facilitate processes of shared decision-making, in which patient and clinician engage in a two-way communication and together decide on a plan of action. In addition, the use of self-report instruments may provide opportunities for patient self-management.
- As in Australia, in the Dutch model the HoNOS is used for outcome assessment in long-term patients and in patients with psychotic disorders. However, the Dutch model adds to this a patient-rated instrument, namely, the Manchester Short Assessment of quality of life (MANSA [10]). Therefore, for this category of patients also, the perspective of the patient in the Dutch ROM model seems to be more strongly implemented.

Having described the Australian and the Dutch ROM models, we can now see the enormous amount of energy devoted to the development of national ROM databases. These databases are a spearhead of the government, as far as mental health care is concerned. However, national databases are in fact of limited value in the efforts to improve quality of mental health care. The real power of ROM lies in its use in the daily practice of health-care services, in the primary process of treatment where clinicians and patients are at work.

Outline of the Groningen online ROM application (RoQua)

Since the implementation of ROM was practically forced by insurance companies, mental health-care services had to look for workable ways to integrate ROM into clinical practice. The University Center for Psychiatry, part of the University Medical Center Groningen, therefore started a non-profit project called Routine Outcome and Quality Assessment (RoQua). The main aim of this project was to develop a ROM tool that could computerise the ROM assessment and feedback procedures. The specifications for the development of this RoQua tool included the following:

- It should be web-based and operated by an IT team in the University Medical Center Groningen. The yearly budget for the team is paid for by the participating mental health-care organisations.

- The ROM tool should be fully integrated into the electronic patient file systems of all mental health-care services participating in the project. As the health-care services use electronic patient file systems from different IT providers, the ROM tool should be able to communicate with all those different systems.
- The tool should be able to create and present digital versions of all sorts of instruments (patient-rated and clinician-rated), to calculate scores (e.g. sum scores of scales) and to compare these with norm scores.
- The ROM tool should be able to present immediate feedback of each ROM assessment at patient level. Because the ROM tool is integrated into the electronic patient file, the ROM result will be directly available there.
- Patients should have access to the ROM tool, in order to complete self-report instruments online. In addition, it should be possible to send ROM invitation emails to patients, including an introductory letter with a login code to enter the ROM website.
- The ROM databases (each institution has its own database) should be hosted at the University data centre according to state-of-the-art safety principles.

The RoQua tool is principally directed towards providing immediate feedback to clinicians of ROM outcome data at the patient level. As such, RoQua supports the use of ROM assessments in the daily treatment practice. The tool has been developed for four years now and will be developed further continuously. One of the greatest struggles has been its integration with the electronic patient files. We use a Health Level 7 (HL7) connection, which is the medical international standard for exchange and integration of electronic health information (http://www.hl7.org). Through this HL7 connection, ROM data can be sent to and be extracted from the existing electronic patient file systems. This connection simplifies data processing, but it also has the advantage that the ROM data can be directly linked to other data in the electronic patient file, such as data about care utilisation (the DTC data). By means of this linkage, automatically generated data sets can be produced for deliverance to the national ROM database.

Clinicians form the primary group of RoQua end users. They can start the RoQua tool by clicking the button 'ROM' in the electronic patient file. This button is only activated when the file of a specific patient is selected so as to ensure that the data are connected to the right internal patient number. In the RoQua environment, clinicians and/or administrative planners can create an invitation for patients to complete the self-report instruments. This invitation consists of an automatically generated standard invitation letter that includes a login code with which patients can access the RoQua environment from any place with a computer and internet connection. Depending on the patient's diagnosis and treatment, a pre-specified set of ROM instruments (a ROM protocol) can be chosen, or clinicians can compose their own set of instruments. Subsequently, clinicians can immediately complete the clinician-rated instruments. When a ROM assessment is complete, clinicians can view the results in the 'Outcome' section in RoQua. This section shows outcome scores for a particular patient, presented in tables and graphics. The graphics visualise progress (or lack of it) during a treatment episode, depending on the frequency of assessments. (A short video demonstration of RoQua can be seen at http://roqua.nl/about/.)

In addition, the RoQua technology offers the possibility of generating ROM reports or letters that summarise the assessment outcomes in words and figures. This functionality has been put into effect for the ROM protocol for people with psychotic disorders. This protocol is called Phamous, which stands for Pharmacotherapy monitoring and outcome survey (www.phamous.nl), and consists of a psychiatric, psychosocial and physical assessment. From these data, two reports are generated: one for the clinician and a shortened version for the general practitioner. Clinicians can print this report, discuss it with their patients in an evaluation meeting and decide whether or not the course of treatment needs readjustment.

One of the contributions of a ROM tool such as RoQua to the improvement of the quality of mental health care is that it stimulates (re)structuring of service delivery. The implementation of a ROM feedback system facilitates mental health services in planning treatment evaluations and in discussing patient progress at fixed points in time. It also stimulates services to more strictly organise treatments based on (ROM) goals to be reached. Most of the treatment modules that are currently being developed have integrated ROM into the treatment trajectory.

An example is the treatment module cognitive-behavioural therapy (CBT) for depression. This module consists of 16 weekly sessions of CBT with a monthly ROM assessment with the Inventory of Depressive Symptomatology-Self Report (IDS-SR [11]). The goal of this treatment is remission, which is a total score below 13 on this instrument. During the treatment trajectory, the clinician can follow the assessment outcome and see whether this goal is likely to be achieved.

ROM implementation

In the past years, we have gained experience with the implementation of ROM in the Dutch mental health-care services. From this experience, a number of implementation guidelines can be derived.

In general, ROM will fail if it is not well integrated in daily practice. In the Dutch model, insurance companies impose penalties on mental health budgets when services do not use ROM. One of the unfortunate consequences is that ROM sometimes serves merely as an administrative process that has to be implemented to prevent these penalties. In such a scenario, ROM, as a tool to improve the quality of mental health care, will fail because outcomes are not used. However, from good practices developed throughout recent years, we have learnt that ROM works best when

- Each ROM assessment has a clear goal and according consequences for clinical decision-making.
- Services work with well-structured treatment protocols in which ROM assessments are clearly integrated and in which outcomes are discussed with patients. An example was given earlier in this chapter.
- Clinicians are trained in the use of clinical ratings, such as the HoNOS, which provides a good opportunity for implementation of ROM instruments. The training we offer in the RoQua project is within treatment teams on the spot, using real patients from their caseloads. During the training, the teams learn to score their patients, work with the RoQua application and interpret the ROM outcomes. In addition, the trainers discuss with the team how it wants to implement regular HoNOS assessments and how it will relate these assessments to treatment evaluations.

Clinician-rated instruments

The gamut of ROM instruments on a national and international level is enormous. In fact, all available assessment instruments which have been successfully tested in psychometric research might be used. Although it does not make sense to give an overview of ROM instruments, we can make some distinctions.

The first distinction that is useful to make is between clinician-rated and patient-rated instruments. Well-known and widely used clinician-rated instruments are the family of HoNOS instruments, introduced earlier in this chapter, and the Camberwell Assessment of Needs-Short Version (CANSAS [12]). Both instruments are designed for use in ROM for the severely mentally ill. One of the main reasons is that self-report in this category of patients has been considered less feasible. Outcome scores of the CANSAS are the number of needs and the number of unmet needs. The sum score of the HoNOS is a measure of global severity of dysfunctioning. There are HoNOS versions for specific groups, like the HoNOSCA for children and adolescents and the HoNOS65+ for elderly patients. They are widely used in England, Australia and the Netherlands. Both the HoNOS and the CANSAS can be rated within ten minutes.

Patient-rated instruments

Patient-rated instruments can be subdivided into global and disorder-specific instruments. Widely used global instruments in ROM are, for example, the Strengths and Difficulties Questionnaire (SDQ [13]) for children and the Outcome Questionnaire-45 (OQ-45 [14]) for adults. One of the prerequisites for successful ROM is not to overload the patient. A rule of thumb could be that 30 minutes of time for ROM assessment is the maximum. Therefore, there is a tendency to create shorter questionnaires. Well-known instruments like the Child Behavior Checklist (CBCL) and the Symptom Checklist-90 (SCL-90) are not very suitable in ROM, because they are too long and time-consuming.

Disorder-specific instruments measure symptom severity of diagnostic disorders, like depression, anxiety disorders, alcohol/drug dependency, eating disorders, personality disorders and so on.

We believe that it is often useful to include both a global and a disorder-specific measure in a ROM protocol when a treatment is designed for a specific diagnostic category. In case of treatments for depression, this may be the OQ-45 and the IDS-SR. The IDS-SR reports on the depressive symptoms the patient experiences, while the OQ-45 adds information about problems caused by these depressive symptoms.

In fact, the OQ-45 may be a useful global patient-rated ROM instrument for many patients. This instrument is based on problems psychotherapy patients put forward in their therapy sessions, regardless of diagnosis or disorder. Although these patients might suffer from depression, they not only talk about depressive symptoms but primarily about problems caused by these symptoms, like problems in relationships or stress at work. The OQ-45 has subscales for symptom distress interpersonal relationships, and the functioning in social roles, like work or school. So, by including these scales, not only is the reduction in symptom severity of depression measured but also progress made in other areas relevant for the patient. By adding the OQ-45 to a disorder-specific instrument, we can create a more complete insight into the effectiveness of psychotherapy, which is probably more closely related to the needs or unmet needs of patients.

High-frequency assessments

An additional category of ROM instruments that can be distinguished is the category of 'high-frequency assessment' instruments. A ROM strategy based on high-frequency assessment with very short scales is Scott Miller's 'feedback-informed treatment' (see www.scottdmiller.com for information and references). At the start of each session of psychotherapy, the Outcome Rating Scale is completed by the patient, which includes four questions about well-being. At the end of each session, the Session Rating Scale is completed by the patient, including four questions about working alliance. Results of the latter are shortly discussed by clinician and patient at the last minutes of the session. In this strategy, ROM is more than a monitor to follow the course of treatment; it is an integral part of the treatment. We believe that short and frequent assessments will become prominent in the future, with the increasing availability of smart phones and tablets.

ROM outcomes for clinicians

Reliable clinical change and clinically significant change

Clinicians use outcome data at the patient level for clinical decision-making. One of the problems clinicians are confronted with is how to interpret the data.

Useful statistics have been proposed by Jacobson and Truax [15, 16]. One is the 'reliable change index' (RCI). This is the number of points of improvement on a scale that has to be realised to consider it a reliable (not due to measurement error) change. The RCI algorithm is based on the reliability of a scale (test–retest reliability or internal consistency) and the pooled standard deviation of two assessments. For example, the RCI of the symptom distress scale of the OQ-45 (which has a range from 0 to 100) is 14, meaning that a patient should have a decrease of 14 points on this scale between two assessments to be considered reliably improved. The other statistic is 'clinically significant change' (CSC). This is a cut-off score between normal and clinical functioning. To calculate this statistic, normative data are needed from both normal populations and from clinical populations. For example, the CSC of the symptom distress scale of the OQ-45 is 36, meaning that scores above 36 are scores in the clinical range, and scores including and below 36 are considered as scores in the normal range. To calculate RCI and CSC, software applications are available on the internet (http://www.psyctc.org/stats/rcsc1.htm).

The RCI and CSC can be part of the feedback of ROM outcomes for clinicians as they are fairly easy to interpret. For example, a clinician may set the goal of treatment for his or her patient on symptom recovery, which is measured by scores below 36 on the symptom distress scale of the OQ-45. However, he or she can also monitor the treatment progress during treatment by using the RCI. For instance, after six sessions of psychotherapy, the clinician can conclude that the patient reliably improved when the score dropped from the initial 70 points to a current 51 (RCI of the symptom distress scale=14).

The effect of feedback of ROM data on quality of care in psychotherapy was studied by Lambert [17, 18], who conducted a controlled study among 1020 university students, treated at the counselling centre for psychological distress, using the OQ-45 total score as the outcome measure [19]. The OQ-45 was completed once every week. In the experimental condition (N=528 students), therapists received feedback, and in the control condition (N=492), they did not. The feedback system included a graphic showing consecutive scores, but also a coloured card giving an indication of the most likely treatment outcome, based on RCI and CSC statistics. This card system is interesting because it is simple and directly linked to clinical decision-making. The following four cards were available:

- White=patient is functioning in the normal range; consider termination
- Green=rate of change is adequate; no change in treatment plan recommended
- Yellow=rate of change less than adequate; consider altering the treatment plan
- Red=not making the expected level of progress; may drop out of treatment prematurely or have a negative treatment outcome

The therapists in the trial were given free choice in what to do with the feedback information, and they were allowed to share it with their patients. Every treatment was followed from start to finish. There were a number of interesting outcomes. First, all treatment trajectories were divided into 'on track' (white or green cards) and 'not on track' (yellow and red cards). In the 'not on track' group without feedback, 18% reached 'reliable or clinically significant change'. In the 'not on track' group with feedback, this percentage was 32%. This suggests that such a warning sign, including advice, might improve treatment result. No effect of feedback was found in the 'on track' group. This makes sense as there is no signal to change. One might have expected that the white card would show earlier termination of treatments, but it did not. In a regression analysis, three factors were significantly related to change in outcome: (a) initial OQ score (higher initial scores give more change in outcome), (b) course qualification ('on track'/'not on track'), (c) feedback (feedback gives more change in outcome).

Dose response analysis and expected treatment response

The RCI and CSC index enable us to evaluate change in a patient's health status by making use of ROM data on an individual level. However, a patient's treatment course can also be evaluated by using ROM data on an aggregated level. A first example is the dose response approach. A dose response analysis answers the question: How much therapy is needed in order to achieve a meaningful treatment outcome? The outcome is obtained by calculating the number or proportion of patients that have reached a clinical reliable change in health status at a certain point in time. In one such study, again from the Lambert group, the OQ-45 was assessed at each session of psychotherapy. The study included 75 patients. It showed that 25% of patients reached reliable clinical change after 5 sessions, 50% after 9 sessions and 75% after 17 sessions. These figures can be used to evaluate how individual patients relate to what can be expected on group level.

Another promising approach of analysing ROM data at an aggregated level is expected treatment response (ETR) analysis. ETR answers the question: What treatment response can we expect, based on clinical patient characteristics? In the ETR model, growth modelling is used to predict course of treatment progress (measured by a ROM instrument) in time. This might result in one or more profiles, depending on initial case mix data. These profiles can then be used as a benchmark to evaluate progress of an individual patient. First, the likely course of a new patient is selected from these profiles. During treatment, the predicted profile is compared with the actual score of the patient. From this, it can be decided if the patient is 'on track' (actual score and predicted score are comparable) or 'not on track' (actual score is worse than the predicted score). In the latter case, treatment might be reconsidered.

ROM and health-care consumers

The introduction of ROM has been accompanied by a heated debate about its relevance. On the one hand, sceptics labelled ROM a bureaucratic exercise with little value for the practice of mental health care, arguing that ROM was of little benefit to patients. ROM was said to be unable to capture individual differences between patients, and it was criticised for not measuring the aspects of mental health care that patients considered valuable. On the other hand, ROM believers stated that ROM was an opportunity for patients to be more involved in the care planning process and to keep track of their own functioning in a structured way [20–22].

The truth is that ROM can be a useful and meaningful instrument for consumers when implemented meticulously and in the right way. To start with, ROM has to incorporate the consumer's perspective by including self-report measures that allow for self-assessment. Ideally, consumers are involved in the decision-making about the content of a ROM protocol, for clinicians and consumers disagree with each other as to what outcomes are most vital. In general, clinicians tend to concentrate on those ROM measures that provide information about clinical symptoms and functioning [20, 23], whereas consumer-oriented approaches promote a focus on personal recovery, which reflects the importance of finding meaning and giving value to personal experiences [23]. Moreover, regarding ROM results, clinicians are usually more interested in disturbing values, in what goes wrong and to what extent their clients are 'off track', while consumers are usually more interested in what goes well and on which measures they have made progress. The implication is that all ROM results should be considered important and made available to consumers.

A national voice to the consumers' perspective

In the Netherlands, a ROM expert group was formed, which consisted of 20 users from the Dutch national platform of patient and family members in mental health care (called LPGGZ), to give a national voice to the consumers' perspective on ROM. This expert group set themselves the task of critically evaluating ROM, starting from the question: 'How can ROM effectively contribute to the recovery of mental health-care clients?'. A vision document was also published, listing the following eight quality criteria for ROM implementation [24]:

1 Patients will be adequately informed about the content and the aim of various assessments included in ROM.
2 Patients will have the opportunity to decide whether or not to complete assessments and in what way (online, on paper, with the help of a family member).
3 The ROM procedure will form an integrated part of the treatment context.
4 Assessments will be conducted periodically (twice for patients with severe mental illness, four times a year for people in short-term care).
5 ROM results will be fed back to patients.
6 ROM results will be discussed with patients.
7 Patients will be given the opportunity to compare their ROM results with ROM results based on a group level.
8 Patients own the ROM data, meaning that they can take the ROM data with them to other health-care organisations.

Furthermore, the expert group has stressed the idea that ROM functions as a valuable contribution to recovery-oriented care only when it is embedded in a four-step Plan–Do–Check–Act cycle of (a) creating a treatment plan (Plan), (b) executing the treatment plan (Do), (c) measuring the results of the treatment plan by ROM (Check) and (d) adaptating the treatment plan (Act) [24].

Although this four-step cycle may seem obvious, in some health-care organisations it is yet to become a common routine. Care teams have to adjust their way of working so that regular treatment plan evaluations coincide with the evaluation of ROM results. This is quite a challenge. While most clinicians are familiar with the use of questionnaires and assessments in the treatment process, interpreting and comparing outcomes in a meaningful way can be time-consuming. The feeling that time spent on ROM is time not spent on patient contact appears to be persistent [20, 25]. Therefore, not all clinicians are yet accustomed to discussing ROM results with their patients [25], which precludes consumers from optimally benefiting from ROM.

A web-based ROM support system for patients

One way of encouraging discussion about ROM results between clinicians and patients is to convince clinicians about its importance and to provide them with practical means (e.g. a summary letter) to do so. Another approach consists of enabling patients to access their ROM results and to reflect upon their implications. An example of an attempt which represents this latter approach is the Dutch project called Wegweis, which focuses on the development of online tools to support self-management for people with severe mental illness (http://development.wegweis.nl). Wegweis is a collaboration between the Dutch Northern mental health institutions, the University Psychiatry Center and the University of Groningen. As part of the project, a web-based ROM support system for patients has been created that provides patients with an overview of their ROM results and personalised advice based on these results [26, 27].

The support system has the form of a website, which can be accessed by entering user name and password and can be used by consumers at home or in a clinical setting. Clinicians can invite patients to the support system by sending an automatically generated email from within the electronic patient file. After logging in, consumers are provided with an overview of their ROM results, including their score on several questionnaires and interviews. These results are accompanied by a short explanation of the ROM evaluation (the aims of ROM), the included measures (e.g. what they measure, by whom it was completed) as well as the scores. Linked to the ROM results, the website offers personalised advice about various topics related to psychiatric treatment, rehabilitation and personal recovery. The content of this advice consists of information derived from evidence-based research (e.g. the Dutch multidisciplinary guideline), clinical expertise and consumer experiences. The support system identifies specific health-care problems and matching advice for each individual consumer, based on item scores of ROM measures, using algorithms and combined with ontological reasoning. Patients can print the ROM results as well as the advice and take this along with them to the ROM evaluation meeting with their clinician. A usability study with patients with a psychotic disorder showed that they could work with the system easily and that the content of the advice was considered meaningful and supportive [27].

Self-management

A system like Wegweis allows for processes of self-management and shared decision-making in which consumers can empower themselves and take more responsibility for their own care. Consumers are no longer dependent upon their clinicians to access their ROM results and to explore what their options are if they feel action must be taken. Self-management opportunities with ROM become even more apparent when using high-frequency assessments, as mentioned earlier. Apart from Miller's Outcome Rating Scale and Session Rating Scale, we can also think of short online diary questionnaires and health-care-related smart phone apps to collect and feed back information. These high-frequency assessments provide an opportunity to create a more continuous and ecologically valid data flow, which may be used to discern certain patterns in functioning. If patterns are present, ROM data may be used to predict possible future outcome and to support relapse prevention.

Conclusion

ROM might give a boost to improve the quality of mental health care in a number of ways. First, ROM data are of vital importance in the primary health-care process. ROM provides an opportunity for both clinicians and patients to evaluate treatment progress on an individual level and to adjust the course of treatment if needed. Second, ROM data can inform us about the effectiveness of mental health treatments in a way that is far closer to real life than data collected in randomised controlled trials (which always use 'ideal' patients). Third, transparency in outcome of treatments will produce an incentive for mental health services to restructure and improve treatments.

As the patient perspective in ROM (and in mental health care in general) gains importance, we believe that ultimately patients may become the driving force in the proper implementation and continuation of ROM. As a consumer of mental health products, they might want to be informed about treatment results. They may also want to know whether progress during treatment is 'on track', and if not, it is in their interest that clinical decisions are taken.

We are more doubtful about benchmarking at a global (national) level, as has been argued in this chapter. A comparison between services will be biased by many factors. The matrix model of Tansella and Thornicroft shows the complexity of interpreting results.

References

[1] Trauer T (ed.). (2010) *Outcome Measurement in Mental Health: Theory and Practice*, 1st edn. Cambridge: Cambridge University Press.

[2] Lasalvia A, Ruggeri M. (2007) Assessing the outcome of community-based psychiatric care: building a feedback loop from 'real world' health services research into clinical practice. *Acta Psychiatrica Scandinavica Supplementum* **437** (437): 6–15.

[3] Tansella M, Thornicroft G. (1998) A conceptual framework for mental health services: the matrix model. *Psychological Medicine* **28** (3): 503–508.

[4] Pirkis J, Burgess P, Coombs T et al. (2005) Routine measurement of outcomes in Australia's public sector mental health services. *Australia and New Zealand Health Policy* **2** (1): 8.

[5] Pirkis J, Callaly T. (2010) Mental health outcome measurement in Australia. In: Trauer T (ed.), *Outcome Measurement in Mental Health*. Cambridge: Cambridge University Press, pp. 15–25.

[6] Coombs T, Stapley K, Pirkis J. (2011) The multiple uses of routine mental health outcome measures in Australia and New Zealand: experiences from the field. *Australasian Psychiatry* **19** (3): 247–253.

[7] Orrell M, Yard P, Handysides J et al. (1999) Validity and reliability of the Health of the Nation Outcome Scales in psychiatric patients in the community. *British Journal of Psychiatry* **174**: 409–412.

[8] Rosen A, Hadzi-Pavlovic D, Parker G. (1989) The life skills profile: a measure assessing function and disability in schizophrenia. *Schizophrenia Bulletin* **15** (2): 325–337.

[9] Van Os J, Kahn R, Denys D et al. (2012) ROM: gedragsnorm of dwangmaatregel? Overwegingen bij het themanummer over routine outcome monitoring. *Tijdschrift voor psychiatrie* **54** (3): 245–253.

[10] Priebe S, Huxley P, Knight S et al. (1999) Application and results of the Manchester short assessment of quality of life (MANSA). *International Journal of Social Psychiatry* **45** (1): 7–12.

[11] Trivedi MH, Rush AJ, Ibrahim HM et al. (2004) The Inventory of Depressive Symptomatology, Clinician Rating (IDS-C) and Self-Report (IDS-SR), and the Quick Inventory of Depressive Symptomatology, Clinician Rating (QIDS-C) and Self-Report (QIDS-SR) in public sector patients with mood disorders: a psychometric evaluation. *Psychological Medicine* **34** (1): 73–82.

[12] Phelan M, Slade M, Thornicroft G et al. (1995) The Camberwell assessment of need: the validity and reliability of an instrument to assess the needs of people with severe mental illness. *British Journal of Psychiatry* **167** (5): 589–595.

[13] Ford T, Hutchings J, Bywater T et al. Strengths and Difficulties Questionnaire Added Value Scores: evaluating effectiveness in child mental health interventions. *British Journal of Psychiatry* **194** (6): 552–558.

[14] Vermeersch DA, Lambert MJ, Burlingame GM. (2000) Outcome Questionnaire: item sensitivity to change. *Journal of Personality Assessment* **74** (2): 242–261.

[15] Jacobson NS, Truax P. (1991) Clinical significance: a statistical approach to defining meaningful change in psychotherapy research. *Journal of Consulting and Clinical Psychology* **59** (1): 12–19.

[16] Lambert MJ, Ogles BM. (2009) Using clinical significance in psychotherapy outcome research: the need for a common procedure and validity data. *Psychotherapy Research* **19** (4–5): 493–501.

[17] Lambert MJ, Hansen NB, Finch AE. (2001) Patient-focused research: using patient outcome data to enhance treatment effects. *Journal of Consulting and Clinical Psychology* **69** (2): 159–172.

[18] Lambert MJ, Harmon C, Slade K et al. (2005) Providing feedback to psychotherapists on their patients' progress: clinical results and practice suggestions. *Journal of Clinical Psychology* **61** (2): 165–174.

[19] Lambert MJ, Whipple JL, Vermeersch DA et al. (2002) Enhancing psychotherapy outcomes via providing feedback on client progress: a replication. *Clinical Psychology & Psychotherapy* **9** (2): 91–103.

[20] Lakeman R. (2004) Standardized routine outcome measurement: pot holes in the road to recovery. *International Journal of Mental Health Nursing* **13** (4): 210–215.

[21] Happell B. (2008) Meaningful information or a bureaucratic exercise? Exploring the value of routine outcome measurement in mental health. *Issues in Mental Health Nursing* **29** (10): 1098–1114.

[22] Black J, Lewis T, McIntosh P et al. (2009) It's not that bad: the views of consumers and carers about routine outcome measurement in mental health. *Australian Health Review* **33** (1): 93–99.

[23] Guthrie D, McIntosh M, Callaly T et al. Consumer attitudes towards the use of routine outcome measures in a public mental health service: a consumer-driven study. *International Journal of Mental Health Nursing* **17** (2): 92–97.

[24] Makkink S, Cliënten KL. (2011) Herstellen doe je zelf. In: Van Hees S, Van der Vlist P, Mulder N (eds.), *Van weten naar meten. ROM in de GGZ*. Amsterdam: Boom, pp. 97–107.

[25] Schaefer B, Nijssen Y, Van Weeghel J. (2011) Behandelaars. Van meten naar oplossingsgericht werken. In: Van Hees S, Van der Vlist P, Mulder N (eds.), *Van weten naar meten. Rom in de GGZ*, Amsterdam: Boom, pp. 89–96.

[26] van der Krieke L, Emerencia AC, Sytema S. (2011) An online portal on outcomes for Dutch service users. *Psychiatric Services* **62** (7): 803.

[27] van der Krieke L, Emerencia AC, Aiello M et al. (2012) Usability evaluation of a web-based support system for people with a schizophrenia diagnosis. *Journal of Medical Internet Research* **14** (1): e24.

CHAPTER 17

Psychiatric case registers: Their use in the era of global mental health

Povl Munk-Jørgensen and Niels Okkels

Department of Organic Psychiatric Disorders and Emergency Ward, Aarhus University Hospital, Risskov, Denmark

Introduction

The following statements can all be easily verified in any country with a well-functioning case register: 'The mortality among the severely mentally ill compared with the background population has not decreased', 'the length of hospitalisation periods continues to decrease' and 'readmission rates are still on the increase'. What we cannot demonstrate by means of registers is why the mortality is still high, or whether the decreasing length of hospitalisations is due to increasing quality of treatment, or if it is merely because of administrative decisions. The registers can also not help us in answering why readmission rates are still increasing.

Register research, in its present form, is based on the ability to process large, if not enormous, data sets and, most of all, society's acceptance of the registration of identifiable personal data and acceptance of data being used for research and administrative purposes.

Definition

In a 2009 editorial published in the *British Journal of Psychiatry*, Perera and co-authors [1] revived the now more than 25-year-old definition by Ten Horn [2] of 'a patient-centred longitudinal record of contacts with a defined set of psychiatric services originating from a defined population'. This definition originates from a 1983 World Health Organization (WHO) working group from Mannheim, Germany [3].

This is a very broad, but useful, definition, which highlights the two principal requirements:

1 Following a patient on his or her way through a variety of treatment institutions.
2 Covering a well-defined population, that is, a well-defined administrative catchment area, for example, a health service district, municipality, county or country, which, until now, is the largest area registered.

Improving Mental Health Care: The Global Challenge, First Edition.
Edited by Graham Thornicroft, Mirella Ruggeri and David Goldberg.
© 2013 John Wiley & Sons, Ltd. Published 2013 by John Wiley & Sons, Ltd.

Under this umbrella definition, each register must operationalise the requirements, for example, as done for the Psychiatric Case Register Middle Netherlands by Smeets et al. [4] or for the Danish Psychiatric Central Register [5–7], the latter fitting the following criteria:

- Clearly defined variables.
- Data are person-identifiable through a unique person-identifiable number, making it possible to follow the patients through psychiatry, somatic health service, primary care, social registers, taxation register, etc.
- Data are exhaustive, for example, when a register covers a defined type of institution in a catchment area, it must report all institutions of that type in the catchment area covered.
- The register is data-excluding, that is, if a certain variable, for example, auxiliary diagnosis or somatic diagnosis, is not reported from all institutions reporting to the register, those reported will be excluded.
- Data are collected continuously – there are no time limits for the existence of the register; every time a patient enters one of the reporting institutions, his or her present data are added to his or her record in the register.

Types of use

More attempts to classify the use of modern health registers for research and clinical purposes have been launched, for example, by Mortensen in 1995 [8] and Tansella and Ruggeri [9], and summarised by Tansella [10] and, more recently, by Wierdsma et al. [11].

We shall not propose yet another classification or grouping of the use of registers but will restrict ourselves to presenting and discussing some examples of the most frequent types of research. These will be *health service research, outcome studies, identification of representative clinical cohorts, follow-up of clinical cohorts* and *linkage to bio-banks*.

As the majority of health registers are established, processed and used for administrative purposes, they are used mainly for descriptive/administrative research. However, registers are most useful when used in health service research.

Health service research

The simplest forms of health service research, or, perhaps, better medical statistics, are prevalence and incidence studies. It is in the interest of professionals and not least of administrators and politicians to see how psychiatric services are used. For example, the regular description of diagnostic profiles in each hospital obtained by sending out questionnaires to every department in a huge catchment area (e.g. Denmark) and then collecting the data, validating them and analysing them was an enormous effort 50 years ago [12]. This has now become very easy and can be done almost automatically within hours with the help of electronic registers – a technical possibility that was already available in the 1970s [12].

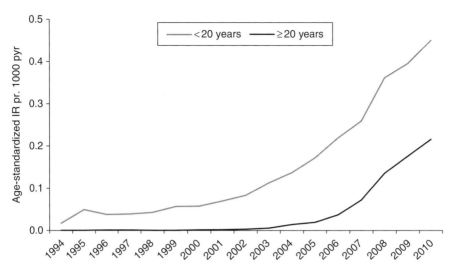

Figure 17.1 Age-standardised incidence of rate of ADHD [16].

Through modern statistical methods, we can achieve a high-quality overview of, for example, the development of a changing diagnostic profile, with work by Lay and colleagues from Canton Zürich [13] finding a 50% reduction in the length of inpatient episodes for patients with psychosis from 1977 to 2004, a 100% increase of inpatient admissions and, parallel to this, a mere 50% reduction in the proportion of schizophrenia among inpatients from 1977 to 1993 – this on a background of a two-to-threefold increase in other patient groups.

A thorough review of the prevalence of schizophrenia by Saha et al. [14] includes many papers based on register studies.

Pharmaco-epidemiological studies indicate different treatment principles in different diagnostic and treatment cultures; for example, the use of pharmaceutical compounds prescribed for the treatment of attention deficit hyperactivity disorder (ADHD) by using prescription databases shows a sevenfold variation among the five Nordic countries [15]. However, is this perhaps caused by variation in the incidence of ADHD? This question illustrates the most important limitation of administrative health service registers: that we cannot add anything about the causes from our findings. Is the variation due to different treatment cultures? Is it due to different diagnostic habits? Is it due to variations in identification rates of the disease? Or is it due to true differences in the population of incidence/prevalence of the disease?

Incidence studies represent a register research discipline producing data in the grey zone between health service research for administrative and political use on the one side and causative research on the other.

As recent examples, a few simple studies can be mentioned, for example, an increase in new cases of ADHD over a certain period of time (Figure 17.1) [16] or in the use of schizophrenia diagnosis in children and adolescents [17].

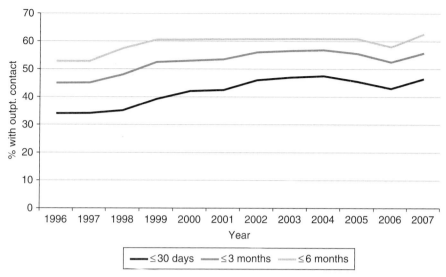

Figure 17.2 Time from latest schizophrenia discharge to contact [5].

Changes in incidence over time or differences in incidence in different environments lead us to question the causes for these differences. The problem is that the incidences we can identify in health service registers are not population incidences – which is what we need for performing causative research – they are treated incidences, that is, they are dependent on how many cases pass the threshold from the population and primary care into secondary care, a pathway that is dependent on the capacity of secondary care and competences, as well as the willingness of primary care to refer and the willingness of the population to be treated in secondary care. After having passed these thresholds [18], the patient then faces different diagnostic cultures and traditions among services and over geography, to mention but a few of the most common causes for heterogeneity found in the registers.

The question about how many cases in the population are reaching secondary health care and therefore enter the psychiatric registers has been a topic of debate during the entire 50 years of electronic-based register research. Weiser et al. [19] have validated this by using data from a population survey in Israeli registers and comparing their findings with the Israeli National Psychiatric Hospitalization Registry 24 years later, identifying 93% of the cases from the survey.

Figure 17.2 shows a classic example of medical statistics/health service research. It illustrates the percentage of patients discharged from inpatient treatment diagnosed with schizophrenia until their first appearance in an out-patient service within 30 days, 3 months and 6 months, respectively. The diagram shows an increase of 10–15% over a ten-year period, reaching close to 70% registered as outpatients within a six-month period following discharge from inpatient treatment. This type of result must never be used without being discussed or commented upon. At first glance, there is a positive trend – the percentage of patients continuing in an outpatient setting within a maximum of six months of discharge is increasing. But what is discouraging is the result that fewer than 70% reach an outpatient treatment programme within six months of discharge – a result that has not seen considerable improvement since 2001/2002. However, there are many reservations about the results that need to be dealt with before definitive conclusions can be drawn.

- We do not know what kinds of patients have been investigated. The statistical data in the register only inform us that someone in clinical psychiatry has diagnosed a person with schizophrenia and reported it to the register; they do not reveal any further details.
- We do not know how severely ill each patient is.
- We do not know if they are mildly ill.
- We do not know what has happened to them, in particular for the more than 30% not initiating an outpatient treatment programme within six months of discharge from inpatient treatment. Have some of them dropped out from treatment? Have some of them died? Are some of them in good care in social psychiatric institutions, in sheltered living accommodations or in hostels (not reporting to health registers in Denmark)?
- Are they homeless and living on the streets or are they living with elderly parents?
- Are they well-treated by their general practitioner (GP) or by a practising psychiatric specialist (none of them reporting to the psychiatric register in Denmark)?
- Or has something else happened?

Our sole conclusion is that between 65% and 70% of those discharged from a psychiatric inpatient treatment having been diagnosed with schizophrenia are showing up in the secondary health-care outpatient setting within six months of discharge. The basic nature of the data does not allow us to come to a conclusion on other issues such as what kind of treatment they get, what is the quality of this treatment and what has happened to those not included. Making a regular health service research effort, linking the psychiatric register to the causes of death register, to the register on where people are living, to the GP and practising psychiatric specialist register identifying days of consultations, to the prescription register to see if they have obtained the medicine prescribed, to social registers to see if they have been in contact with any social welfare systems, etc., would be of help. However, the quality of treatment and quality of living of those not in any identifiable treatment cannot be ascertained. As to the question about the validity of data from registers, we must conclude that no matter how clear the clinical information seems, it is still very sparse.

The more severe a disease, the higher is the possibility of finding the patient again in the register. In contrast, the milder a case, the lower is the possibility of finding the person in the register. This severe limitation may hinder our understanding of a disease like schizophrenia, because we have very limited knowledge about possible mild cases of schizophrenia if, indeed, they exist. We tend to define schizophrenia based on the cases seen in secondary-health-care-identifiable cases in the registers.

Concerning affective disorders, in particular major depressive disorders, the picture is somewhat different, because it is so obvious that only 5–10% (maximum) of the cases reach secondary health care [18]. That, however, implies that the value of register research on major depressive disorders is of very little use for the treatment of the 90–95% of major depressive disorders in the population, of which only approximately half reach treatment level in primary health care, thus introducing bias into the case register system. When considering Denmark, it should be noted that outpatient visits were included in 1995 and that Denmark shifted from International Classification of Diseases (ICD)-8 to ICD-10 in 1994.

Revisiting schizophrenia incidence (which is, in fact, treated incidence) has shown tremendous oscillations from around 10 and 5 per 100 000 male and female, respectively, in the early 1970s to approximately 6 and 4, respectively, in the early 1980s, and is now around 20 in total for both sexes in the 2000s [20, 21, The Danish Psychiatric Central Research Register, personal communication].

Outcome and prediction of outcome

Suicidology has for many years now been a major discipline within register research, perhaps because the event – suicide – is a catastrophic incident. It may also be because the validity of the variable is very high in operating registers. The first steps taken 50 years ago in register-based research mostly described incidences of suicide, and changes in these incidences and methods of suicide (poisoning, shooting, hanging, and so on). The cases of suicide could be identified in national mortality statistics, and, subsequently, could be searched in health registers and vice versa. The next step after mere description of changes in incidence was prediction analysis, which was made possible by linking two or more registers. An early study from Mortensen's group [22] shows the benefits derived from linking several registers using modern computer technology that is able to handle very large data sets, and modern epidemiology and biostatistics. Later, high-quality examples from Sweden from Reutfors et al.'s group [23], which investigated more than 20 000 suicides, replicated Rosseau and Mortensen's [22] findings of the immediate phase after discharge from psychiatric hospitalisation as the most high-risk period [23]. Furthermore, Nordentoft et al. [24] identified the important finding that a decrease in suicide rates in patients with schizophrenia is proportional to a decrease in the background population.

These studies illustrate the importance of linking registers, perhaps the most dramatic progress in epidemiological research, which may even be comparable to the most revolutionary breakthrough in biological medicine, such as brain imaging techniques and nanotechnology.

Regrettably, the predictors identified in this kind of suicide register research are of limited value in directly preventing clinical and public health interventions because suicide is, however tragic, a very rare event resulting in the predictors receiving a low predictive value; for example, it is not of any clinical use to know that the odds ratio of men committing suicide as compared with women is 2:1 – a 100% doubling. A further limitation in predictive register research is the predictor variables available. We can only very rarely use those variables which, from a theoretical point of view, could test our hypothesis. Instead, we are restricted to using the variables already in the registers, mostly for administrative purposes; that is, our analysis will be predominantly exploratory instead of hypothesis testing.

In contrast to suicide research, register research aimed at predicting mortality rates in psychiatrically ill patients with physical illnesses has a much higher impact because of the very high occurrence of physical illnesses in the mentally ill. This research started peaking in the years following Harris and Barraclough's benchmarking study in 1998 [25], which showed increased mortality in patients with mental illness because of physical diseases.

Register-linking studies are a unique tool for mapping this issue, for example, the study by Munk-Jørgensen et al. [26], which followed an exploratory model examining a broader spectrum of physical diseases in schizophrenia. More specifically, association studies have been performed between schizophrenia and autoimmune diseases [27] and between autoimmune diseases and severe infections as risk factors for schizophrenia [28], acute myocardial infarction in depression, anxiety and schizophrenia [29], and hypertension in bipolar disorder, anxiety and schizophrenia [30].

However, having access only to those variables already in the registers and not to those which would be most relevant is still a problem.

Identification of representative clinical cohorts

As we will further discuss in this chapter, the major advantages of register research are its high level of representativeness and, therefore, generalisability of results. The price to pay, however, is the low data validity and reliability. Combining registers with clinical data helps to maximize the benefits. This is done by identifying a representative cohort years back and following it in a register, and then contacting the identified people for further clinical research interview and investigation. An example of this method has been used by Munk-Jørgensen et al. [31]. Such a cohort, however, suffers from low data quality at index.

If the purpose is to create a representative cohort which actually has its first contact with the health service system 'now' for future personal research-based interviews and examination, we have almost created the highest-quality situation benefitting from a high level of representativeness as well as a high level of data quality. In this situation of high representativeness and high data quality, we lose one of the advantages of register research: the historical prospective follow-up in the register; that is, we have the disadvantages of the high costs of long-term personal research follow-up, and we still have to rely on retrospective data.

From Sweden, we find a classical example of combining identification of probands in registers followed by collection of detailed clinical data *in casu* from case records when analysing the diagnostic profile among suicide cases [32].

Follow-up of clinical cohorts

Clinically established cohorts suffer from two limitations when followed up: first, because of being clinically established, they can, in the vast majority of situations, have only local representativeness and therefore limited generalisability; second, they suffer from loss to follow up because of death, moving out of the catchment area, dropping out of treatment/research programme, and so on.

When using registers to supplement a personal follow-up, it is possible to identify the addresses and re-establish a personal contact with some of the probands who have dropped out and those who have left the catchment area. As for those who have died, immigrated or in other ways 'disappeared', it is possible to identify some data, but this is not of great quality: for example, the number of hospitalisations, the prescriptions picked up and the number of visits to GPs or practising specialists. A fine example of this is the five-year follow-up of a first episode psychosis cohort by Bertelsen et al. [33].

Some very large sample clinical databases designed for long-term follow-up studies, which, however, cannot be defined as registers, are more valuable for cause-searching research than (administrative) health registers, for example, the New Zealand Christchurch cohort [34], the UK 1946 birth cohort [35] and the Finland 1966 birth cohort [36]. When using these databases, researchers have the opportunity to supplement clinical follow-up data with nationwide register data, improving data compilation and, through that, generalisability [36].

More examples of this using a very large sample database followed up in registers can be obtained in the Swedish conscript database, which is linked to national registers by Allbeck's group. This has given us invaluable information on cannabis as a risk factor – direct or indirect – for suicide [37]. The same database has also used the principle of linking with national registers, drawing the conclusion that psychiatric diagnosis given in adolescents increases the risk for suicide not only in the immediate future but also in the years to come [38].

Linkage to bio-banks

As mentioned at the beginning of this chapter, traditional psychiatric register research can describe the medical statistics of any given psychiatric illness, and can predict course and outcome to a very detailed degree. Over the past 50 years, the methodology for doing research linking several registers has become increasingly sophisticated, and, when using modern computer technology, there are no upper limits on the size of the data sets that can be handled, or on the number of registers that can be linked.

However, there is one unbreakable limit: traditional (administrative) register research cannot answer the 'whys'. While it can predict who is at risk of developing a given disease, it cannot identify the cause of the disease, that is, the pathogenesis. Therefore, we have to investigate the unique patient, and as soon as we do so, we are in danger of losing the representativeness. We can, to some extent, retain a certain degree of representativeness by using the methods described earlier, identifying a cohort for research by means of registers, but we are still down to a limited number of probands. There is a limitation both in terms of finance and time as to how many patients we can identify and examine personally. However, this can, to a vast degree, be overcome by using the very large bio-banks established in recent years. Therefore, when linking traditional health service registers with bio-banks, it is possible to bypass the time-consuming and expensive part of a research programme by identifying the patients, approaching them, examining them and collecting blood samples or other biological samples. An early example of this is the identification of *Toxoplasma gondii* as a risk factor for early-onset schizophrenia by Mortensen's group [39].

Strengths and limitations

We have touched upon the question of strengths and limitations connected to register research earlier. This will now be discussed further, in particular in so far as it concerns register research when attempting to answer clinical questions.

Psychiatric register research deals with that part of a total population which has (a) been identified as having a psychiatric illness and (b) has overcome the threshold for being offered treatment by an institution covered by registers useable for research.

The registers give no information about the entire population, only about individuals admitted, and, furthermore, we know nothing about their diseases; the only information is that a group of individuals has been given a certain diagnosis. This fact is very often forgotten and the studies are at risk of drawing hasty conclusions. Examples of this are seen in research about suicide among psychiatric patients/former psychiatric patients compared with suicide in the general population never admitted to psychiatric institutions. The reasons for possible differences/no differences discussed are almost pure guesswork: we know nothing about the mental status of those who have committed suicide in the portion of the population that have never been recorded in a psychiatric register or that have never been in contact with a psychiatric institution. These individuals may well have been mentally ill without being treated or may have been treated in services not reporting to the register, but are, however, defined as not mentally ill in the analyses.

Table 17.1 Strengths and limitations in register studies compared with some clinical types of studies.

	Naturalistic follow-up	Case-control study	Historical register follow-up study	Health service register research
Validity of explanatory variables	↑↑	↓	↓	↑↑
Validity of outcome variables	↑↑	↑↑	↓	↑↑
Representativeness	↓	↓↓	↑	↑↑
Time consumption	↓↓	↑	↑↑	↑↑
Expenses	↓↓	↑	↑↑	↑↑

↑, strength; ↑↑, important strength; ↓, limitation; ↓↓, severe limitation.

Also, measuring changes in length of stay over time gives meaning only to those institutions covered by registers. The length of stay may easily decline in a monitored psychiatric hospital but may remain long, and maybe even increase, in a neighbouring private hospital not reporting to the register in question.

A clinical naturalistic follow-up study, for example, the Copenhagen High Risk Study [40], has a very high data validity of both explanatory variables and outcome variables because the researchers have followed the probands throughout the entire study collecting data only for research purposes. The representativeness may be questionable, as it includes a certain group of probands selected from what is available. It is also a very time-consuming and expensive process and requires extensive manpower (Table 17.1).

The clinical case-control study sampling patients at the time of 'outcome' has very limited data quality with regard to explanatory variables, because they must be collected from data sources such as case records and retrospective interviews. The validity of the outcome data is high because the researchers have the possibility of collecting data directly from the patient about variables designed for the study. The representativeness is low because the probands represent only those patients who are alive and present, for example, schizophrenia patients alive and in contact with the service performing the study. The data for patients who have died or have dropped out and who should have been included is lost. The time consumption is a relative limitation because it takes time to dig up data from the various data sources. This makes the expenses rather high, because all patients should be interviewed for collecting outcome data; however, they are not as high as in the long-term follow-up (Table 17.1).

In contrast to the two methods (the clinical long-term follow-up and the clinical retrospective case-control study), a historical prospective register follow-up study has limited data quality concerning both explanatory variables and outcome variables. As these are indeed clinical data, they are in fact heterogeneous, changing clinical trends and approaches over time, as well as geography and psychiatric schools.

The high representativeness is one of the strengths, because the probands are identified in the registers when they were all present years ago at registration. After their indexed admission, they are followed in one or more registers, and it is even possible to supplement the register follow-up with a personal follow-up of those still alive and identified by public civil registers. It is not optimal because they are representative only of those groups of patients included in the register. Time consumption is minimal and expenses are limited, which are also strengths (Table 17.1).

To do justice to register research, it must be underlined that if the purpose is certain areas of administrative health service research, such as the number of bed days or outpatient visits, the average length of stay and readmission rates, the register study is second to none. Indeed, all the items listed in Table 17.1 – validity of both explanatory and outcome variables, representativeness, time consumption and expenses – should be given maximum rating for strengths.

The dubious quality of the validity of data in the large (nationwide) administrative health registers calls for a continuous validation of register data when used for research. Mors et al. [6] identified five validation studies of diagnoses in the Danish Psychiatric Register compared to case notes. Jörgensen et al. [41] documented that register-originated incidence studies of non-affective psychosis from Sweden would be severely underestimated if they did not include outpatient services.

Few studies validate register data against research interviews of patients. This method is exemplified by Hansen et al.'s validation study from 2000 [42], which examined newly admitted patients for substance use disorders and compared their findings first to clinical case notes and then to register data. They found a high concordance between case notes and register data, but a severe under-reporting of diagnoses in case notes summarising the clinical findings. These findings point to the importance of keeping case records on a high-quality level as they are otherwise a weak link in the process of data collection.

Byrne and colleagues [43] found only 14 studies in a systematic review of validity studies in psychiatric register research. Based on this review, Parker [44] argued strongly for 'representative constituent dataset examined for validity at appropriate intervals'. Five years earlier, Tansella [10], the founder of the South Verona Psychiatric Case Register, predicted that there will 'probably' be a need for psychiatric case registers and pointed at the lack of 'direct evidence' for register cost-effective tools 'for improving our understanding of the causes, course and outcome of mental disorders as well for making more rational use of mental health services'.

In an overview article on case registers, Allebeck [45] argues for further utilisation of registers in research and underlines the importance of the critical consideration of quality with a specific focus on *coverage, attrition, representativeness* and *validity* of registers. The debate about registers supports the continuing use of registers in psychiatric research, but points to different aspects of validity problems which, in the future, must attract attention.

Ethics

Povl Munk-Jørgensen (the senior author of this chapter) remembers a time in the late 1970s and early 1980s when at least in Scandinavia the instances of control at the administrative and political level related to granting permission for the use of data from registers became overwhelming, and in some research milieus was considered to be obstructive. The reality now, however, is quite the opposite – it is now very easy to get permission to use register data. In practice, the public, through its representatives the politicians, is no longer part of the process. One should anticipate a massive (read: political and/or media created) reaction against the use of public registers and databases within either a shorter or longer period of time. Twenty-five years ago, important results were obtained in Denmark by including the leading patients and relatives' organisation at the time as an official collaborator in the use of the Danish Psychiatric Register for research. A massive resistance to the register over a period of two to three years changed into positive collaboration and support. Perhaps it would be fruitful to revitalise a public debate about the extensive use of register research in certain countries.

The future for psychiatric register research

Where should psychiatric case register research go in the future?

We have exemplified some authors' arguments for the continuous use of registers in psychiatric research, but under the condition of an intensified validation of data [10, 43–45] and evaluation of cost-effectiveness [10]. Wierdsma et al. [11] point out the severe lack of serving health-care stakeholders with sufficient information for evaluating health-care policies and cooperation between mental health care and public service, despite a wide range of research carried out with the registers. One wonders if the politicians would have given as much financial priority to treatment of first-episode psychosis if they had been fully informed about the 12–15-fold difference in admission of first-episode psychoses and readmission of schizophrenia [46], the latter being a severely burdened group with high public expenses, both direct and indirect (Figure 17.3).

Perera and colleagues [1] made a list of recent advantages in modern registers, which should facilitate the use of psychiatric case registers. One way to go about this would be to continue the classical linking strategy. However, instead of ad hoc linking for each research project, linking could be done electronically, giving the researcher direct and immediate access to all the data sets needed; a super-register could also be created if technological advances allow this. However, no matter how many administrative registers we link, it will not solve the problem of the lack of clinical and biological data, though with case notes becoming increasingly electronic, it gives us access to full text case notes. This is being used in the South London and Maudsley NHS Foundation Trust Biomedical Research

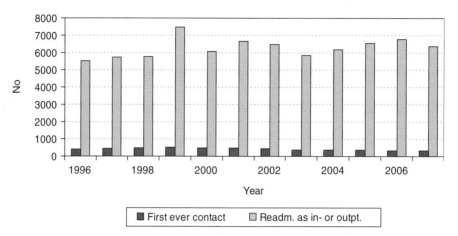

Figure 17.3 First ever contact/readmitted with schizophrenia in Denmark, IDD-10 F20 [46].

Centre (SLAM BRC) Case Register [47], which covers a 1 000 000+ catchment area. Similar ideas are being discussed presently in Denmark (P. Munk-Jørgensen, personal communication), which would cover 5.5 million inhabitants. This model calls for a revitalised public–political debate about the ethical and juridical aspects of using person-identifiable data to such an extreme extent.

Another way to go about this would be to make better use of the classical local case register [48], a model sophisticated in, for example, the South Verona Psychiatric Case Register, as will be discussed later. This model could, along with the super-register, present electronic full text case notes. It has several advantages: it is integrated in clinical daily practice, clinical working professionals will gain an epidemiological overview of their activities and research will be driven by relevant clinical problems and hypothesis. Additional patient-focused research activities will not be removed from the daily clinical treatment of patients, and it will be inspired by clinical problems.

A third model may be an intensifying of hypothesis-driven research based on linking between data from administrative registers and bio-banks. This would benefit the biological cause-seeking research in maintaining a high level of representativeness. Another advantage would be the possibility of a close connection to population's representatives, the ethical committees, the data surveillance authorities, politicians and the population in general, making these bodies able to follow and discuss progress in psychiatric (register) research.

The clinically focused register revisited

Some minor registers such as the Italian South Verona Psychiatric Case Register can be defined as a continuation of the pioneering local registers presented in *Psychiatric Case Registers in Public Health* [48].

The South Verona Psychiatric Case Register has been in operation since 1979. It covers a population of 75 000 and is therefore able to collect several detailed data about psychiatry and somatic and social variables, with high validity and reliability. This register has contributed continuously to the international literature over a span of more than 30 years, documenting the importance of smaller, intensive clinical registers. Examples of this are studies about highly relevant topics: mortality among psychiatric patients [49], avoidable mortality [50] and health economic aspects of community psychiatry [51].

The South Verona Psychiatric Case Register was established as part of the South Verona Community Mental Health Service. It has, therefore, contributed to the ongoing and comprehensive evaluation of the service from its very beginning over the consolidating years into routine [52, 53] and further development over more than 30 years, and it is gradually also being used for more cause-seeking research.

The establishment of the register as an integrated part of a new service is an ideal model for any new service that would like to establish itself responsibly in a political, organisational and academic context.

Academic articles published by this service show how well clinical research benefits from using the register (http://www.psychiatry.univr.it); for example, Tansella et al. [54] used data from the register to provide illustrative documentation of the shift from inpatient to outpatient and day-patient treatment over 25 years of the service's treatment profile.

Final remarks

When rereading Ten Horn and co-editors' benchmarking book from 1986 [48], it is striking how the authors communicated their messages clearly and presented data of high educational quality. This was also recently done by, for example, Amaddeo et al. [53].

Keeping these examples in mind, one notices how the language in today's register-generated health research has shifted towards epidemiological/statistical jargon and, consequently, is at great risk of losing the average clinical working reader or the public health service worker, both of whom should be the key readers of the articles.

As the authors of this chapter, we should be the first to acknowledge the impressive progress in theory, methodology and information technology capacity, which have characterised the development of register research since the early 1970s. However, a consequence – a side effect, so to say – has been that register research is progressively being hidden away in epidemiological centres, health service research institutes and register research centres staffed with epidemiologists, statisticians and software engineers, some with only a few medically educated people with no, or only homoeopathic, clinical experience. This is necessary in order to handle and develop methods and techniques, but we are in danger of losing those colleagues who should benefit from the research.

In this process, the research is in danger of losing the feeling for the clinical topics and losing the prime audience. This could be a challenge to modern register-based research in the coming years.

Over the past 50 years, register research has developed from the local, pioneering, clinically based register, established after World War II, until now, where we have the possibility of handling enormous data sets in super-registers. The main trend in how these opportunities should be used in the future should not be left to single groups, register researchers and epidemiologists, health trust administrators, politicians or any other group. We conclude in strong support of Wierdsma et al. [11] when they call for 'join[ing of] the forces' and suggest a renewal of the WHO initiative which organised a workgroup on psychiatric case register in Mannheim 30 years ago in 1983.

References

[1] Perera G, Soremekun M, Breen G et al. (2009) The psychiatric case register: noble past, challenging present, but exciting future. *British Journal of Psychiatry* **195**: 191–193.

[2] Ten Horn GHMM. (1986) Definitions and classifications: introduction. In: Ten Horn GHMM, Giel R, Gulbinat WH et al. (eds.), *Psychiatric Case Registers in Public Health: A Worldwide Inventory 1960–1985*, 1st edn. Amsterdam: Elsevier Science Publishers B.V., pp. 170–174.

[3] Ten Horn GHMM. (1983) *Psychiatric Case Registers*. Report on a WHO working group, Mannheim, Copenhagen: World Health Organization.

[4] Smeets HM, Laan W, Engelhard IM et al. (2011) The psychiatric case register middle Netherlands. *BMC Psychiatry* **11**: 106.

[5] Munk-Jorgensen P, Mortensen PB. (1997) The Danish psychiatric central register. *Danish Medical Bulletin* **44**: 82–84.

[6] Mors O, Perto GP, Mortensen PB. (2011) The Danish psychiatric central research register. *Scandinavian Journal of Public Health* **39** (Suppl. 7): 54–57.

[7] Munk-Jørgensen P, Østergaard SD. (2011) Register-based studies of mental disorders. *Scandinavian Journal of Public Health* **39** (Suppl. 7): 170–174.

[8] Mortensen PB. (1995) The untapped potential of case registers and record-linkage studies in psychiatric epidemiology. *Epidemiologic Reviews* **17**: 205–209.

[9] Tansella M, Ruggeri M. (1996) Monitoring and evaluating a community-based mental health service: the epidemiological approach. In: Peckham M, Smith R (eds.), *Scientific Basis of Health Services*. London: BMJ Publishing Group, pp. 160–169.

[10] Tansella M. (2000) Do we still need psychiatric case registers? *Acta Psychiatrica Scandinavica* **101**: 253–255.

[11] Wierdsma AI, Sytema S, van Os J et al. (2008) Case registers in psychiatry: do they still have a role for research and service monitoring? *Current Opinion in Psychiatry* **21**: 379–384.

[12] Munk-Jorgensen P, Weeke A, Jensen EB et al. (1986) Changes in utilization of Danish psychiatric institutions. II. Census studies 1977 and 1982. *Comprehensive Psychiatry* **27**: 416–429.

[13] Lay B, Nordt C, Rossler W. (2007) Trends in psychiatric hospitalisation of people with schizophrenia: a register-based investigation over the last three decades. *Schizophrenia Research* **97**: 68–78.

[14] Saha S, Chant D, Welham J et al. (2005) A systematic review of the prevalence of schizophrenia. *PLoS Medicine* **2**: e141.

[15] Zoega H, Furu K, Halldorsson M et al. (2011) Use of ADHD drugs in the Nordic countries: a population-based comparison study. *Acta Psychiatrica Scandinavica* **123**: 360–367.

[16] Kjeldsen BV, Jensen SO, Munk-Jorgensen P. (2012) Increasing number of incident ADHD cases in psychiatric treatment. *Acta Psychiatrica Scandinavica* **126**: 151–152.

[17] Okkels N, Vernal DL, Jensen SO et al. (2012) Changes in the diagnosed incidence of early onset schizophrenia over four decades. *Acta Psychiatrica Scandinavica* **127**: 62–68.

[18] Goldberg G, Goodyer I. (2005). *The Distribution of Common Mental Disorders. The Origins and Course of Common Mental Disorders*, 1st edn. New York: Routledge, pp. 16–32.

[19] Weiser M, Werbeloff N, Dohrenwend BP et al. (2012) Do psychiatric registries include all persons with schizophrenia in the general population? A population-based longitudinal study. *Schizophrenia Research* **135**: 187–191.

[20] Munk-Jorgensen P, Mortensen PB. (1992) Incidence and other aspects of the epidemiology of schizophrenia in Denmark, 1971–87. *British Journal of Psychiatry* **161**: 489–495.

[21] Tsuchiya KJ, Munk-Jorgensen P. (2002) First-admission rates of schizophrenia in Denmark, 1980–1997: have they been increasing? *Schizophrenia Research* **54**:187–191.

[22] Rossau CD, Mortensen PB. (1997) Risk factors for suicide in patients with schizophrenia: nested case-control study. *British Journal of Psychiatry* **171**: 355–359.

[23] Reutfors J, Brandt L, Ekbom A et al. (2010) Suicide and hospitalization for mental disorders in Sweden. A population-based case-control study. *Journal of Psychiatric Research* **44**: 741–747.

[24] Nordentoft M, Munk Laursen T, Agerbo E et al. (2004) Changes in suicide rates for patients with schizophrenia in Denmark, 1981–97: nested case control. *BMJ* **329**: 261.

[25] Harris EC, Barraclough B. (1998) Excess mortality of mental disorder. *British Journal of Psychiatry* **173**: 11–53.

[26] Munk-Jørgensen P, Mors O, Mortensen PB et al. (2000) The schizophrenic patients in the somatic hospital. *Acta Psychiatrica Scandinavica* **102** (Suppl. 407): 96–99.

[27] Eaton WW, Byrne M, Ewald H et al. (2006) Association of schizophrenia and autoimmune diseases: linkage of Danish medical registers. *American Journal of Psychiatry* **163**: 521–528.

[28] Benros ME, Nielsen PR, Nordentoft M et al. (2011) Autoimmune diseases and severe infections as risk factors for schizophrenia: a 30-year population-based register study. *American Journal of Psychiatry* **168**: 1303–1310.

[29] Jakobsen AH, Foldager L, Parker G et al. (2008) Quantifying links between acute myocardial infarction and depression, anxiety and schizophrenia using case register databases. *Journal of Affective Disorder* **109**: 177–181.

[30] Johannessen L, Strudsholm U, Foldager L et al. (2006) Increased risk of hypertension in patients with bipolar disorder and patients with anxiety compared to background population and patients with schizophrenia. *Journal of Affective Disorders* **95**: 13–17.

[31] Munk-Jørgensen P, Mortensen PB, Machón RA. (1991) Hospitalization patterns in schizophrenia. A 13-year follow-up. *Schizophrenia Research* **4**: 1–9.

[32] Reutfors J, Bahmanyar S, Jönsson EG et al. (2010) Diagnostic profile and suicide risk in schizophrenia spectrum disorder. *Schizophrenia Research* **123**: 251–256.

[33] Bertelsen M, Jeppesen P, Petersen L et al. (2008) Five-year follow-up of a randomized multicenter trial of intensive early intervention vs standard treatment for patients with a first episode of psychotic illness. *Archives of General Psychiatry* **65**: 762–771.

[34] Gibb SJ, Fergusson DM, Horwood LJ. (2011) Relationship separation and mental health problems: findings from a 30-year longitudinal study. *Australian and New Zealand Journal of Psychiatry* **45**: 163–169.

[35] Colman I, Ploubidis GB, Wadsworth ME et al. (2007) A longitudinal typology of symptoms of depression and anxiety over the life course. *Biological Psychiatry* **62**: 1265–1271.

[36] Moilanen K, Jokelainen J, Jones PB et al. (2010) Deviant intrauterine growth and risk of schizophrenia: a 34-year follow-up of the Northern Finland 1966 Birth Cohort. *Schizophrenia Research* **124**: 223–230.

[37] Price C, Hemmingsson T, Lewis G et al. (2009) Cannabis and suicide: longitudinal study. *British Journal of Psychiatry* **195**: 492–497.

[38] Lundin A, Lundberg I, Allebeck P et al. (2011) Psychiatric diagnosis in late adolescence and long-term risk of suicide and suicide attempt. *Acta Psychiatrica Scandinavica* **124**: 454–461.

[39] Mortensen PB, Norgaard-Pedersen B, Waltoft BL et al. (2007) *Toxoplasma gondii* as a risk factor for early-onset schizophrenia: analysis of filter paper blood samples obtained at birth. *Biological Psychiatry* **61**: 688–693.

[40] Mednick SA, Parnas J, Schulsinger F. (1987) The Copenhagen high-risk project, 1962–86. *Schizophrenia Bulletin* **13**: 485–495.

[41] Jörgensen L, Ahlbom A, Allebeck P et al. (2010) The Stockholm non-affective psychoses study (snaps): the importance of including out-patient data in incidence studies. *Acta Psychiatrica Scandinavica* **121**: 389–392.

[42] Hansen SS, Munk-Jørgensen P, Guldbæk B et al. (2000) Psychoactive substance use diagnoses among psychiatric in-patients. *Acta Psychiatrica Scandinavica* **102**: 432–438.

[43] Byrne N, Regan C, Howard L. (2005) Administrative registers in psychiatric research: a systematic review of validity studies. *Acta Psychiatrica Scandinavica* **112**: 409–414.

[44] Parker G. (2005) Register now: validity later. *Acta Psychiatrica Scandinavica* **112**: 407–408.

[45] Allebeck P. (2009) The use of population based registers in psychiatric research. *Acta Psychiatrica Scandinavica* **120**: 386–391.

[46] Munk-Jørgensen P, Nielsen J, Nielsen RE et al. (2009) Last episode psychosis. *Acta Psychiatrica Scandinavica* **119**: 417–418.

[47] Stewart R, Soremekun M, Perera G et al. (2009) The South London and Maudsley NHS Foundation Trust Biomedical Research Centre (SLAM BRC) case register: development and descriptive data. *BMC Psychiatry* **9**: 51.

[48] Ten Horn GHMM, Giel R, Gulbinat WH et al. (eds.) (1986) *Psychiatric Case Registers in Public Health*, 1st edn. Amsterdam: Elsevier Science Publishers.

[49] Grigoletti L, Perini G, Rossi A et al. (2009) Mortality and cause of death among psychiatric patients: a 20-year case-register study in an area with a community-based system of care. *Psychological Medicine* **39**: 1875–1884.

[50] Amaddeo F, Barbui C, Perini G et al. (2007) Avoidable mortality of psychiatric patients in an area with a community-based system of mental health care. *Acta Psychiatrica Scandinavica* **115**: 320–325.

[51] Donisi V, Jones J, Pertile R et al. (2011) The difficult task of predicting the costs of community-based mental health care. A comprehensive case register study. *Epidemiology and Psychiatric Sciences* **20**: 245–256.

[52] Lasaliva A, Ruggeri M. (2007) Assessing the outcome of community-based psychiatric care: building a feedback loop from 'real world' health services research into clinical practice. *Acta Psychiatrica Scandinavica* **116** (Suppl. 437): 6–15.

[53] Amaddeo F, Burti L, Ruggeri M et al. (2009) Long-term monitoring and evaluation of system of community-based psychiatric care. Integrating research, teaching and practice at the University of Verona. *Annali dell'Istituto Superiore di Sanità* **45**: 43–53.

[54] Tansella M, Amaddeo F, Burti L et al. (2006) Evaluating a community-based mental health service focusing on severe mental illness. The Verona experience. *Acta Psychiatrica Scandinavica* **113** (Suppl. 429): 90–94.

CHAPTER 18

Can brain imaging address psychosocial functioning and outcome in schizophrenia?

Marcella Bellani[1], Nicola Dusi[1] and Paolo Brambilla[2,3]

[1] Department of Public Health and Community Medicine, Section of Psychiatry and Section of Clinical Psychology, Inter-University Center for Behavioural Neurosciences (ICBN), University of Verona, Verona, Italy

[2] Department of Experimental & Clinical Medical Sciences (DISM), Inter-University Center for Behavioural Neurosciences (ICBN), University of Udine, Udine, Italy

[3] Department of Psychiatry and Behavioral Sciences, University of Texas Medical School at Houston, USA

Introduction

Psychiatric diagnoses are still made using clinical interview and observation, without any specific contribution from instrumental and radiological investigations [1]. Towards the end of the twentieth century, several studies highlighted that there were some organic features of psychiatric conditions like schizophrenia [2]. Currently, imaging research mainly focuses on discovering cerebral 'biomarkers' and could help move to an aetiological and/or pathophysiological definition of the disease. Indeed, the progressive amelioration and advance of brain imaging is producing scientific advances in understanding schizophrenia and has potential applications as support to clinical definition of diagnosis, prognosis and clinical/psychosocial outcome [3]. In this regard, schizophrenia has always been considered a disease that severely affects cognitive and social functioning [4, 5]. Patients with schizophrenia report several limitations in daily living, such as self-care, employment and social life, regardless of their psychopathology or clinical state [6]. Social disability might be observed in patients before clinical manifestations of the disease and might not be influenced by effective pharmacological treatment [7]. Also, altered social functioning has been reported in patients at high risk of developing schizophrenia and in relatives of patients with schizophrenia [8]. Therefore, poor social outcome is a trait feature of the illness.

Starting from the 1970s, computerised tomography found ventricular enlargement and a generalised loss of brain tissue in patients with schizophrenia as compared to healthy controls [9]. In the following decades, structural magnetic

Improving Mental Health Care: The Global Challenge, First Edition.
Edited by Graham Thornicroft, Mirella Ruggeri and David Goldberg.
© 2013 John Wiley & Sons, Ltd. Published 2013 by John Wiley & Sons, Ltd.

resonance imaging (sMRI) has replicated those findings and convincingly demonstrated additional volume deficits in the prefrontal and temporal lobes, although it is still not clear whether these changes are progressive, and whether they may normalise after medication [10].

In addition, there is robust evidence that white matter pathology is implicated in schizophrenia [11]. Microstructural disruption of inter- and intra-hemispheric white matter has indeed been demonstrated by several imaging studies using diffusion weighted imaging, which is a technique examining the fine organisation of brain tissue, specifically of white matter [12, 13]. In this regard, connectivity disturbances have been suggested to play a major role in schizophrenia [14, 15], potentially being sustained by two main different mechanisms, the *hyper-connectivity hypothesis*, in which synapses are supposed not to be eliminated during brain development [16], and the *hypo-connectivity hypothesis*, in which too many synapses are eliminated during development because of abnormal interactions between neurons [17]. Moreover, other connectivity theories have focused on *aberrant neural timing* in schizophrenia [18–20], which could be caused by conduction delays arising from structural damage to the white matter fasciculi that physically connect spatially different populations of neurons [19, 21].

Thus, there is reason to suspect that schizophrenia is associated with aberrant inter- and intra-hemispheric connectivity, which has been suggested to ultimately affect cognition and, finally, psychosocial functioning of patients suffering from this illness.

In this regard, David proposed abnormal inter-hemispheric integration as a 'plausible model for a range of psychiatric phenomena from alexithymia to delusions and hallucinations' [22]. Indeed, white matter disruption may alter inter-hemispheric communication and functional brain lateralisation in patients with schizophrenia [23, 24], as also suggested by results from our group showing widespread abnormal fronto-temporal and callosal white matter coherence in a large epidemiological-based sample of subjects with schizophrenia [25, 26]. In this perspective, it has recently been shown that better performance in declarative memory and executive functions correlated with higher coherence of white matter in hippocampus, parahippocampus and corpus callosum in schizophrenia [27]. Also, abnormal white matter integrity has been found in poor-outcome patients suffering from the disorder [28]. With regard to corpus callosum, it is already well known that it is crucial for the development of structural brain asymmetry, which has been found to be reduced in schizophrenia [23, 24, 29]. Moreover, it is generally well accepted that cerebral asymmetry, which is the anatomical substrate of the functional lateralisation, occurs with decreased callosal connectivity [30]. Although this may be an oversimplification [31], the current models of inter-hemispheric communication in humans suggest that the correlation between cerebral asymmetry and callosal connectivity is inversed, and that cortical areas are topographically mapped in the corpus callosum [32]. Therefore, exchange of inter-hemispheric information decreases with increasing cerebral asymmetry, leading to hemispheric independence/dominance of the human brain [33–35].

In the last decades, it has been consistently found that hemispheric asymmetries are abnormal in schizophrenia [36] and the overall balance indicates a left hemisphere abnormality [37]. This picture clearly suggests white matter abnormalities in schizophrenia, mainly located in the corpus callosum and involving size reduction and microstructural disorganisation. This white matter disruption may ultimately alter the fasciculi that connect, in particular, the frontal and temporal lobes [21]. A meta-analysis by Ellison-Wright and Bullmore [38] of 15 voxel-based diffusion imaging studies confirmed the presence of abnormalities in frontally projecting fasciculi in patients with schizophrenia. In this perspective, in a longitudinal study an abnormal developmental trajectory for the splenium of the corpus callosum was shown in patients with childhood-onset schizophrenia during adolescence and early adulthood [39]. However, it is unclear whether these alterations result from faulty neurodevelopment or constitute compensatory changes that may develop over the course of the illness. It indeed needs to be elucidated whether microstructure alterations of white matter fibres is due to dys-/demyelination, variation of membrane permeability to water, less dense packing of fibres and/or disruption of internal axonal integrity (reduced intra-axonal microtubular density). Since white matter is mostly composed of myelinated axons, the density of axonal membranes and myelin should play a major role. Postmortem studies also support this evidence, describing reductions in white matter cells, and in expression of myelin- and oligodendrocyte-related genes [40–42].

In this context, oligodendrocytes may play a major role for the white matter alterations in schizophrenia, since they are the myelin-producing cells in the central nervous system [43]. Therefore, dysfunctional oligodendrocytes may lead to impaired myelination and synaptic transmission, which ultimately result in altered connectivity and cognition. Moreover, abnormalities in the expression of genes and proteins associated with the integrity of the nodes of Ranvier also support the role of oligodendrocytes for the dysconnectivity syndrome in schizophrenia [43]. Nonetheless, the origin of such abnormalities is still largely unknown.

In this regard, the role of inflammation may be crucial in schizophrenia [44–46]. There is in fact evidence that some pro-inflammatory cytokines (e.g. IFN-γ, IL-1β, IL-6, IL-18) have a potential pathogenic role for the CNS, causing cell damage, affecting myelin structures or activating macrophages [47]. Cytokines and chemokines are indeed the most promising markers of chronic immune demyelinating diseases, such as multiple sclerosis [48]. Moreover, astrocytes and microglia secrete cytokines that can influence oligodendrocyte physiology and pathology, ultimately inducing white matter alterations [47]. Potentially, oligodendroglial dysfunction induced by inflammation may subsequently lead to abnormalities in myelin maintenance and repair, possibly explaining white matter pathology in schizophrenia. In this context, a disbalance in the immune response associated with a slight inflammatory process of the CNS has been proposed as the 'mild encephalitis' hypothesis for schizophrenia [49].

It is important to note, at this level, that brain imaging studies will be crucial not only to further clarify the role of white matter disruption for the pathophysiology of schizophrenia but also to explore the possible role of connectivity in sustaining psychosocial functioning deficits and other outcome measures [50]. In this perspective, imaging studies have started exploring the neuroanatomical underpinnings of schizophrenia in accordance to symptom severity and psychosocial outcome [51, 52]. For instance, progressive brain changes affecting the frontal lobes and white matter [53] have been proposed to potentially support functional impairment and disability in schizophrenia. However, the identification of the neural markers of such psychosocial features will require long-term imaging studies evaluating prognosis, social functioning and cognitive performance [54, 55].

In this context, different characterizations of poor and good psychosocial outcome have been proposed across studies [56–58]. For instance, Keefe et al. defined poor-outcome patients according to a *Kraepelinian* conceptual frame, based on the following criteria lasting for at least five years prior to study contact: (a) continuous hospitalisation or complete dependence on others for daily life, (b) no employment and (c) no evidence of symptom remission [53]. Also, poor outcome has been defined by the persistency of delusions and hallucinations, which influence the behaviour of the patient, along with severe negative symptoms, such as social isolation and poor self-care. In contrast, good outcome has been defined by the absence of delusions, hallucinations or thought disturbances, negative symptoms and a preserved social functioning [59]. Furthermore, patients with more than 15-year illness duration have been described as having a good outcome if they were (a) hospitalised less than 10% of total illness duration and (b) not hospitalised in the previous year. On the contrary, poor-outcome subjects with schizophrenia had hospitalisations for longer than 50% than total illness duration or continuous hospitalisation for the previous three years [60].

Some structural MRI and diffusion tensor imaging studies, both cross-sectional and longitudinal, have been conducted to get some understanding of the correlation between biological variables and psychosocial functioning. In cross-sectional studies, imaging data and clinical or functioning assessments are obtained during the same evaluation. Early TC studies reported increased ventricle/brain ratio in patients with poor-outcome measures, such as longer hospitalisations [61–64], low Global Assessment of Functioning (GAF) scores or Strauss–Carpenter scale rates [59, 65] (or severe positive and negative symptoms [59, 61, 66–71]. Successively, structural MR studies have confirmed that ventricular enlargement is associated with low GAF scores, higher severity of negative symptoms [72, 73] or unemployment [74, 75], and have also pointed out the role of cortical shrinkage, particularly involving the prefronto-temporal cortex, and of subcortical structures such as the putamen and thalamus [60, 76–81]. The involvement of cortical and subcortical regions in sustaining psychosocial outcome in schizophrenia suggests that the white matter fibres connecting these areas may play a role as well. For instance, extensive connectivity disruption including corpus callosum, fronto-occipital fasciculus, left optic radiation and fronto-temporal white matter [82] has been reported in poor-outcome patients with schizophrenia, defined according to the aforementioned *Kraepelinian* criteria [53].

Longitudinal brain imaging studies have also been conducted to correlate structural markers with the progression of illness and related outcome measures. For instance, it has been shown that larger ventricular volumes and (frontal) cortical atrophy [83–89] predict poor clinical and social outcome. Also, it has been reported that *Kraepelinian* patients with poor cognitive performance [90] are characterised by a progressive reduction over time of frontal grey and white matter, basal ganglia and the limbic system, with parallel enlargement of ventricles [91–97]. Moreover, in poor-outcome patients, reduced corpus callosum and frontal white matter volumes have been reported to be associated with negative symptoms and cognitive deficits over time [92, 98].

Most of the available structural imaging studies have been conducted in chronic patients, being therefore biased by several confounding factors having potential effects on brain anatomy, such as psychotropic drug administration, psychotic episodes, length of illness and physical health [99, 100]. In this perspective, some studies have also been performed in first-episode patients, showing that patients with cortical atrophy and increased ventricle volumes have a severe course of illness, higher number of hospitalisations, low social functioning and poor response to pharmacological treatment [85, 101–105].

In conclusion, there is evidence that white matter dysconnectivity plays a major role in the pathophysiology of schizophrenia, potentially sustaining poor psychosocial outcome. In particular, a dysfunctional neural network involving the corpus callosum, fronto-temporal regions and basal ganglia is apparently associated with poor clinical and psychosocial functionality in schizophrenia. In this context, future brain imaging studies should further clarify whether white matter dysconnectivity may predict worse prognosis and social functioning in schizophrenia. This would help in detecting homogenous subgroups of patients sharing clinical and biological features who could undergo more tailored therapeutic and rehabilitative strategies. Specific treatment strategies may indeed potentially preserve or normalise white matter connectivity and, ultimately, lead to better clinical and social outcome in patients suffering from schizophrenia.

Acknowledgements

We thank all the subjects for participating in our projects during these last ten years and the patient families for the support to our research programme. We also thank Dr Cinzia Perlini for her thoughtful comments.

References

[1] Kendell RE, Jablensky A. (2003) Distinguishing between the validity and utility of psychiatric diagnoses. *American Journal of Psychiatry* **160**: 4–12.

[2] Keshavan MS, Tandon R, Boutros NN et al. (2008) Schizophrenia, "just the facts": what we know in 2008. Part 3: neurobiology. *Schizophrenia Research* **106**: 89–107.

[3] Lawrie SM, Olabi B, Hall J et al. (2011) Do we have any solid evidence of clinical utility about the pathophysiology of schizophrenia? *World Psychiatry* **10**: 19–31.

[4] Rose D, Willis R, Brohan E et al. (2011) Reported stigma and discrimination by people with a diagnosis of schizophrenia. *Epidemiology and Psychiatric Sciences* **20**: 193–204.

[5] Van OJ. (2003) Is there a continuum of psychotic experiences in the general population? *Epidemiologia e Psichiatria Sociale* **12**: 242–252.

[6] Schaub D, Brune M, Jaspen E et al. (2011) The illness and everyday living: close interplay of psychopathological syndromes and psychosocial functioning in chronic schizophrenia. *European Archives of Psychiatry and Clinical Neuroscience* **261**: 85–93.

[7] Andreasen NC. (2006) Standardized remission criteria in schizophrenia. *Acta Psychiatrica Scandinavica* **113**: 81.

[8] Velthorst E, Nieman DH, Linszen D et al. (2010) Disability in people clinically at high risk of psychosis. *British Journal of Psychiatry* **197**: 278–284.

[9] Lawrie SM, Abukmeil SS. (1998) Brain abnormality in schizophrenia. A systematic and quantitative review of volumetric magnetic resonance imaging studies. *British Journal of Psychiatry* **172**: 110–120.

[10] Brambilla P, Bellani M. (2010) Limited evidence that antipsychotic drug treatment is associated with reduced brain volume. *Evidence Based Mental Health* **13**: 64.

[11] Uranova NA, Vostrikov VM, Orlovskaya DD et al. (2004) Oligodendroglial density in the prefrontal cortex in schizophrenia and mood disorders: a study from the Stanley Neuropathology Consortium. *Schizophrenia Research* **67**: 269–275.

[12] Diwadkar VA, De Bellis MD, Sweeney JA et al. (2004) Abnormalities in MRI-measured signal intensity in the corpus callosum in schizophrenia. *Schizophrenia Research* **67**: 277–282.

[13] Andreone N, Tansella M, Cerini R et al. (2007) Cortical white-matter microstructure in schizophrenia. Diffusion imaging study. *British Journal of Psychiatry* **191**: 113–119.

[14] Crow TJ. (1998) Schizophrenia as a transcallosal misconnection syndrome. *Schizophrenia Research* **30**: 111–114.

[15] Hoffman RE, McGlashan TH. (1998) Reduced cortico-cortical connectivity can induce speech perception pathology and hallucinated 'voices'. *Schizophrenia Research* **30**: 137–141.

[16] Feinberg I. (1982) Schizophrenia: caused by a fault in programmed synaptic elimination during adolescence? *Journal of Psychiatric Research* **17**: 319–334.

[17] Friston KJ, Frith CD. (1995) Schizophrenia: a disconnection syndrome? *Clinical Neuroscience* **3**: 89–97.

[18] Andreasen N, Nopoulos P, O'Leary D et al. (1999) Defining the phenotype of schizophrenia: cognitive dysmetria and its neural mechanisms. *Biological Psychiatry* **46**: 908–920.

[19] Bartzokis G. (2002) Schizophrenia: breakdown in the well-regulated lifelong process of brain development and maturation. *Neuropsychopharmacology* **27**: 672–683.

[20] Stephan K, Friston K, Frith C. (2009) Dysconnection in schizophrenia: from abnormal synaptic plasticity to failures of self-monitoring. *Schizophrenia Bulletin* **35**: 509–527.

[21] Whitford TJ, Kubicki M, Schneiderman JS et al. (2010) Corpus callosum abnormalities and their association with psychotic symptoms in patients with schizophrenia. *Biological Psychiatry* **68**: 70–77.

[22] David AS. (1993) Callosal transfer in schizophrenia: too much or too little? *Journal of Abnormal Psychology* **102**: 573–579.

[23] Bleich-Cohen M, Sharon H, Weizman R et al. (2012). Diminished language lateralization in schizophrenia corresponds to impaired inter-hemispheric functional connectivity. *Schizophrenia Research* **134**: 131–136.

[24] Falkai P, Bogerts B, Schneider T et al. (1995) Disturbed planum temporale asymmetry in schizophrenia A quantitative post-mortem study. *Schizophrenia Research* **14**: 161–176.

[25] Brambilla P, Cerini R, Gasparini A et al. (2005) Investigation of corpus callosum in schizophrenia with diffusion imaging. *Schizophrenia Research* **79**: 201–210.

[26] Andreone N, Tansella M, Cerini R et al. (2007) Cerebral atrophy and white matter disruption in chronic schizophrenia. *European Archives of Psychiatry and Clinical Neuroscience* **257**: 3–11.

[27] Lim KO, Ardekani BA, Nierenberg J et al. (2006) Voxelwise correlational analyses of white matter integrity in multiple cognitive domains in schizophrenia. *American Journal of Psychiatry* **163**: 2008–2010.

[28] Mitelman SA, Newmark RE, Torosjan Y et al. (2006) White matter fractional anisotropy and outcome in schizophrenia. *Schizophrenia Research* **87**: 138–159.

[29] Crow TJ, Colter N, Frith CD et al. (1989) Developmental arrest of cerebral asymmetries in early onset schizophrenia. *Psychiatry Research* **29**: 247–253.

[30] Galaburda AM, Rosen GD, Sherman GF. (1990) Individual variability in cortical organization: its relationship to brain laterality and implications to function. *Neuropsychologia* **28**: 529–546.

[31] Luders E, Rex DE, Narr KL et al. (2003) Relationships between sulcal asymmetries and corpus callosum size: gender and handedness effects. *Cerebral Cortex* **13**: 1084–1093.

[32] Jarbo K, Verstynen T, Schneider W. (2012) In vivo quantification of global connectivity in the human corpus callosum. *Neuroimage* **59**: 1988–1996.

[33] Brambilla P, Tansella M. (2007) The role of white matter for the pathophysiology of schizophrenia. *International Review of Psychiatry* **19**: 459–468.

[34] Bellani M, Marzi CA, Savazzi S et al. (2010) Laterality effects in schizophrenia and bipolar disorder. *Experimental Brain Research* **201**: 339–344.

[35] Tettamanti M, Paulesu E, Scifo P et al. (2002) Interhemispheric transmission of visuomotor information in humans: fMRI evidence. *Journal of Neurophysiology* **88**: 1051–1058.

[36] Caligiuri MP, Hellige JB, Cherry BJ et al. (2005) Lateralized cognitive dysfunction and psychotic symptoms in schizophrenia. *Schizophrenia Research* **80**: 151–161.

[37] Crow TJ. (2008) The 'big bang' theory of the origin of psychosis and the faculty of language. *Schizophrenia Research* **102**: 31–52.

[38] Ellison-Wright I, Bullmore E. (2009) Meta-analysis of diffusion tensor imaging studies in schizophrenia. *Schizophrenia Research* **108**: 3–10.

[39] Keller A, Jeffries NO, Blumenthal J et al. (2003) Corpus callosum development in childhood-onset schizophrenia. *Schizophrenia Research* **62**: 105–114.

[40] Chambers JS, Perrone-Bizzozero NI. (2004) Altered myelination of the hippocampal formation in subjects with schizophrenia and bipolar disorder. *Neurochemical Research* **29**: 2293–2302.

[41] Flynn SW, Lang DJ, Mackay AL et al. (2003) Abnormalities of myelination in schizophrenia detected in vivo with MRI, and post-mortem with analysis of oligodendrocyte proteins. *Molecular Psychiatry* **8**: 811–820.

[42] Hof PR, Haroutunian V, Friedrich VL Jr et al. (2003) Loss and altered spatial distribution of oligodendrocytes in the superior frontal gyrus in schizophrenia. *Biological Psychiatry* **53**: 1075–1085.

[43] Roussos P, Katsel P, Davis KL. (2012) Molecular and genetic evidence for abnormalities in the nodes of Ranvier in schizophrenia. *Archives of General Psychiatry* **69**: 7–15.

[44] Hanson DR, Gottesman II. (2005) Theories of schizophrenia: a genetic-inflammatory-vascular synthesis. *BMC Medical Genetics* **6**: 7.

[45] Garver DL, Tamas RL,. Holcomb JA. (2003) Elevated interleukin-6 in the cerebrospinal fluid of a previously delineated schizophrenia subtype. *Neuropsychopharmacology* **28**: 1515–1520.

[46] Mittleman BB, Castellanos FX, Jacobsen LK et al. (1997) Cerebrospinal fluid cytokines in pediatric neuropsychiatric disease. *Journal of Immunology* **159**: 2994–2999.

[47] Schmitz T, Chew LJ. (2008) Cytokines and myelination in the central nervous system. *Scientific World Journal* **8**: 1119–1147.

[48] Martino G, Adorini L, Rieckmann P et al. (2002) Inflammation in multiple sclerosis: the good, the bad, and the complex. *Lancet Neurology* **1**: 499–509.

[49] Müller N, Myint AM, Schwarz MJ. (2012) Inflammation in schizophrenia. *Advances in Protein Chemistry and Structural Biology* **88**: 49–68.

[50] Dusi N, Perlini C, Bellani M et al. (2012) Searching for psychosocial endophenotypes in schizophrenia: the innovative role of brain imaging. *Rivista di Psichiatria* **47**: 76–88.

[51] Roy MA, Merette C, Maziade M. (2001) Subtyping schizophrenia according to outcome or severity: a search for homogeneous subgroups. *Schizophrenia Bulletin* **27**: 115–138.

[52] Bellani M, Perlini C, Brambilla P. (2009) Language disturbances in schizophrenia. *Epidemiologia e Psichiatria Sociale* **18**: 314–317.

[53] Keefe RS, Mohs RC, Davidson M et al. (1988) Kraepelinian schizophrenia: a subgroup of schizophrenia? *Psychopharmacology Bulletin* **24**: 56–61.

[54] Priebe S, Warner R, Hubschmid T et al. (1998) Employment, attitudes toward work, and quality of life among people with schizophrenia in three countries. *Schizophrenia Bulletin* **24**: 469–477.

[55] Weinmann S, Roick C, Martin L et al. (2010) Development of a set of schizophrenia quality indicators for integrated care. *Epidemiologia e Psichiatria Sociale* **19**: 52–62.

[56] Bellani M, Dusi N, Brambilla P. (2010) Longitudinal imaging studies in schizophrenia: the relationship between brain morphology and outcome measures. *Epidemiologia e Psichiatria Sociale* **19**: 207–210.

[57] Figueira ML, Brissos S. (2011) Measuring psychosocial outcomes in schizophrenia patients. *Current Opinion in Psychiatry* **24**: 91–99.

[58] Minzenberg MJ, Laird AR, Thelen S et al. (2009) Meta-analysis of 41 functional neuroimaging studies of executive function in schizophrenia. *Archives of General Psychiatry* **66**: 811–822.

[59] Kolakowska T, Williams AO, Ardern M et al. (1985) Schizophrenia with good and poor outcome. I: early clinical features, response to neuroleptics and signs of organic dysfunction. *British Journal of Psychiatry* **146**: 229–239.

[60] Staal WG, Hulshoff Pol HE, Schnack HG et al. (2001) Structural brain abnormalities in chronic schizophrenia at the extremes of the outcome spectrum. *American Journal of Psychiatry* **158**: 1140–1142.

[61] Kemali D, Maj M, Galderisi S et al. (1987) Clinical, biological, and neuropsychological features associated with lateral ventricular enlargement in DSM-III schizophrenic disorder. *Psychiatry Research* **21**: 137–149.

[62] Weinberger DR, Torrey EF, Neophytides AN et al. (1979) Lateral cerebral ventricular enlargement in chronic schizophrenia. *Archives of General Psychiatry* **36**: 735–739.

[63] Kanba S, Shima S, Masuda Y et al. (1987) Selective enlargement of the third ventricle found in chronic schizophrenia. *Psychiatry Research* **21**: 49–53.

[64] Gattaz WF, Rost W, Kohlmeyer K et al. (1988) CT scans and neuroleptic response in schizophrenia: a multidimensional approach. *Psychiatry Research* **26**: 293–303.

[65] DeLisi LE, Schwartz CC, Targum SD et al. (1983) Ventricular brain enlargement and outcome of acute schizophreniform disorder. *Psychiatry Research* **9**: 169–171.

[66] Weinberger DR, Bigelow LB, Kleinman JE et al. (1980) Cerebral ventricular enlargement in chronic schizophrenia. An association with poor response to treatment. *Archives of General Psychiatry* **37**: 11–13.

[67] Boronow J, Pickar D, Ninan PT et al. (1985) Atrophy limited to the third ventricle in chronic schizophrenic patients. Report of a controlled series. *Archives of General Psychiatry* **42**: 266–271.

[68] Andreasen NC, Smith MR, Jacoby CG et al. (1982) Ventricular enlargement in schizophrenia: definition and prevalence. *American Journal of Psychiatry* **139**: 292–296.

[69] Pearlson GD, Garbacz DJ, Moberg PJ et al. (1985) Symptomatic, familial, perinatal, and social correlates of Computerized Axial Tomography (CAT) changes in schizophrenics and bipolars. *Journal of Nervous and Mental Disease* **173**: 42–50.

[70] Cullberg J, Nyback H. (1992) Persistent auditory hallucinations correlate with the size of the third ventricle in schizophrenic patients. *Acta Psychiatrica Scandinavica* **86**: 469–472.

[71] Vita A, Giobbio GM, Dieci M et al. (1994) Stability of cerebral ventricular size from the appearance of the first psychotic symptoms to the later diagnosis of schizophrenia. *Biological Psychiatry* **35**: 960–962.

[72] Degreef G, Ashtari M, Bogerts B et al. (1992) Volumes of ventricular system subdivisions measured from magnetic resonance images in first-episode schizophrenic patients. *Archives of General Psychiatry* **49**: 531–537.

[73] Becker T, Elmer K, Schneider F et al. (1996) Confirmation of reduced temporal limbic structure volume on magnetic resonance imaging in male patients with schizophrenia. *Psychiatry Research* **67**: 135–143.

[74] Harvey I, Ron MA, du BG et al. (1993) Reduction of cortical volume in schizophrenia on magnetic resonance imaging. *Psychological Medicine* **23**: 591–604.

[75] Turetsky B, Cowell PE, Gur RC et al. (1995) Frontal and temporal lobe brain volumes in schizophrenia. Relationship to symptoms and clinical subtype. *Archives of General Psychiatry* **52**: 1061–1070.

[76] Buchsbaum MS, Shihabuddin L, Brickman AM et al. (2003) Caudate and putamen volumes in good and poor outcome patients with schizophrenia. *Schizophrenia Research* **64**: 53–62.

[77] Mitelman SA, Brickman AM, Shihabuddin L. (2007) A comprehensive assessment of gray and white matter volumes and their relationship to outcome and severity in schizophrenia. *Neuroimage* **37**: 449–462.

[78] Mitelman SA, Shihabuddin L, Brickman AM et al. (2003) MRI assessment of gray and white matter distribution in Brodmann's areas of the cortex in patients with schizophrenia with good and poor outcomes. *American Journal of Psychiatry* **160**: 2154–2168.

[79] Mitelman SA, Shihabuddin L, Brickman AM. (2005) Volume of the cingulate and outcome in schizophrenia. *Schizophrenia Research* **72**: 91–108.

[80] Losonczy MF, Song IS, Mohs RC et al. (1986) Correlates of lateral ventricular size in chronic schizophrenia, I: behavioral and treatment response measures. *American Journal of Psychiatry* **143**: 976–981.

[81] Brickman AM, Buchsbaum MS, Ivanov Z et al. (2006) Internal capsule size in good-outcome and poor-outcome schizophrenia. *Journal of Neuropsychiatry and Clinical Neurosciences* **18**: 364–376.

[82] Van OJ, Fahy TA, Jones P et al. (1995) Increased intracerebral cerebrospinal fluid spaces predict unemployment and negative symptoms in psychotic illness. A prospective study. *British Journal of Psychiatry* **166**: 750–758.

[83] Katsanis J, Iacono WG, Beiser M. (1991) Relationship of lateral ventricular size to psychophysiological measures and short-term outcome. *Psychiatry Research* **37**: 115–129.

[84] Vita A, Dieci M, Giobbio GM et al. (1991) CT scan abnormalities and outcome of chronic schizophrenia. *American Journal of Psychiatry* **148**: 1577–1579.

[85] DeLisi LE, Stritzke P, Riordan H et al. (1992) The timing of brain morphological changes in schizophrenia and their relationship to clinical outcome. *Biological Psychiatry* **31**: 241–254.

[86] Goldman M, Tandon R, DeQuardo JR et al. (1996) Biological predictors of 1-year outcome in schizophrenia in males and females. *Schizophrenia Research* **21**: 65–73.

[87] Prasad KM, Sahni SD, Rohm BR et al. (2005) Dorsolateral prefrontal cortex morphology and short-term outcome in first-episode schizophrenia. *Psychiatry Research* **140**: 147–155.

[88] van Haren NE, Cahn W, Hulshoff Pol HE et al. (2003) Brain volumes as predictor of outcome in recent-onset schizophrenia: a multi-center MRI study. *Schizophrenia Research* **64**: 41–52.

[89] Wood SJ, Berger GE, Lambert M et al. (2006) Prediction of functional outcome 18 months after a first psychotic episode: a proton magnetic resonance spectroscopy study. *Archives of General Psychiatry* **63**: 969–976.

[90] Gur RE, Cowell P, Turetsky BI et al. (1998) A follow-up magnetic resonance imaging study of schizophrenia. Relationship of neuroanatomical changes to clinical and neurobehavioral measures. *Archives of General Psychiatry* **55**: 145–152.

[91] Davis KL, Buchsbaum MS, Shihabuddin L et al. (1998) Ventricular enlargement in poor-outcome schizophrenia. *Biological Psychiatry* **43**: 783–793.

[92] Mitelman SA, Nikiforova YK, Canfield EL et al. (2009) A longitudinal study of the corpus callosum in chronic schizophrenia. *Schizophrenia Research* **114**: 144–153.

[93] Mitelman SA, Canfield EL, Brickman AM et al. (2010) Progressive ventricular expansion in chronic poor-outcome schizophrenia. *Cognitive and Behavioral Neurology* **23**: 85–88.

[94] Mitelman SA, Canfield EL, Chu KW et al. (2009) Poor outcome in chronic schizophrenia is associated with progressive loss of volume of the putamen. *Schizophrenia Research* **113**: 241–245.

[95] van Haren NE, Hulshoff Pol HE, Schnack HG et al. (2008) Progressive brain volume loss in schizophrenia over the course of the illness: evidence of maturational abnormalities in early adulthood. *Biological Psychiatry* **63**: 106–113.

[96] van Haren NE, Hulshoff Pol HE, Schnack HG et al. (2007) Focal gray matter changes in schizophrenia across the course of the illness: a 5-year follow-up study. *Neuropsychopharmacology* **32**: 2057–2066.

[97] Mathalon DH, Sullivan EV, Lim KO et al. (2001) Progressive brain volume changes and the clinical course of schizophrenia in men: a longitudinal magnetic resonance imaging study. *Archives of General Psychiatry* **58**: 148–157.

[98] Mitelman SA, Torosjan Y, Newmark RE et al. (2007) Internal capsule, corpus callosum and long associative fibers in good and poor outcome schizophrenia: a diffusion tensor imaging survey. *Schizophrenia Research* **92**: 211–224.

[99] Madsen AL, Keidling N, Karle A et al. (1998) Neuroleptics in progressive structural brain abnormalities in psychiatric illness. *Lancet* **352**: 784–785.

[100] McCrone P, Knapp M, Henri M et al. (2010) The economic impact of initiatives to reduce stigma: demonstration of a modelling approach. *Epidemiologia e Psichiatria Sociale* **19**: 131–139.

[101] Lieberman JA, Alvir JM, Koreen A et al. (1996) Psychobiologic correlates of treatment response in schizophrenia. *Neuropsychopharmacology* **14**: 13S–21S.

[102] Lieberman J, Chakos M, Wu H et al. (2001) Longitudinal study of brain morphology in first episode schizophrenia. *Biological Psychiatry* **49**: 487–499.

[103] Cahn W, Hulshoff Pol HE, Lems EB et al. (2002) Brain volume changes in first-episode schizophrenia: a 1-year follow-up study. *Archives of General Psychiatry* **59**: 1002–1010.

[104] DeLisi LE, Sakuma M, Maurizio AM et al. (2004) Cerebral ventricular change over the first 10 years after the onset of schizophrenia. *Psychiatry Research* **130**: 57–70.

[105] Rais M, Cahn W, Van HN et al. (2008) Excessive brain volume loss over time in cannabis-using first-episode schizophrenia patients. *American Journal of Psychiatry* **165**: 490–496.

CHAPTER 19

Statistics and the evaluation of the effects of randomised health-care interventions

Graham Dunn

Institute of Population Health, Centre for Biostatistics, University of Manchester, Manchester, UK

Introduction

> There could not be worse experimental animals on earth than human beings; they complain, they go on vacations, they take things they are not supposed to take, they lead incredibly complicated lives, and, sometimes, they do not take their medicine [1].

We are all aware of the pitfalls of relying on anecdote and unstructured observational studies when drawing inferences concerning the efficacy or effectiveness of health-care interventions. And most of us believe that the gold standard to aim for is the randomised controlled health-care trial. We have in mind the idealisation of the randomised experiment where treatment receipt is masked from everyone in the trial – especially the person responsible for assessing outcome – and, in particular, all of the participants receive the treatment or management option to which they have been randomly allocated. But all too frequently the gold is alloyed – it is not 23 carat. Not all participants receive the treatment as intended. Some fail to turn up for their therapy, others might get access to the treatment meant for another arm of the trial, and still others receive a treatment that is not in any part of the trial protocol, either in addition or instead of the intended intervention. Being aware of these complications, many investigators might shy away from the randomised trial and believe that they have to rely on routinely collected observational data (increasingly in the form of eHealth records). But this would be a mistake. Even with protocol violations, the randomised trial has many advantages over unstructured observational data. Great care needs to be exercised in the interpretation of the results, however, and statistical methods to cope with all of the possible problems are only now being actively developed. Their application to mental health trials is in its infancy.

Improving Mental Health Care: The Global Challenge, First Edition.
Edited by Graham Thornicroft, Mirella Ruggeri and David Goldberg.
© 2013 John Wiley & Sons, Ltd. Published 2013 by John Wiley & Sons, Ltd.

In this chapter, we are concerned with the statistical issues involved in the estimation of treatment effects from less than perfect randomised trials, always keeping the technical details to a minimum. We start by clarifying what we mean by a treatment effect. We then define average treatment effects (ATEs) and consider how these might be estimated from data arising from a perfect randomised controlled trial or RCT ('perfect' indicating that there are no protocol violations – specifically that participants get the treatment or intervention they are allocated to receive) and the problems we face when trying to make causal inference concerning treatment effects from uncontrolled observational data. Returning to the randomised trial, we then move on to consider in some detail how we might deal with data from a 'broken' [2] RCT; that is, how we might estimate treatment effects (and interpret what they might mean) in a trial in which a considerable number of the participants do not receive the treatment or intervention to which they were allocated. This leads to the definition and estimation of the complier-average causal effect (CACE). We explain and illustrate its estimation using data from an actual trial. We discuss the assumptions that are necessary for CACE estimation and stress that interpretation of the results of a CACE analysis should always be accompanied by a critical appraisal of the validity of these assumptions.

What do we mean by a treatment effect?

We start with a motivating example described in Dunn [3]. We have just been informed that Joe, a young male patient, has committed suicide. Although he was suffering from an acute episode of psychotic symptoms, it had been decided that he should be treated as a day patient in the community, rather than being admitted to hospital. Could the clinical service have been better? Could we have treated him in another way that would have avoided such a tragic outcome? Would admission to hospital have been helpful? Would he have committed suicide in any event? In other words: 'we ask whether Joe's death occurred *because* of the treatment, *despite* the treatment, or *regardless* of the treatment' (4, p. 33). A similar patient, Michael, who had actually received intensive inpatient care a few months ago, has now relapsed and has attacked and injured his girlfriend. Could a different approach to Michael's care have prevented this relapse or, if not, have prevented the attack on his girlfriend? Yet, a third patient, Mary, had recently been very severely disturbed but has responded so well to treatment as a day patient that she has managed to return to work. Is this the effect of the way we provided care, or would she have got better anyway? Would the outcome been as good if she had been admitted as an inpatient?

In the use of the word 'treatment', we mean any form of intervention such as particular forms of patient management, education, care, medication, psychotherapy and so on. What is a treatment effect? It is the comparison of what is and what might have been. It is counterfactual. We are interested in comparing the outcome of psychotherapy in a given individual with what it might have been if they had not received this treatment. Comparison is essential: without comparison, the causal effect of treatment does not make sense.

Keeping life simple, let us consider two options. A particular individual suffering from psychosis (schizophrenia or a similar diagnosis) may receive a course of cognitive-behavioural therapy (CBT) (the treatment condition, T) in addition to routine care. Alternatively, they may receive routine care alone (the control condition, C). We measure the patient's outcome by measuring the severity of their symptoms (using the total score on the Positive and Negative Syndrome Scale, PANSS [5], say) at a fixed time after the treatment decision is made (ignoring the difficulties over deciding when this is in the context of an observational study). Before the treatment choice is made, there are two poten-tial outcomes: the PANSS total after choosing the treatment condition, which we will represent by $P(T)$, and the PANSS total after choosing the control condition, represented by $P(C)$. The impact or effect of receiving treatment is some form of comparison of $P(T)$ with $P(C)$, the simplest being the arithmetic difference $P(T) - P(C)$. Given that a higher PANSS score implies more severe symptoms, we would hope that this difference would be a negative number. We refer to this individual treatment effect (ITE) by use of the Greek letter Δ. So, for the ith participant in a study,

$$\Delta_i = P(T)_i - P(C)_i \qquad (19.1)$$

The problem is that this treatment effect can *never* be observed. Depending on the patient's treatment history, we observe $P(T)_i$ or $P(C)_i$, but not both. If we observe $P(T)_i$, then $P(C)_i$ is a counterfactual, and *vice versa* [6]. Holland [7] has referred to this as the fundamental problem of causal inference. But, provided we are prepared to make various assumptions, we can solve this problem by dealing with averages (see following text).

Treatment-effect heterogeneity

It would appear to be self-evident that the treatment effect for one individual may be quite different from that for another, that is, that there will always be treatment-effect heterogeneity. We can attempt to 'smooth over' this problem by dealing with overall averages (essentially, ignoring it), or we might wish to capitalise on this heterogeneity in order to optimise treatment decisions for individual patients (as in personalised or stratified medicine). In the following section, we introduce various definitions for ATEs, and their interpretation is vitally dependent on what we are prepared to assume concerning the existence of treatment-effect heterogeneity. It is beyond the scope of the chapter to pursue the sources of this heterogeneity (as in the search for treatment-effect moderators), but we will pause to point out a very common error in much of this work: correlating prior patient characteristics or characteristics of the therapeutic process with outcomes in a cohort of treated patients. We would like to look at sources of variability in the Δ_is, but from Equation (19.1), it should be clear that the outcome of treatment is measured by the sum of Δ_i and $P(C)_i$. By claiming, for example, that the outcome of therapy (i.e. $\Delta_i + P(C)_i$) is positively related to the strength of the therapeutic alliance, we are not making a valid claim about the effect of the alliance on the treatment effects (the Δ_is). We cannot distinguish the effects of alliance on the Δ_is (effects of treatment) from its relationship with the $P(C)_i$s (treatment-free prognosis). Having made this point, we will now move on. Interested readers are referred to [8] for a discussion on how this sort of investigation might be done properly.

Average treatment effects

If there is no treatment-effect heterogeneity, then much of what follows is fairly trivial. But, if there is heterogeneity, then we have to think carefully about its implications. The problem is one of generalisability. Let us assume that we have estimated an ATE on a particular group of patients. What can we (validly) infer from this about the likely effects of treatments in other groups of patients? In order to get an answer to this, we need to be very careful how we define the relevant target populations.

Let us take our target population as self-evident (the population of depressed patients, say, who would be considered eligible for the receipt of treatment). The ATE relevant to this population is the average of the ITEs (the Δs) taken across everyone in the population (irrespective of whether they actually receive treatment). That is (dropping the i subscripts for simplicity),

$$
\begin{aligned}
\text{ATE} &= \text{Ave}(\Delta) \\
&= \text{Ave}[P(T) - P(C)] \\
&= \text{Ave}[P(T)] - \text{Ave}[P(C)] \qquad (19.2)
\end{aligned}
$$

Now let us assume that the patients' clinicians decide to treat only the worst 10% (i.e. those with the most severe depression) in this population. What is the average effect of the treatment in this severe sub-group. We define the ATE on the treated (ATT) by

$$
\begin{aligned}
\text{ATT} &= \text{Ave}[\Delta \mid \text{Treated}] \\
&= \text{Ave}[P(T) \mid \text{Treated}] - \text{Ave}[P(C) \mid \text{Treated}] \qquad (19.3)
\end{aligned}
$$

where '|' means 'given that'. We could also define an ATE in those that are not treated in a similar way. *If* and *only if* treatment effects have no heterogeneity would these three average effects be the same. Homogeneity of treatment effects is extremely unlikely. We would be extrapolating beyond reason to assume that an estimate of the effect of treatment on the treated would be a good predictor of treatment effects on those not chosen from treatment. Here we have chosen a rather extreme case for illustrative purposes, but it is important that the distinction is always kept in mind.

Now let us consider something a little more subtle. Suppose we have an RCT to compare the outcome after hospital admission with the outcome of community care in patients suffering from an acute episode of psychosis (1:1 allocation). We randomise eligible patients to hospital admission or community care. Some (say, 40%, i.e. 20% of all those in the trial) of the patients allocated to hospital admission fail to be admitted because of a lack of beds. A similar proportion of those allocated to community care have to be admitted because they became too ill and were a threat to either themselves or to others. This leaves about 60% of those allocated who actually receive the allocated treatment condition. These patients we refer to as Compliers – but note that non-compliance is not necessarily due to any 'delinquent' behaviour on behalf of the patients. So, we might assume that we have three classes of patients in this trial:

1 Compliers who receive hospital care if and only if allocated to hospital care,

2 Those who are Always Admitted (AA), irrespective of treatment allocation and

3 Those who are Never Admitted (NA), irrespective of treatment allocation.

Again, let us assume that the outcome is measured using the total PANSS score. We use T to indicate hospital admission and C care in the community. This gives rise to three possible ATEs:

$$\text{Ave}[\Delta|\text{Complier}] = \text{Ave}[P(T)|\text{Complier}] - \text{Ave}[P(C)|\text{Complier}]$$
$$\text{Ave}[\Delta|\text{AA}] = \text{Ave}[P(T)|\text{AA}] - \text{Ave}[P(C)|\text{AA}]$$
$$\text{Ave}[\Delta|\text{NA}] = \text{Ave}[P(T)|\text{NA}] - \text{Ave}[P(C)|\text{NA}] \tag{19.4}$$

Although the latter two ATEs make sense in principle, we have no hope of estimating either Ave[Δ|AA] or Ave[Δ|NA] because we never observe $P(C)$ in any of the AA group and we never observe $P(T)$ in any of the NA group. No comparison of what was and what might have been is ever possible here. The only group for which we can estimate an ATE is the Compliers. This ATE is defined as the CACE of treatment [9]. Details of how we might estimate the CACE are given later.

Now let us move on to a second trial of hospitalisation versus community care. Our patient population is similar to that of the first trial, but the hospital administration is considerably more efficient, and only, say, 2% of those allocated to hospitalisation fail to get admitted. And, for whatever reason, the treating clinicians are a bit more relaxed about having to admit patients in a crisis (or are a bit more selective in recruiting seriously ill patients into the trial in the first place), and, say, only 5% of those allocated to community care are admitted. Would we expect the CACE to be the same as in our previous trial? Probably not.

The change in the proportion of the NA should have little if any impact because failure to be admitted is an administrative problem that is completely independent of the characteristics of the patient (but, then again). It is clear, however, that relaxing the criteria for admission in those allocated to community care is changing the characteristics of the Compliers. The CACE is likely to change accordingly. This also has implications for implementing community care in routine practice. The rate of non-compliance will inevitably change with the setting and the relevance of a given trial's CACE estimate to the new setting open to challenge.

Estimating average treatment effects from a perfect randomised trial

Consider a randomised CBT trial for psychotic patients. We randomly allocate patients to receive CBT plus routine care (T) or routine care alone (C). Everyone receives the treatment condition to which they were offered, and everyone provides a measure of the severity of their psychotic symptoms at the end of the trial (i.e. there is perfect compliance with treatment allocation, and there are no missing outcome measurements). We also assume that all of the other assumptions for a valid trial hold.

We wish to estimate the ATE. Randomisation ensures (on average) the following two equalities:

$$\text{Ave}[P(T) \mid \text{Treated}] = \text{Ave}[P(T) \mid \text{Control}]$$

(i.e. the average outcome that would be observed *if treated* is not dependent on treatment allocation)

and

$$\text{Ave}[P(C) \mid \text{Treated}] = \text{Ave}[P(C) \mid \text{Control}]$$

(i.e. the average outcome that would be observed *if not treated* is not dependent on treatment allocation)

So, it follows that

$$\begin{aligned}
\text{ATE} &= \text{Ave}[P(T) - \text{Ave}(P(C))] \\
&= \text{Ave}[P(T) \mid \text{Treated}] - \text{Ave}[P(C) \mid \text{Control}]
\end{aligned} \tag{19.5}$$

That is, we can estimate the ATE by comparing the average PANSS score in the treated group with the average of the PANSS score in the controls. This is the fundamental characteristic of a randomised experiment and explains why the RCT is so important. Note, also, that in the case of an RCT with full compliance with treatment allocation, the ATE is also the same as the ATT. In general, in an observational study, a quasi-experiment or a trial with non-compliance with treatment allocation, these equalities will *not* hold.

Estimating average treatment effects from observational data

Let us use a hypothetical electronic patient register (eHealth) as a motivating example. We have treatment and routine outcome data on a very large sample of psychotic patients. Some of these will have received a course of CBT; many others would not. What can we learn about ATEs from these data? In general,

$$\text{Ave}[P(\text{T})\,|\,\text{Treated}] \neq \text{Ave}[P(\text{T})\,|\,\text{Control}]$$

(i.e. the average outcome that would be observed *if treated* is not the same for the two groups – they are not comparable)

and

$$\text{Ave}[P(\text{C})\,|\,\text{Treated}] \neq \text{Ave}[P(\text{C})\,|\,\text{Control}]$$

(i.e. the average outcome that would be observed *if not treated* is not the same for the two groups – they are not comparable)

We are not comparing outcomes in similar patients. We are not comparing like with like. Naïve comparison of groups is likely to be severely biased (invalid) as a result of confounding (by omitted factors determining treatment-free prognosis). Using some straightforward algebra,

$$\text{Ave}[P(\text{T})\,|\,\text{Treated}] - \text{Ave}[P(\text{C})\,|\,\text{Control}]$$
$$= \text{Ave}[P(\text{T})\,|\,\text{Treated}] - \text{Ave}[P(\text{C})\,|\,\text{Treated}] + \text{Ave}[P(\text{C})\,|\,\text{Treated}]$$
$$\quad - \text{Ave}[P(\text{C})\,|\,\text{Control}]$$
$$= \text{Ave}[(P(\text{T}) - P(\text{C}))\,|\,\text{Treated}] + \text{Ave}[P(\text{C})\,|\,\text{Treated}] - \text{Ave}[P(\text{C})\,|\,\text{Control}]$$
$$= \text{ATT} + \text{bias due to confounding} \begin{pmatrix} \text{i.e. lack of equality of the average} \\ \text{treatment} - \text{free outcome for the} \\ \text{two groups} \end{pmatrix} \quad (19.6)$$

We are not even estimating the ATE! As readers will be aware, we attempt to solve the confounding problem by measuring as many of the potential confounders as possible and subsequently stratify, match or condition on the confounders in the resulting analysis. A more recent and increasingly popular alternative is the use of propensity scores [10]. Essentially, we achieve balance in treatment-free outcomes by estimating the probability of receipt of treatment given a relatively complex model containing the confounders (complex in the sense of including polynomial effects of quantitative covariates – allowing for deviations from straight line relationships – and possible interactions between the covariates) – this probability being known as the propensity score – and then stratifying, matching, conditioning or producing inverse probability of treatment weights using these propensity scores so that, in essence, we proceed to estimate the ATE *as if* treatment had been randomised. Technical details can be found elsewhere [10]. One point is extremely important, however. We are concerned with the comparison of potential outcomes in patients who could have received either the treatment or the control condition; that is, both options have to be possible. In patients with a propensity score very close to 0 (those to whom CBT would never be offered) or, alternatively (much rarer in this example), very close to 1, such a comparison is not possible. Data from these people are not included in the analysis. We only wish to compare outcomes in patients in which there has been a choice.

What if we either know or suspect that we cannot allow for all confounders? The use of instrumental variables is a possible solution, but it is not always easy to find suitable candidates or to convince oneself that they really do have the properties of instruments. An instrumental variable (or instrument) has to be strongly correlated to treatment receipt but only influence outcome via treatment receipt (i.e. there is no direct causal influence of the instrument on outcome). A valid instrument is not associated with the unmeasured confounders. One possibility for our community care example might be distance from the patient's home to the hospital. This might have a strong influence on a decision to admit, but it is unlikely to influence outcome via a pathway that includes that treatment decision. In the context of a randomised trial with non-compliance, randomisation is a very strong candidate for a role as the instrumental variable. This will be discussed in detail in the following section.

Estimating efficacy in a broken RCT: Complier-average causal effects

Now let's look at an actual trial. Creed et al. [11] describe what we will refer to as the Day Care Trial to compare the effects of day and inpatient treatment of acute psychiatric illness. Randomisation produced 93 inpatients and 94 day patients. We then have the following sequence of events, illustrating that there are two types of non-compliance with the randomised treatment allocation (hence the use of the term 'broken'):

'Eight were excluded because of diagnosis or early discharge, leaving 89 inpatients and 90 day patients. Five randomised inpatients were transferred to the day hospital because of lack of beds, and 11 randomised day patients were transferred to the inpatient unit because they were too ill for the day hospital' ([11], p. 1382).

One of the outcomes for the Day Care Trial was a total score on the Comprehensive Psychiatric Rating Scale (the CPRS [12]); here we only consider outcome at four weeks after entry – a higher score indicating poorer outcome. Table 19.1 shows that there was some loss to follow-up in those patients receiving the intervention to which they had been allocated, but follow-up in the two non-compliant groups was complete. Data from this trial will be used to illustrate the problems of inferring the size of the causal effects and the methodologies used to solve them.

Table 19.1 A randomised trial with two types of non-compliance [11].

	Allocated to day patient treatment		Allocated to inpatient treatment	
	Received day patient treatment	Received inpatient treatment	Received inpatient treatment	Received day patient treatment
Number of patients	79	11	84	5
Number at four-week follow-up	65	11	67	5
Mean (SD) CPRS score	14.338 (11.280)	15.455 (12.517)	9.940 (9.191)	10.200 (10.281)
Probability weight (w) to allow for missing follow-up	79/65	1	84/67	1
Estimated proportion of Compliers (π_c)=79/90 − 5/89=0.822				
ITT effect=[(79 × 14.338)+(11 × 15.455)]/90 − [(84 × 9.940)+(5 × 10.200)]/89=4.520				
CACE=4.520/0.822=5.500				
Per Protocol=14.338 − 9.940=4.398				
As Treated=[(79 × 14.338)+(5 × 10.200)]/84 − [(84 × 9.940)+(11 × 15.455)]/95=3.513				

We first assume (as in most trials) that the outcomes for the individual patients are statistically independent (known as the stable unit treatment value assumption or SUTVA), and also that randomisation does actually have a strong influence on who receives each of the two treatment options. Then, following Angrist et al. [9], we postulate that our RCT comprises up to four potentially latent classes of patients:

1 Subjects who will always be day patients, irrespective of random allocation (Always Day Patients – ADP),

2 Subjects who will never be day patients, irrespective of randomisation (Never Day Patients – NDP),

3 Subjects who will always receive the treatment to which they are allocated. That is, they will be day patients if and only if they are randomly allocated to the day care arm (Compliers) and

4 Subjects who will always defy their allocation – if randomised to be a day patient they will finish up as an inpatient, and *vice versa* (Defiers).

Perhaps we should not take the labels implying never or always too seriously, but they are useful indicators to identify those patients who were either admitted to hospital or treated as a day patient, *despite* the results of the random allocation rather than because of them. Following most authors in this area, we will assume that we do not have any patients of Type D (known as the monotonicity assumption). This leaves Type A (ADP), Type B (NDP) and Type C (Compliers). In the day care arm, those that receive day care are either Compliers or ADPs (we cannot distinguish them). In the inpatient arm, those that were actually admitted were either Compliers or NDPs – again, we cannot distinguish the two types.

Let us denote the proportions of types A, B and C subjects by π_A, π_B and π_C, respectively. Class membership is assumed to be independent of randomisation – that is, the three proportions are the same in the two arms of the trial. This is an important assumption, but follows fairly obviously from the randomisation procedure. The proportion of ADPs (π_A) is estimated by the proportion of subjects receiving day care in the inpatient arm. Similarly, the proportion of NDPs (π_B) is estimated from the proportion of people who were admitted in the day care arm. The proportion of Compliers (π_C) is $1 - \pi_A - \pi_B$. Alternatively, the proportion of patients receiving day care in the day care arm is $\pi_A + \pi_C$, and the proportion of patients receiving day care in the inpatient arm is π_A. The proportion of Compliers in the trial (π_C) is simply estimated by the difference between these two – that is, the effect of randomisation (the *intention-to-treat* or ITT effect) on the proportion of subjects receiving day care.

How do we estimate treatment effects? First, we analyse *as randomised* (the ITT effect). Importantly, this provides us with a valid hypothesis test for the null hypothesis that there is no effect of treatment allocation on outcome. If we assume that treatment allocation (randomisation) has no effect in the ADPs or in the NDPs, then ITT is providing a valid test of the null hypothesis of zero treatment effect in the Compliers (i.e. that there are no effects of treatment allocation in any of the three classes, A, B and C).

Obviously, we wish to go beyond hypothesis testing. We want to know the size of the treatment effect on the outcome, together with a valid estimate of, say, a 95% confidence interval. As we have pointed out before, the treatment effect can only be estimated for those participants whose treatment receipt is determined by the randomised treatment allocation (i.e. in Compliers). Here, the ITT estimate will be a biased estimate of efficacy in the Compliers – it estimates the effect of the management decision, not the effect of actual receipt of treatment. If the ITT effects in the ADPs and the NDPs are zero, then the overall ITT effect will be attenuated as an efficacy estimator (it will be brought closer to zero than it should be). Algebraically, the overall ITT effect will be a weighted average of the ITT effects within each of the three classes:

$$\text{ITT}_{\text{Overall}} = \pi_A \text{ITT}_A + \pi_B \text{ITT}_B + \pi_C \text{ITT}_C \qquad (19.7)$$

Now, assuming that both $\text{ITT}_A = 0$ and $\text{ITT}_B = 0$ (incidentally, these assumptions are often referred to as exclusion restrictions), it follows that

$$\text{ITT}_{\text{Overall}} = \pi_C \text{ITT}_C \qquad (19.8)$$

and, therefore,

$$\text{CACE} = \text{ITT}_C = \frac{\text{ITT}_{\text{Overall}}}{\pi_C} \qquad (19.9)$$

Equation (19.9) implies immediately that the CACE can be estimated by dividing the ITT effect on outcome by the ITT effect on the receipt of day care. So,

$$CACE = \frac{ITT\,effect\,on\,outcome}{ITT\,effect\,on\,treatment\,receipt} \qquad (19.10)$$

Note that in Equation (19.10), we are dividing an ITT effect by an estimated proportion (the latter always being less than or equal to 1.0). The implication of this is that the CACE estimate will always be larger (further from 0 – we ignore the sign here) than the corresponding ITT estimate. If the CACE estimate is an unbiased indicator of the effect of treatment receipt (in the Compliers), then the implication of Equation (19.10) is that the ITT estimate is biased (attenuated). Returning to Table 19.1, the proportion of Compliers (π_C) is estimated to be 0.822. The estimated ITT effect on the CPRS score is 4.520 (i.e. the outcome appears to be a little worse in the day care arm – Creed et al. conclude that recovery is quicker in the day care arm, but by 12 months of follow-up the two groups are very similar) – this has been calculated assuming that the observed average outcomes in each of the four columns of the table are representative of all of those originally randomised (as displayed at the top of the columns) – the arithmetic is illustrated within the table. This is one way of dealing with loss to follow-up – an example of a missing data mechanism called missing at random (MAR) – see [13]. Beware of this phrase – its technical meaning is not what one might think, but we will not go into details here. Finally, the CACE estimate is obtained by dividing the ITT estimate (4.520) by 0.822, that is, 5.500. Is this statistically significant? How precise is it? What is the associated 95% confidence interval? We will leave answering these questions to the next section, in which we introduce instrumental variable regression (using two-stage least squares (2SLS)).

Before we discuss CACE estimation in further detail, we will briefly cover other commonly used options: Per Protocol and As Treated. The Per Protocol estimate compares the outcomes in the two arms, restricting the analysis to those patients who received the treatment option to which they were allocated. In the Day Care Trial, this corresponds to comparison of the mean CPRS scores from the first and third columns. As Treated abandons randomisation altogether and simply compares the outcomes in all those who have received day care with those of all those who were admitted (i.e. treating the trial as an observational study). These calculations are illustrated in Table 19.1. The Per Protocol estimate is 4.398; the As Treated estimate is 3.513. In this example, both are closer to the null than the original ITT effect, but that is not always the case, and, in fact, it is very difficult to interpret either of them in the presence of selection effects (confounding). Do they have any credibility? They are both dependent on the assumption that there are no selection effects (no confounding) – that is, that the treatment crossovers are occurring purely at random. This is extremely unlikely.

Instrumental variable regression

CACE estimation can be shown to be a specific example of the use of instrumental variables [9]. The expression in Equation (19.9) is an instrumental variable estimator. In our example, random allocation is the instrumental variable (or instrument, for short). The instrumental variable has a high correlation with both treatment received (the ITT effect on receipt of day care) and final outcome (the ITT effect on the outcome, the CPRS), but the instrument *only* influences outcome indirectly through treatment receipt. There is no direct effect of randomisation on outcome (another way of describing an exclusion restriction). The path diagram to illustrate this simple instrumental variable model is shown in Figure 19.1.

We do not wish to discuss technical details – that would be well beyond the scope of this chapter and the probable interest of its readers – but simply point out that the parameters of the model in Figure 19.1 (and, in particular, the effect of treatment receipt on outcome) can be estimated through the use of what is called instrumental variable regression, using a two-stage least-squares (2SLS) algorithm that we make no attempt to explain. This regression procedure is available in most general purpose statistical software packages, and its use fairly straightforward. We will illustrate using a simple Stata command (using Stata [14]):

ivregress 2sls cprs4 (treat = rgroup)[pw = w]

'ivregress 2sls' is telling the software to fit an instrumental variable regression model using 2SLS. The final outcome is cprs4, receipt of day care is the variable treat and randomisation to receive day care is rgroup. The final bit of the command '[pw=w]' is a weighting adjustment to take into account that there are missing outcome data. Each person has a weight variable, w, assigned to them (depending on which column of Table 19.1 they belong to – i.e. their compliance status) as calculated in Table 19.1.

This produces a treatment-effect (CACE) estimate of 5.501 with a robust standard error of 2.076 (robust because we a using a weighting adjustment). The corresponding 95% confidence interval is (1.433, 9.570). The *p*-value associated with the test of the null hypothesis (zero treatment effect) is 0.008. For future

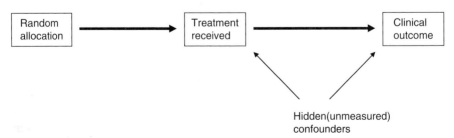

Figure 19.1 A simple instrumental variable model.

reference (see following text), the ITT effect (estimated through the simple command: regress cprs4 rgroup [pw=w]) is 4.520 (s.e. 1.697) with 95% confidence interval (1.167, 7.873). The associated *p*-value is 0.009 (practically identical to that for the ITT effect).

Equivalence and non-inferiority

In the aforementioned Day Care Trial, we are comparing two active treatments in order to decide which might be best. A similar approach might be used to compare two active pharmacotherapies – the *CUtLASS 1* trial, for example, was an open label trial designed to compare the outcomes after treatment of patients with psychosis with second-generation (atypical) antipsychotics with those after treatment with the much less expensive first-generation (typical) antipsychotics [15]. Instead of demonstrating that, for example, day care is more effective than hospital admission, we might be more concerned with the more subtle challenge of demonstrating that the cheaper option (day care) is equivalent to or, more accurately, not inferior to hospital admission. Similarly, we might wish to demonstrate that the outcomes of treatment with the cheaper first-generation drugs are not inferior to those of the newer atypicals.

We have already seen that there is non-compliance (treatment crossovers) in the Day Care Trial. This was also observed in *CUtLASS 1*; many patients starting on first-generation drugs switched to atypicals, and *vice versa*. What are the implications of non-compliance for the evaluation of non-inferiority? We first have to recognise that in an equivalence trial, the roles of the null and alternative hypotheses are reversed: the null is that the two treatments are *not* equivalent; the alternative is that they are. In the usual context (demonstrating relative efficacy), the ITT estimate (and associated confidence interval) is said to be *conservative* (i.e. it is attenuated – biased towards the null – that the two treatments are equally effective and away from the alternative – that one is better than the other), but in an evaluation aimed at evaluating equivalence, the bias is towards the alternative (the outcome we are looking for). The more non-compliance (treatment crossovers) we have, the more similar the outcomes in the two groups are going to be, irrespective of their relative efficacy! The ITT estimate is now said to be *anti*conservative. Many investigators (e.g. cancer trialists) recognise this problem when they are writing their trial protocols and associated analysis plans. To try to get over the problem, they very frequently say that they will supplement their ITT analyses with the Per Protocol approach (and we have already seen that this is potentially flawed). Rather bizarrely, they seem to think that the use of two potentially flawed analyses will lead to safer conclusions! The CACE (or IV) estimator does not have this obvious problem, and its use in the analysis of equivalence/non-inferiority trials ought to be more widely considered. We know of no examples of its use to evaluate non-inferiority in mental health trials, but it has occasionally been used by the present author in applications elsewhere [16, 17].

Let us illustrate the problem using the Creed Day Care Trial. Suppose, for the sake of argument, that we were able to set a non-inferiority limit of 8 points difference in four-month CPRS scores. That is, if the average outcome in the day care group is less than 8 points greater than it is in the admitted group, then we can conclude that day care is no less beneficial than hospital admission (one of the difficulties in designing such a non-inferiority trial is a sensible and defensible choice for this limit). We conclude that we have demonstrated non-inferiority if the 95% confidence interval has its upper limit less than +8. This choice of 8 points is entirely arbitrary in this particular example – chosen simply to illustrate that the different approaches to the analysis (ITT vs CACE) may lead to contradictory conclusions. From the Day Care Trial, our 95% confidence interval (as estimated using ITT) is (+1.167, +7.873) – we are just there – although there seems to be a benefit of hospital admission, we have demonstrated (or think we have!) that it is less than our non-inferiority limit of +8 points. The corresponding 95% confidence interval for the CACE is (+1.433, +9.570) – now covering our limit of +8. We have failed to demonstrate that day care is non-inferior to hospital admission. Again, we see that the ITT approach is producing an attenuated ATE (in terms of the actual impact of receiving the treatment). Do we really wish to conclude that two interventions are equally effective when their equivalence appears to be arising from non-compliance rather than from differences in treatment efficacy? Pragmatic health-care planners might be perfectly justified in doing so (they are assessing the equivalence of two management decisions), but clinical scientists wishing to understand the underlying reasons should be a bit more wary of doing so.

Further discussion and conclusions

The basic rationale of the randomised clinical trial is to compare treatment outcomes that arise *as a result of randomisation*. In a trial with non-compliance, we must distinguish the effects of random allocation on outcome (an ITT analysis) from the effects of treatment receipt in the sub-group of participants (the Compliers) whose treatment receipt is determined by that same randomisation (a CACE analysis). The first evaluates the effect of a management decision; the second the effect of treatment receipt. If treatment receipt has no effect (zero efficacy), then both analyses will lead to identical conclusions, and a test of the null hypothesis of zero efficacy will be identical in the two analyses. If, however, we wish to evaluate the *size* of the treatment effect, we should bear in mind that the only participants who provide information on the effect of treatment receipt (efficacy) are the Compliers. The CACE analysis will provide an unbiased estimate of the treatment effect in this sub-group; the ITT analysis will produce a biased (attenuated) estimate of this same effect. However, we do not advocate abandoning the ITT approach to the primary analysis of an RCT, but we do suggest that the primary analysis is supplemented by a detailed description of the patterns of non-compliance together with evaluation of the effects of treatment receipt in those participants whose treatment was determined by randomisation.

Adjusting for non-compliance using instrumental variable methods (now usually referred to as CACE estimation) is not new – it has a history of nearly 30 years, starting with work by Bloom [18] and independent developments by Newcombe [19], Sommer and Zeger [20] and Cuzick et al. [21]. A key paper, demonstrating that under the correct assumptions the instrumental variable estimate can, indeed, be interpreted as a causal effect of treatment, is that by Angrist et al. [9]. The application of this statistical methodology to the analysis of mental health trials is still quite rare. The report by Dunn et al. [22] appears to be the earliest example, and the method is illustrated in considerable detail in Dunn et al. [23]. Similar, but more complex, models enable us to begin to explore treatment-effect mechanisms [8, 24, 25] with enormous potential for the development of 'stratified' or personalised health care (psychiatry).

After the enthusiasm – now a 'health warning': instrumental variable methods (including CACE estimation) are not a fool-proof panacea [26]. The validity of CACE estimation is vitally dependent on strong assumptions that are frequently unverifiable. One of the great strengths of ITT, and why, along with randomisation, it lies at the very core of trial methodology, is its minimal use of untestable assumptions. Once we move away from ITT and begin to try to estimate more subtle causal effects (including the evaluation of treatment effect mediation [24] or the role of components of therapy in treatment-effect heterogeneity) [25], we are moving into a much less-defensible territory. The CACE analyses we have presented earlier have been completely dependent on exclusion restrictions (i.e. in the non-compliers, randomisation – i.e. treatment allocation – has no effect on outcome). This may be defensible in the case of a double-blind placebo-controlled drug trial (if you do not take the tablets, then it does not matter what is in them), but is it defensible in the case of an open trial of community care? In our example using the Creed et al. Day Care Trial, we have assumed that random allocation in the ADP group has no effect on outcome; that is, in this patient sub-group, the outcomes in those allocated to day care are the same as those allocated to be admitted but fail to be admitted because of failures in the health-care system. It is quite plausible that the outcomes in the latter may actually be worse in those whose care has been disrupted in this way. Similarly, in the NDP group, admission immediately or soon after randomisation may lead to different outcomes to emergency admission after a period of deterioration during day care. Ideally, these exclusion restrictions need testing. Given sufficient information, such testing is possible [23], but frequently it is not. Whatever be the case, readers of research reports using these relatively complex and other statistical methods should hone their critical appraisal skills and always be appropriately sceptical.

Another potential problem is generalisability (or lack of it). CACE is the treatment effect in those patients who have been induced to change their treatment by randomisation. What about the others? We cannot learn anything about them from the data. There is a tendency to think 'We have an estimate of the treatment effect in those who have complied with the treatment allocation (CACE), and that this is an estimate of the treatment effect that would be seen in everyone were they to receive the treatment'. This line of thinking is flawed. We should be very wary of inferring the effects of treatment that might have been seen were the non-compliers, contrary to fact, persuaded to comply with their treatment allocation. There may be scientific/theoretical reasons why we might expect this inference to be safe, but we should always remember that it is not an inference supported by the data (but neither do the data rule it out – the trial says nothing on this issue).

References

[1] Efron B. (1998) Foreword. *Statistics in Medicine* **17**: 249–250.

[2] Barnard J, Du J, Hill JL et al. (1998) A broader template for analysing broken randomised experiments. *Sociological Methods & Research* **27**: 285–317.

[3] Dunn G. (2002) Estimating the causal effects of treatment. *Epidemiologia e Psichiatria Sociale* **11**: 206–215.

[4] Pearl J. (2000) *Causality*. Cambridge: Cambridge University Press.

[5] Kay SR, Opler LA. (1987) The Positive and Negative Syndrome Scale (PANSS) for schizophrenia. *Schizophrenia Bulletin* **13**: 507–518.

[6] Rubin DB. (1974) Estimating causal effects of treatments in randomized and nonrandomized studies. *Journal of Educational Psychology* **66**: 688–701.

[7] Holland PW. (1986) Statistics and causal inference (with discussion). *Journal of the American Statistical Association* **81**: 945–970.

[8] Dunn G, Bentall R. (2007) Modelling treatment-effect heterogeneity in randomized controlled trials of complex interventions (psychological treatments). *Statistics in Medicine* **26**: 4719–4745.

[9] Angrist JD, Imbens GW, Rubin DB. (1996) Indentification of causal effects using instrumental variables (with discussion). *Journal of the American Statistical Association* **91**: 444–472.

[10] D'Agostino RB, Jr. (1998) Propensity score methods for bias reduction in the comparison of a treatment to a non-randomized control group. *Statistics in Medicine* **17**: 2265–2281.

[11] Creed F, Mbaya P, Lancashire S et al. (1997) Cost effectiveness of day and inpatient psychiatric treatment: results of a randomized controlled trial. *BMJ* **314**: 1381–1385.

[12] Asberg M, Perris C, Schalling D et al. (1978) The CPRS – development and applications of a psychiatric rating scale. *Acta Psychiatrica Scandinavica* **57** (Suppl. 271): 5–27.

[13] Little RJA, Rubin DB. (2002) *Statistical Analysis with Missing Data*, 2nd edn. Hoboken: John Wiley & Sons, Inc.

[14] StataCorp. (2009) *Stata Version 11*. College Station: StataCorp.

[15] Jones PB, Barnes TRE, Davies L et al. (2006) Randomised controlled trial of the effect on quality of life of second- vs first-generation antipsychotic drugs in schizophrenia. *Archives of General Psychiatry* **63**: 1079–1087.

[16] Kitchener HC, Dunn G, Lawton V et al. (2006) Laparoscopic versus open colposuspension – results of a prospective randomised controlled trial. *BJOG: An International Journal of Obstetrics and Gynaecology* **113**: 1007–1013.

[17] Beaver K, Tysver-Robinson D, Campbell M et al. (2009) Comparing hospital and telephone follow-up after treatment for breast cancer: randomized equivalence trial. *BMJ* **338**: article number a3147.

[18] Bloom HS. (1984) Accounting for no-shows in experimental evaluation designs. *Evaluation Review* **8**: 225–246.

[19] Newcombe RG. (1988) Explanatory and pragmatic estimates of the treatment effect when deviations from allocated treatment occur. *Statistics in Medicine* **7**: 1179–1186.

[20] Sommer A, Zeger SL. (1991) On estimating efficacy from clinical trials. *Statistics in Medicine* **10**: 45–52.

[21] Cuzick J, Edwards R, Segnan N. (1997) Adjusting for non-compliance and contamination in randomized clinical trials. *Statistics in Medicine* **16**: 1017–1029.

[22] Dunn G, Maracy M, Dowrick C et al. (2003) Estimating psychological treatment effects from an RCT with both non-compliance and loss to follow-up: the ODIN Trial. *British Journal of Psychiatry* **183**: 323–331.

[23] Dunn G, Maracy M, Tomenson B. (2005) Estimating treatment effects from randomized clinical trials with non-compliance and loss to follow-up: the role of instrumental variable methods. *Statistical Methods in Medical Research* **14**: 369–395.

[24] Emsley R, White IR, Dunn G. (2010) Mediation and moderation of treatment effects in randomised controlled trials of complex interventions. *Statistical Methods in Medical Research* **19**: 237–270.

[25] Dunn G, Fowler D, Rollinson R et al. (2012) Effective elements of cognitive behaviour therapy for psychosis: results of a novel type of subgroup analysis based on principal stratification. *Psychological Medicine* **42**: 1057–1068.

[26] Hernan MA, Robins JM. (2006) Instruments for causal inference: an epidemiologist's dream? *Epidemiology* **17**: 360–372.

CHAPTER 20

Service user involvement in mental health research

Diana Rose

Service User Research Enterprise (SURE), Health Services and Population Research, Institute of Psychiatry, King's College London, London, UK

Introduction

This chapter is concerned with service-user-led research in mental health. It is written by a service user researcher, so let me straightaway explain what this means. A 'service user researcher' is not just someone who is a researcher and happens to have experienced distress and used mental health services. He or she is someone who uses their experiences of treatments and services directly to inform their research. Such a researcher has 'insider knowledge' not available to a conventional researcher, and this can be captured by the idea of having a 'double identity'.

The chapter opens with a look at the history of user-led research, and this is crucial because this history has its roots in the user/survivor movement and to some extent continues to do so. Next, I will describe some new methods developed by user-led research organisations focusing very much on my own research team: the Service User Research Enterprise (SURE) at the Institute of Psychiatry, King's College London. But new methods are not enough; we need new concepts and theories. User researchers differ from conventional researchers as they tend to be explicit about the epistemological underpinnings of their work. Conventional university researchers often give the impression that the way they do research is the 'obvious' way to do it. User researchers question themselves and thus are reflective. The United Kingdom is ahead of other countries in promoting (or saying they promote) user-led research, and there are good reasons for this which I will cover in the historical exegesis. However, there is activity internationally which should be mentioned. Finally, user-led research is not without its critics and challenges, and I end with a discussion of these.

Improving Mental Health Care: The Global Challenge, First Edition.
Edited by Graham Thornicroft, Mirella Ruggeri and David Goldberg.
© 2013 John Wiley & Sons, Ltd. Published 2013 by John Wiley & Sons, Ltd.

History of user-led research

Aside from Italy, closure of the old asylums took place relatively early in the United Kingdom. By the early 1980s, people who would have spent their lives institutionalised might be admitted to these hospitals for a brief period of time and then discharged back into the community. Although there had been some patient-organised activity *within* asylum walls, it was people who had been discharged who began to organise and organise for better services or to avoid services altogether (see www.studymore.org for a full description). It could be said that the policy of community care gave birth to the user/survivor movement. For present purposes, there were people active in the user/survivor movement who also had a background in research. Their mission was to provide information to the movement, and they took their research questions from it (see Campbell and Rose [1], for a full description of the history of the user movement).

In the early 1990s, most of this research activity took place in London and Bristol [2]. Sometimes, user groups paired up with voluntary organisations to undertake research. This was the case in an early study when Camden Mental Health Consortium, a local user group, joined forces with the voluntary organisation 'Good Practices in Mental Health' to survey experiences of the transition of acute provision from the old asylums to wards in a district general hospital [3].

The next development took place in the mid-1990s when two London-based charities set up user research units in their organisations. The Mental Health Foundation hosted the Strategies for Living project (S4L; [4]), whilst the Sainsbury Centre for Mental Health was home to a peer-led evaluation model of local services known as User-Focused Monitoring (UFM; [5]). S4L was concerned with the strategies people employed to live with distress either in concert with or without statutory services. UFM involved trained user researchers interviewing their peers about local services. In both cases, the argument was that the interview situation would be more comfortable for a participant knowing that the interviewer shared their experiences, and that this would lead to more open discussion and so different results.

A quite separate spur to the development of user research came from the Department of Health, which in 1996 set up a unit called Consumers in NHS Research. This signalled an interest in involving service users across health research. Later, the remit was broadened to include social care and public health, and when the National Institute of Health Research (NIHR) came into being, the unit was renamed INVOLVE and became a programme for promoting patient and public involvement (PPI) in research across the NHS (www.invo.org.uk). INVOLVE has always had a strong mental health membership.

Throughout the last 15 years, user involvement in research has developed. There are now many service users who have written PhDs from a user/survivor standpoint, and some of these are in universities, notably Suresearch in Birmingham (http://www.suresearch.org.uk/) and SURE, which was mentioned earlier and which the current author co-leads. Others work on an independent, freelance basis. Whether we have all remained true to the grass roots where we began is a moot point, and some argue that those who moved into higher education institutions compromised their political integrity.

Developing new methods: The case of outcome measures

In this section, I will describe a new way of developing outcome measures for use in large studies. The method was developed in SURE so I will refer to it as the 'SURE model'. It starts from the premises of action research [6] which state that research questions should come from involved communities, and that these communities should be part of the research itself. When this is well done, it is sometimes called 'emancipatory research' [7]. The intention is to level the power relation between researcher and researched, although Mason and Boutilier [8] caution that this is not easily achieved. In the traditional model, the researcher comes from outside the community to assist them in research. The SURE model attempts to equalise the power relation between researcher and researched further by having the *researchers* as 'insiders'. So, the researcher is not brought in from the outside; rather, he or she is part of the community in the sense of having experienced the treatments and services that are being evaluated.

The SURE model starts with focus groups [9] with participants who have or still are having the treatment or service at issue. The facilitators also have this experience as described earlier. The focus groups meet twice, and in between the two meetings the researchers analyse the results of the first. These findings are then fed back to the second meeting to make sure we have captured what was said and whether any amendments need to be made [10]. Both sets of discussions, which are digitally recorded and fully transcribed, are subject to a thematic analysis [11]. From this, the researchers develop a mixed methods scale consisting of Likert items and open text boxes.

The next step is to subject the measure to further scrutiny by presenting it to 'expert panels'. There are two of these: one drawn from focus group members and the second a completely independent one (but still having the relevant experience) to look at the measure afresh. The task of the expert panels is to amend the measure and pay particular attention to issues such as language, layout and format. Usually this results in quite a few changes. Finally, the measure goes through a feasibility study. This is an iterative process with approximately 50 service users showing in vivo where the measure may be difficult or unclear so that it can ultimately be as acceptable as possible.

The final part of the SURE model for developing outcome measures is psychometric testing as it is for any other measure. We follow the precepts of the Health Technology Assessment [12] using both quantitative and qualitative psychometric testing. However, there is another reason for doing this. That is to compare measures generated by the SURE model to more traditional measures of the same or similar domains to see how they are different, the argument being that they will better reflect the concerns of service users.

There is much talk at the moment about patient-reported outcome measures (PROMs). However, it has been argued that these are not of clinical significance because they do not change practice [13]. It is argued that current PROMs are clinician-driven and not patient-valued. We therefore call our measures PG-PROMs: patient-generated, patient-reported outcome measures. Examples of PG-PROMs are continuity of care [14], satisfaction with cognitive-behavioural therapy for psychosis [15] and users' perceptions of acute wards [16]. The latter is being used as the main outcome measure in a large randomised controlled trial, and we can assess whether it is more sensitive to change and has better completion rates than conventionally produced measures. This is a rigorous test of user-produced outcome measures. A fuller account of the method can be found in Rose et al. [17].

International developments

As far as I am aware, there is no unit like SURE elsewhere in Europe, and in North America there are fledgling moves to develop user-led research. It can be argued that the existence of INVOLVE in relation to research funded by NIHR has played a major role here because user involvement is now required in research protocols and the conduct of research. However, there are initiatives in Europe and Australia. In Australia, Cath Roper is a prominent user researcher who, amongst other things, has done research around users' views of medication [18] and she has an academic position. In Europe, there are several service users working in universities, but they tend to be lone voices and do not have the support of peers. Norway is an exception with a team deploying a method which they call 'user ask user', which was developed from the model of UFM mentioned earlier (Heidi Westerlund, personal communication).

Notable is the Mental Disability Advocacy Group (MDAC), which is a human rights organisation based in Budapest, Hungary (http://www.mdac.info/en). MDAC frequently employs service users to carry out research. For example, in collaboration with the Health Services and Population Department at the Institute of Psychiatry, a large project was undertaken to assess compliance with the Convention on the Rights of People with Disabilities in institutions across both western and eastern Europe. The project aimed to develop a 'toolkit' [19]. To ensure that the toolkit was tailored to the concerns of service users, focus groups were held in each country with participants who had spent time in institutions. In most cases, the facilitator had also spent time in such places, and the findings of the focus groups were fed into the toolkit [20].

Concepts

There is interest today, especially on the part of NIHR, in examining the extent to which PPI in research has an impact both on the process of research itself and, critically, on health outcomes [21]. However, there are also those who argue that impact is not relevant because the involvement of patients and the public in research is an *ethical* matter. Talk of ethics can be concretised around the idea that PPI is a form of civic participation and citizenship. Callon et al. [22] have argued that new modes of participatory engagement can open up the 'secluded spaces' of knowledge production to dispute and reformation by the actors who are involved or will be affected by the research and its implications. They propose a move from 'delegative science' to 'dialogic science' which can be brought about by scientists, politicians and laypeople coming together in 'hybrid forums' to make decisions in situations of uncertainty. Similarly, De Vries et al. [23] propose 'democratic deliberation' as a way of involving lay people in decisions about medical science and particularly in setting the research agenda. The discourse of public engagement with science also has relevance to the ethical argument, especially the move from a 'deficit model' (which could be argued to be the default position of many) towards notions of lay expertise.

These are ethical arguments which aim to make science more democratic. However, there are also arguments that changing the knowledge producer changes the knowledge. This makes sense in terms of the argument that service user researchers have 'insider knowledge' of mental health conditions and treatments as this knowledge should lead to different scientific results. We may start with the relevance of feminist theory to mental health. What is called 'feminist standpoint epistemology' argues that women have been excluded from science (or at least that science has a masculine slant) because they are on the wrong side of key Enlightenment oppositions: intellect/emotion; culture/nature and reason/unreason [24, 25]. Since then, writers have extended their initial focus on feminism to analysing both the exclusion from science of marginalised groups and the special contribution they can nonetheless make. People with mental health problems have not been considered by standpoint theorists, but the model can hold especially since the same oppositions which characterise women in the Enlightenment seem highly applicable to those designated mad. If marginalised groups produce different knowledge to conventional scientists, then the importance of user involvement in mental health research is not only ethical, it is transformative of knowledge itself. A further development by Harding [24] is worth mentioning. She argues that feminist academics, and by extension other academics who identify as marginalised, can produce knowledge characterised by 'strong objectivity'. This means that we have access not just to our own knowledge but to conventional knowledge as well, thus making for a fuller picture.

Challenges to user-led research

User-led research in mental health is neither without its critics nor sceptics. These days, it is considered inappropriate to give voice explicitly to the view that such research will lead to the death of science. I used to have a favourite quotation to put here. However, it dates from 2002, and I know the person concerned has changed his mind so it would seem churlish to repeat the quotation. Nonetheless, not all conventional university researchers by any means are on board with user involvement in research even if they do not say it openly.

A milder version of outright scepticism is to say that what we do is 'biased, anecdotal and over-involved'. Indeed, when I was asked to write a theme piece on user-led research, the editor explicitly asked me to address these issues [26]. I hope, in the earlier discussion of standpoint epistemology, to have addressed the question of bias. There is no such thing as science without methodological underpinnings which should be transparent and open to scrutiny. The difficulty with much mainstream science is that its practitioners think that what they do is 'obvious' – the obvious way to go about science. But all research comes from a certain standpoint; it is just that some research is more critically reflective of its own practice than others. User-led research belongs in the latter camp.

Linked to this is the structure of knowledge as pursued by those of a positivist persuasion. The so-called Cochrane hierarchy privileges the randomised controlled trial as it is argued to be neutral (therefore obviously scientific). However, the outcome measures in trials reflect the concerns of conventional researchers and of clinicians and may not be what matters to service users [27]. This is why SURE takes a different approach to the construction of outcome measures as described earlier.

A further factor in the Cochrane hierarchy concerns the place of qualitative research. It does not have one. It will not have escaped the reader's attention that most of the examples of user-led research I have described are qualitative or mixed methods. Although it seems that qualitative research is gaining a little ground now, quantitative methods still predominate, and it is easy to dismiss qualitative research as 'anecdotal'. It is difficult to persuade many researchers that qualitative work is just as rigorous and difficult as quantitative. Even more so, it is difficult to persuade most mainstream university researchers that qualitative work gives a much richer reflection of the experiences of service users than the use of a dozen scales.

The weakest level of evidence according to such hierarchies is 'expert opinion', which immediately begs the question, 'Who are the experts?' They are people (usually men) deciding, on the basis of their professional opinion, the answers to certain questions. The updates of DSM and ICD are a case in point. But service user researchers have a different expertise, and it is one that should be brought to the table. Clearly, in the last few paragraphs I am arguing for some rethinking of knowledge hierarchies.

The final challenge we face can be starkly put – power. Mental health is a hierarchical world, and user researchers usually cannot command the same kind of resources and status as conventional researchers. The structure of research means that usually only professors can be chief investigators on grants and user researchers have to work under them. This much is common throughout academia, and Thornicroft and Tansella [28] have argued that user research needs to be better resourced. However, there is a more subtle level to this. For a psychiatrist, a user researcher is someone with a diagnosis and so is on a par with patients he or she treats as a clinician. It may be tempting to see the patient and know the researcher or at least to see the user researcher through a double lens – at once patient and researcher. This is not an *ad hominem* argument – I am not saying that clinicians come to the encounter unthinkingly. But that the structure of training and the nature of research make this likely to occur. And, of course, people with mental health diagnosis are held to lack reason [25], which means being on guard for anything untoward in the practice of science by service user researchers. Patient researchers in other specialities may be denigrated on account of their 'lay' status but not because they are inherently irrational, and so patient involvement in general health research may be easier than in mental health. The paradox is that, on the whole, user-led research in mental health is ahead of other specialities, which may have something to do with the history I described at the outset.

Conclusion

This is not an argument that user-led research should replace conventional mental health research. SURE is actually a collaboration, and I am involved in research with many colleagues who are not service users. I am arguing two things. First, that user-led research is a crucial part of the jigsaw. And second, that most research in mental health would benefit from an inflection by a user researcher perspective.

References

[1] Campbell P, Rose D. (2011) Action for change in the UK: thirty years of the user/survivor movement. In: Pilgrim D, Rogers A, Pescosolido B (eds.), *The Sage Handbook of Mental Health and Illness*. Los Angeles, London, New Delhi, Singapore, Washington, DC: Sage, pp. 452–470.

[2] Lindow V. (2001) Survivor research. In: Newnes C, Holmes G, Dunn C (eds.), *This Is Madness Too*. Ross on Wye: PCCS Books, pp. 135–146.

[3] Good Practices in Mental Health/Camden Mental Health Consortium. (1998) *Treated Well: A Code of Practice for Psychiatric Hospitals*. London: GPMH.

[4] Faulkner A, Layzell S. (2003) *Strategies for Living: A Report of User-Led Research into Peoples Strategies for Living with Mental Distress*. London: Mental Health Foundation.

[5] Rose D. (2001) *Users' Voices: The Perspectives of Mental Health Service Users on Community and Hospital Care*. London: Sainsbury Centre for Mental Health.

[6] Cornwall A, Jewkes R. (1995) What is participatory research? *Social Science & Medicine* **41** (11): 1667–1676.

[7] Beresford P, Wallcraft J. (1997) Psychiatric system survivors and emancipatory research: issues, overlaps and differences. In: Barnes C, Mercer G (eds.), *Doing Disability Research*. Leeds: Disability Press/University of Leeds, pp. 67–87.

[8] Mason R, Boutilier M. (1996) The challenge of genuine power sharing in participatory research: the gap between theory and practice. *Canadian Journal of Community Mental Health* **15** (2): 145–151.

[9] Morgan D. (1993) *Successful Focus Group Interviews: Advancing the State of the Art*. Thousand Oaks: Sage Publications.

[10] Lincoln Y, Guba E. (1985) *Naturalistic Inquiry*. Thousand Oaks: Sage Publications.

[11] Braun V, Clarke V. (2006) Using thematic analysis in psychology. *Qualitative Research in Psychology* **3**: 77–101.

[12] Fitzpatrick R, Davey C, Buxton M et al. (1998) Evaluating patient based outcome measures for use in clinical trials. *Health Technology Assessment* **2** (14): 1–86.

[13] Greenhalgh J, Long AF, Flynn R. (2005) The use of patient reported outcome measures: lack of impact or lack of theory? *Social Science & Medicine* **60** (4): 833–843.

[14] Rose D, Sweeney A, Leese M et al. (2009) Developing a user-generated measure of continuity of care: brief report. *Acta Psychiatrica Scandinavica* **119** (4): 320–324.

[15] Greenwood KE, Sweeney A, Williams S et al. (2010) CHoice of Outcome In Cbt for psychosEs (CHOICE): the development of a new service user-led outcome measure of CBT for psychosis. *Schizophrenia Bulletin* **36** (1): 126–135.

[16] Evans J, Rose D, Flach C et al. (2012) VOICE: developing a new measure of service users' perceptions of inpatient care, using a participatory methodology. *Journal of Mental Health* **21** (1): 57–71.

[17] Rose D, Evans J, Sweeney A et al. (2011) A model for developing outcomes measures from the perspective of mental health service users. *International Review of Psychiatry* **23** (1): 41–46.

[18] Happell B, Manias M, Roper C. (2004) Wanting to be heard: mental health consumers' experiences of information about medication. *International Journal of Mental Health Nursing* **13** (4): 242–248.

[19] Randall J, Thornicroft G, Burti L et al. (in press) Development of the ITHACA Toolkit for monitoring human rights and general health care in psychiatric and social care institutions. *Epidemiology and Psychiatric Science*.

[20] Russo J. (2009) Service User Focus Groups for the ITHACA study, internal research report. London: Health Services and Population Research Department, Instituted of psychiatry, King's College London.

[21] Staley K. (2009) *Exploring Impact: Public Involvement in NHS, Public Health and Social Care Research*. London: NIHR/INVOLVE.

[22] Callon C, Lascoumes P, Barthe Y. (2001) *Acting in an Uncertain World: An Essay on Technical Democracy*. Cambridge, MA/London: MIT Press.

[23] De Vries R, Stanczyk A, Wall IF et al. (2010) Assessing the quality of democratic deliberation: a case study of public deliberation on the ethics of surrogate consent for research. *Social Science & Medicine* **70** (12): 1896–1903.

[24] Harding S. (1993) Rethinking standpoint epistemology: what is "strong objectivity". In: Alcoff L, Potter E (eds.), *Feminist Epistemologies*. London: Routledge.

[25] Foucault M. (2006) *A History of Madness*. London: Routledge.

[26] Rose D. (2003) Having a diagnosis is a qualification for the job. *BMJ* **326**: 1331.

[27] Crawford MJ, Rowbotham D, Thana L et al. (2011) Selecting outcome measures in mental health: the views of service users. *Journal of Mental Health* **20** (4): 336–346.

[28] Thornicroft G, Tansella M. (2005) Growing recognition of the importance of service user involvement in mental health service planning and evaluation. *Epidemiologia e Psichiatria Sociale* **14** (1):1–3.

SECTION 4

Delivering better care in the community

CHAPTER 21

Psychotropic drug epidemiology and systematic reviews of randomised clinical trials: The roads travelled, the roads ahead

Andrea Cipriani, Michela Nosè and Corrado Barbui
Department of Public Health and Community Medicine, Section of Psychiatry, University of Verona, Verona, Italy

The roads travelled

The experimental world of randomised evidence

Evidence-based medicine is the integration of the best *research evidence* with *clinical expertise* and *patient values*. When these three elements are integrated, clinicians and patients form a diagnostic and therapeutic alliance which optimises clinical outcomes and quality of life [1].

The term *best research evidence* often refers to results from the basic sciences of medicine, but more recently the relevance of clinical research, especially patient-centred clinical research, in better informing clinical practice has been emphasised because it materially affects accuracy and precision of diagnostic or prognostic tests (including the clinical examination), and the efficacy and safety of therapeutic, rehabilitative and preventive regimens. The term *best research evidence* also means *updated evidence*. New evidence from clinical research both invalidates previously accepted diagnostic tools and treatments and replaces them with new ones that are more powerful, more accurate, more efficacious and safer.

Clinical expertise is linked to the ability to use clinical skills and past experience to rapidly identify each patient's unique health state and diagnosis, their individual risks and benefits of potential interventions.

Patient values refer to the unique preferences, concerns and expectations each patient brings to a clinical encounter and which must be integrated into clinical [2].

These ideas have been around for a long time; however, they were consolidated and named *evidence-based medicine* in 1992 by a group led by Gordon Guyatt at McMaster University in Canada. Since then, the number of articles about

Improving Mental Health Care: The Global Challenge, First Edition.
Edited by Graham Thornicroft, Mirella Ruggeri and David Goldberg.
© 2013 John Wiley & Sons, Ltd. Published 2013 by John Wiley & Sons, Ltd.

evidence-based practice has grown exponentially and rapidly (from one publication in 1992 to about a thousand in 1998). Nowadays, over two million articles are published each year in more than 20 000 biomedical journals. Some form of summary of this information is clearly essential. Even if a clinician restricted his or her reading to the most important psychiatry journals, he or she would need to read over 5000 articles a year. There is an obvious need, with such a wealth of information, for reliable reviews of the literature. Systematic reviews attempt to address this need for reliable summaries of primary research.

The history of synthesising research is inextricably bound up in the history of evidence-based medicine. The pioneer in the field was James Lind, a Scottish naval surgeon, who is credited with having produced one of the early records of a scientific trial and having written one of the first systematic reviews of evidence [3]. In 1747, Lind took 12 patients with scurvy, whose cases 'were as similar as I could have them' and divided them into six groups of two. According to his planned intervention, Lind administered different treatments to each pair of sufferers: cider, elixir vitriol, vinegar, seawater, a combination of oranges and lemons and mixture of garlic, mustard seed and balsam of Peru. Six days later, Lind's findings were clear: 'The result of all my experiments was that oranges and lemons were the most effectual remedies for this distemper at sea' (www.jameslindlibrary.org). The results of this study were published six years later, and interestingly Lind wrote, 'As it is no easy matter to root out prejudices … it became requisite to exhibit a full and impartial view of what had hitherto been published on the scurvy … by which the sources of these mistakes may be detected. Indeed, before the subject could be set in a clear and proper light, it was necessary to remove a great deal of rubbish'. To gather the available research, get rid of the 'rubbish', and summarise the best of what remains is essentially the science of a properly conducted systematic review. It took a while to understand the value and the methodological implications of Lind's attitude; however, in the past century, there were eminent figures, like Archie Cochrane, a British epidemiologist, who persuasively advocated the scientific evaluation of commonly used medical therapies through objective sources of information [4]. Even though the importance of evidence synthesis in medicine was recognised since the 1970s, the widespread use of these systematic reviews and meta-analyses did not occur until two decades later, when it became clear that the judgements and opinions of experts were often biased.

Systematic review and meta-analysis

The terms systematic review, overview and meta-analysis are often used interchangeably but actually refer to different things. Systematic review is a review of primary research studies in which specific methodological strategies that limit bias are used and clearly described in the systematic identification, assembly, critical appraisal and synthesis of all relevant studies on a specific topic. By contrast, meta-analysis is a systematic review that employs statistical methods to combine and summarise the results of several studies. It is worthwhile to acknowledge here that the first use of the term *meta-analysis* was by Smith and Glass in their systematic review of the effects of psychotherapy [5].

A methodologically sound systematic review helps to avoid *systematic error* (or bias) and can be contrasted with traditional reviews (the so-called *narrative reviews*), which often have no method section and a number of methodological flaws. Nevertheless, when used appropriately, meta-analysis provides a method of pooling research data from more than one study to provide an estimate of effect size, which has greater power than any of the constituent studies. This has obvious advantages for clinical research and practice because it provides a method of minimising *random error* and producing more precise, and potentially more generalisable, results. It is worth emphasising that meta-analyses should only be undertaken following systematic review; however, meta-analyses are not an essential part of a systematic review because it may sometimes be inappropriate to proceed to statistical summary of the individual studies (i.e. when included studies are too heterogeneous in terms of patient populations or interventions). As a research tool, a systematic review of the literature can be applied to any form of research question. Results of systematic reviews, with or without meta-analyses, can reliably and efficiently provide the information needed for rational clinical decision-making. However, in our experience, the results of a review are rarely unequivocal and require careful appraisal and interpretation.

Why do reviews need to be systematic?

In non-systematic reviews, the methods for identifying and appraising relevant studies are not explicit, and it cannot be assumed that the methodology is adequate. The conclusions of such reviews must be viewed with suspicion as they may be misleading, though the extent to which they are unreliable is usually difficult to judge. In contrast, systematic reviews use explicit, and therefore reproducible, methods to limit bias and improve the reliability and accuracy of the conclusions [6]. The rationale for systematic review is the same for all questions – the avoidance of random error and systematic bias.

The first stage in conducting a systematic review is the formulation of a clear question. The nature of the questions determines the type of research evidence to be reviewed and allows for the *a priori* specification of inclusion and exclusion criteria. For instance, to answer a question about therapy, such as: 'In the treatment of depressive disorder, are dual action drugs more effective than selective serotonin reuptake inhibitors?', the most reliable study design would be a randomised controlled trial (RCT). Randomisation avoids any systematic tendency to produce an unequal distribution of prognostic factors between the experimental and control treatments that could influence the outcome. However, RCTs are not the most appropriate research design for all questions. Systematic review has been useful in synthesising primary research results in both aetiology and diagnosis. A question such as 'Do obstetric complications predispose to schizophrenia?' could not feasibly be answered by an RCT because it would neither be possible nor ethical to randomise subjects to be exposed to obstetric complications. This is a form of aetiological question and would be best addressed by primary cohort and case control studies. Likewise, a diagnostic question such as 'How well can brief screening questions identify patients with depressive disorder?' would be best answered by a cross-sectional study of patients at risk of being depressed. Systematic reviews of these other study designs have their own methodological problems, and guidelines exist for undertaking reviews and meta-analyses of diagnostic tests and the observational epidemiological designs used in aetiological research [7].

The sources of bias in systematic reviews

Despite their potential to avoid bias, a number of factors can adversely affect the conclusions of a systematic review. When conducting a primary study, it is important to ensure that the sample recruited is representative of the target population; otherwise, the results may be misleading (*selection bias*). The most significant form of bias in systematic reviews is analogous to selection bias in primary studies, but applies to the selection of primary studies, rather than participants. There are various forms of selection bias including *publication bias, language of publication bias* and biases introduced by an over-reliance on electronic databases.

Publication bias is the tendency of investigators, reviewers and editors to differentially submit or accept manuscripts for publication based on the direction or strength of the study findings. The conclusions of systematic reviews can be significantly affected by publication bias. The potential pitfalls of publication bias are obvious: if only studies which demonstrate a treatment benefit are published, the conclusions may be misleading if the true effect is neutral or even harmful. As early as 1959 it was noted that 97.3% of articles published in four major journals had statistically significant results, although it is likely that many studies were conducted which produced non-significant results – but these were less likely to be published [8].

Various strategies have been proposed to counter publication bias. These include methods aimed at detecting its presence and preventing its occurrence. It is generally accepted that prevention is likely to be the most effective strategy, and it has been proposed that the most effective method would be to establish trial registries of all studies. This would mean that a record of the trial or study would exist regardless of whether or not it was published and should reduce the risk of *negative* studies disappearing. Registries of ongoing research have been slow to establish – perhaps because it is not clear who should take a lead or fund them – although some have been established (e.g. www.controlled-trials.com or www.clinicaltrials.gov). Whilst such registries may be useful prospectively, they do not solve the problem of retrospectively identifying primary studies. A number of methods for estimating the likelihood of presence of publication bias in a sample of studies have been developed. One commonly used way of investigating publication bias is the funnel plot [9]. In a funnel plot, the study-specific odds ratios are plotted against a measure of the study's precision – such as the inverse of the standard error or the number of cases in each study. There will be more variation in the results of small studies because of their greater susceptibility to random error, and hence the results of the larger studies, with less random error, should cluster more closely around the *true value*. If publication bias is not present, the graphical distribution of odds ratios should resemble an inverted funnel. If there is a gap in the region of the funnel where the results of small negative studies would be expected, then this would imply that the results of these studies are missing. This could be due to publication bias or mean that the search failed to find small negative studies.

Strenuous attempts to avoid publication bias can cause other problems because it may require the incorporation of unpublished data. Unpublished data are difficult to retrieve and can be problematic as they may not have been subject to peer review, and the data supplied may not be a full or representative sample. However, reliance only on published data may also be problematic and likely to produce biased estimates [10]. Nowhere is the impact of publication bias more obvious than in a meta-analysis. The *trim and fill* method adjusts for any asymmetry in a funnel plot in calculating the pooled estimate of effect.

Restricting a search to one language – for example, searching only for English-language papers – can be hazardous. It has been shown that studies which find a treatment effect are more likely to be published in English-language journals, whilst opposing studies may be published in non-English-language journals. *Language of publication bias* has also been called the *Tower of Babel* bias.

With the increasing availability of convenient electronic bibliographic databases, there is a danger that reviewers may rely on them unduly. This can cause bias because electronic databases do not offer comprehensive or unbiased coverage of the relevant primary literature. For instance, investigating the adequacy of Medline searches for RCTs in mental health care, it has been shown that the optimal Medline search had a sensitivity of only 52%. Sensitivity can be improved by searching other databases in addition to Medline, for example, Embase, PsycLit, Psyndex, CINAHL and Lilacs. To avoid the limitations of relying on electronic databases – or any other resource – for the identification of primary studies, reviews seek to use optimally sensitive, over-inclusive searches to identify as many studies as possible with a combination of electronic searching, hand-searching, reference checking and personal communications.

Meta-analysis: Strengths and limitations

The technique of meta-analysis has been controversial, and this is perhaps because it is potentially so powerful, but it is also particularly susceptible to abuse. A number of key issues should be borne in mind when assessing or carrying out a meta-analysis.

Many trials, especially in psychiatry, are small. There are many difficulties in recruiting patients to randomised trials, although some of these difficulties have been minimised in other areas of medicine by simplification of trial procedures, allowing large-scale, effectiveness trials. Although there is a need for larger randomised trials in psychiatry, it is also important to make the most efficient use of the trials that have been completed. Meta-analysis is a tool that can increase sample size and consequently statistical power by pooling the results of individual trials. Increasing the sample size also allows for more precision – that is, a pooled estimate with narrower confidence intervals [11].

Combining studies, however attractive, may not always be appropriate. The inappropriate pooling of disparate studies can be likened to combining oranges and apples – the result is meaningless. To avoid this, it is necessary to ensure that the individual studies are really looking at the same clinical or research question. Individual studies might vary with respect to study participants, intervention, duration of follow-up and outcome measures. Such a decision will usually require a measure of judgement, and for this reason, a reviewer should always pre-specify the main criteria for including primary studies in the review protocol. Having decided that the primary studies are investigating the same – or a close enough – question, an important role of meta-analysis is to investigate variations between the results of individual studies (heterogeneity). When such variation exists, it is useful to estimate if more heterogeneity exists than can be reasonably explained by the play of chance alone. If so, attempts should be made to identify the reasons for such heterogeneity, and it may then be decided that it is not reasonable to combine the studies, or that it is, but that the overall pooled estimate needs to take the variation into account.

Individual studies vary in their methodological quality. Most has been written about the factors which impact on the quality of randomised trials. It has been shown that allocation concealment and randomisation, blinding or masking and whether or not the study participants were considered in the groups to which they were randomly allocated (intention to treat) can all effect the direction of the results. Studies, which are deficient in any of these areas, tend to over-estimate the effect of the intervention. This presents a dilemma to the meta-analyst, who must determine to what extent the variations in methodological quality threaten the combinability of the data. Many scales and tools have been developed to assess the methodological quality of randomised trials. The scores on these quality assessment scales may be incorporated into the design of a meta-analysis with a *quality weight* applied to the study-specific effect estimate. Although a huge number of quality scales are available, the current consensus is that their use is problematic because of uncertain validity, as it has been shown that using different scales leads to substantial differences in the pooled estimate [12]. The optimal approach at present is to assess qualitatively those aspects of trial design that affect its internal validity (allocation concealment, blinding, study attrition and method of analysis) and investigate the effect of excluding poor-quality trials on treatment outcomes, by conducting pre-planned sensitivity analyses.

The main treatment effect of a trial gives an indication of the average response for an average patient meeting the inclusion criteria. Individual patients in real-life clinical practice deviate from the average to greater or lesser degrees. To tailor the results of a trial to an individual patient, it is tempting to perform a subanalysis of the trial participants with a specific characteristic, or set of characteristics. As many trials conducted in psychiatry are small, further subdivision of these trials into subgroups reduces the sample size and the statistical power of the results even more. Inevitably, estimates of the treatment in subgroups of patients are more susceptible to random error – and therefore imprecision – than the estimate of the average effect for all patients' overall effect. Furthermore, unless the randomisation was initially stratified according to the important subgroups, the protection from confounding afforded by randomisation will not apply, and any observed subgroup difference in treatment effect may be due to confounding. Meta-analysis pools data from individual studies, with a consequent increase in power, and this may make subgroup analyses more reliable – however, it should be emphasised that meta-analysis on its own cannot prevent systematic error in the analysis of subgroups (subgroup analyses should therefore always be viewed cautiously).

The Cochrane Collaboration and evidence-based medicine journals

The recognition of the need for systematic reviews of RCTs and the development of the scientific methodology of reviews have been among the most striking developments in health services research over the last decades. The Cochrane Collaboration, established in 1993, is an international network of more than 28 000 dedicated people from over 100 countries. They work together to help health-care providers, policymakers, patients, their advocates and carers make well-informed decisions about health care, based on the best available research evidence, by preparing, updating and promoting the accessibility of Cochrane Reviews – over 4600 so far, published online in *The Cochrane Library* [13]. In January 2011, the World Health Organization (WHO) awarded the Collaboration a seat on the World Health Assembly, to give the Collaboration an opportunity to promote evidence-based health care at the highest levels of international health-care policy-setting. The Cochrane Collaboration is registered as a charity in the United Kingdom. To tie the organisation together, there are a number of overarching structures, led by the Steering Group, which provides policy and strategic leadership for the organisation. Within the Cochrane Collaboration, there are several collaborative review groups in areas of practice relevant to mental health clinicians. Members of this group are democratically elected from, and by, our contributors. There are active collaborative review groups in the field of mental health including the Cochrane Schizophrenia Review Group and the Cochrane Depression, Anxiety and Neurosis Group. Within psychiatry, there are now over 900 Cochrane reviews.

International interest on systematic reviews and meta-analyses has led to the development of dedicated evidence-based journals (published in many languages) that summarise the most relevant studies for clinical practice and published articles relevant to the study and practice of evidence-based medicine. These journals, like *Evidence-Based Medicine* (ebm.bmj.com) or *Evidence-Based Mental Health* (ebmh.bmj.com), systematically search a wide range of international medical journals applying strict criteria for the validity of research. Experts critically appraise the validity of the most clinically relevant articles and comment on their clinical applicability.

The real world of clinical practice

Psychotropic drug epidemiology is a discipline developed to study the *use* and the *effects* of drugs in large numbers of individuals [14]. It describes how drugs are prescribed and utilised, investigates reasons underlying prescriptions and monitors outcomes and variables which may affect these outcomes. This discipline can constitute a permanent link between the experimental world of clinical trials and the real world of clinical practice. The evidence generated in clinical practice, by means of pharmaco-epidemiological studies, should be used to develop and suggest innovative research hypotheses to be subsequently tested in pragmatic trials.

Drug consumption and expenditure

At the national level, policymakers, administrators and clinicians monitor drug consumption and expenditure for different purposes. Whilst policymakers and administrators are interested in cost-containment issues, clinicians are more interested in analysing changes in prescribing behaviours over time, in making comparisons between countries and in studying whether specific trends in prescribing behaviours positively affect public health measures. Drug consumption and expenditure are usually monitored using drug sales data. These are routinely collected by independent sources on nationally representative samples of wholesalers and community pharmacies. In Italy, for example, data from 251/256 (98%) Italian wholesalers are gathered, and then extrapolated for the whole country; this prescribing information is then provided to manufacturers and health-care providers. Usually, the number of packages of each agent sold is recorded, and data on total prescribing and expenditure are calculated. However, in order to allow comparisons to be made independent of differences in price, preparation and quantity per prescription, data are subsequently converted into defined daily doses (DDDs) per 1000 inhabitants per day (DDD/1000/day). The DDD is the international unit of drug utilisation approved by the WHO for drug use studies [15]. The DDD is a theoretical unit of measurement defined as the assumed average maintenance daily dose for a drug, used for its main indication in adults. The DDD/1000/day indicates how many people per 1000 of the population have in theory received a standard dose (i.e. the DDD) of a particular medication or category of medication daily. For each new therapeutic agent introduced in the market, the WHO calculates the appropriate DDD, and a regularly updated list of all medications with the corresponding DDDs is accessible at www.whocc.no/atcddd. Since this methodology has the advantage of considering entire countries, psychotropic drug prescribing before and after major national changes can be analysed. For example, in Italy psychotropic drug sales data were examined before and after the 1978 psychiatric reform, with the aim of documenting trends in psychotropic drug prescribing alongside the 'Italian experience' of providing psychiatric care with comprehensive and integrated community services [16]. Intriguingly, data showed a marked regional variation in psychotropic drug prescribing, as well as in service provision, with an overall progressive increase in sales [17].

More recently, psychotropic drug prescribing before and after the introduction of new drug classes has been documented. In Italy, from 1995 to June 2003, prescriptions for first-generation antipsychotics progressively decreased from 2.54 to 2.0 DDD/1000/day; in contrast, prescriptions for second-generation anti-psychotics progressively rose up to 1.75 DDD/1000/day in 2003 [18]. In 2003, the antipsychotic drug most frequently used was haloperidol, followed by olan-zapine and risperidone. In 2003, the use of second-generation antipsychotics accounted for nearly 50% of overall DDD/1000/day of antipsychotic agents. From a clinical/epidemiological perspective, these data provide interesting insights. Comparisons between countries reveal that antipsychotic consumption was lower in Italy than in other countries. In Italy, there might have been fewer subjects who received antipsychotic treatment, or subjects might have been treated at lower-dose regimens. The first speculation is difficult to sustain, since epidemiological data have consistently shown that there are similarities in Western countries in the prevalence and distribution of psychotic disorders, and no data support under-recognition and/or under-treatment. In contrast, there are various pharmaco-epidemiological findings suggesting that antipsychotic agents are used at lower doses in Italy than in other countries [19].

Similar analyses have been carried out in the field of antidepressants and ben-zodiazepines. For example, since selective serotonin-reuptake inhibitors were suggested not only in the treatment of major depression but also in the treatment of other psychiatric conditions, including obsessive-compulsive disorder, panic disorder, generalised anxiety disorder, eating disorder, somatoform disorder, premenstrual syndrome, subthreshold depression and other mild depressive states that used to be treated with benzodiazepines, it can be hypothesised that the increasing use of antidepressants would be reflected in a decreased use of benzodiazepines. A recent analysis of actual quantities of benzodiazepines and antidepressants dispensed in Italy from 1995 to June 2003 failed to confirm this hypothesis [20]. During the study period, benzodiazepine consumption remained substantially stable, accounting for 50 DDDs/1000/day in 2003. In the same period, antidepressant consumption dramatically rose, from 9 DDDs/1000/day in 1995 to 26 DDDs/1000/day in 2003, an increase of nearly three times.

It seems, therefore, that selective serotonin-reuptake inhibitors and newer antidepressant availability have been exerting an additive effect over benzodiazepines: in 2003, the use of these two classes of agents reached the enormous estimate of 76 people per 1000 of the population.

Epidemiology of psychotropic drug users

The DDD methodology measures drug consumption, but cannot provide information on subjects receiving a particular category of drugs. These analyses are in fact based on aggregate and not individual data. It is therefore not possible to draw individual-level inferences without giving rise to errors in interpretation, the so-called *ecological fallacy* [21]. Simply stated, the error is to assume that phenomena that are correlated at a gross population level are necessarily correlated within a population of individuals. To overcome these limitations, analyses of databases with individual-level data have increasingly been performed. These databases, usually developed for managements, claims, administration and planning, cover large groups of individuals and generate data that are of value in pharmaco-epidemiological research.

In Italy, a study carried out in the area of Rome in 1989, before the introduction of second-generation antipsychotics, estimated that about 1.3% of a population of slightly less than four million subjects received at least one antipsychotic agent during a 12-month period [22]. Interestingly, this study found that the prevalence of prescribing progressively increased with the increasing age, with the highest rates in those aged 80 years or more. In another Italian survey, very similar patterns of antipsychotic prescribing were recorded, with about 4% of subjects aged 80 years or more receiving these agents [23]. Moreover, the analysis of the mean number of antipsychotics prescribed during the 12-month period showed that the use of antipsychotic agents was not occasional in late life, thus indicating that an epidemiologically relevant proportion of elderly individuals are annually exposed to antipsychotics. In the United Kingdom, information extracted from the General Practice Research Database revealed that the annual use of antipsychotic agents increased from 10.5 per 1000 in 1991 to 12.2 per 1000 in 2000, an overall increase of 1.7 per 1000 [24]. Adjusted for age, the annual use of antipsychotics increased by an average of 2.8% per year in men and 0.3% per year in women. These high rates of antipsychotic exposure in elderly individuals have recently raised the hypothesis that in late life antipsychotics may be widely prescribed for conditions that do not correspond to the diagnostic labels for schizophrenia only but also for a heterogeneous category of subjects with behavioural and cognitive problems associated with the increasing age. Clearly, this has implications for everyday practice, since it highlights that elderly individuals with behavioural abnormalities, tackled by physicians with antipsychotics, represent a clinical problem with no evidence base of optimal care.

Similarly, pharmaco-epidemiological analyses showed a progressive rise in the prevalence of individuals receiving antidepressant treatment with age [25].

Apparently, this finding is in contrast with data on the epidemiology of depression, which showed lower prevalence rates of major depression in the elderly than in young and adult people. It is therefore likely that, similar to what has been observed for antipsychotic agents, in late life antidepressants are widely prescribed in clinically undefined grey areas, constituted by elderly subjects, followed by general practitioners, suffering from medical conditions requiring the use of medications and suffering from depressive *symptoms* which probably do not fulfil current criteria of depressive *disorders*, and therefore cannot be detected by epidemiological studies focusing on the prevalence of depression. Intriguingly, these patient characteristics exactly correspond to clinical trial exclusion criteria, where subjects older than 65 years are usually not included, those taking medicines for medical conditions are never studied, those failing to take antidepressant agents are rarely followed up and those with mild depressive symptoms are considered epidemiologically less important than those suffering from major depression [26]. Although administrative databases with individual-level data are usually employed to describe the epidemiology of psychotropic drug use, they can additionally be used to investigate plausible associations between drug exposure and adverse or beneficial outcomes, linking different databases (e.g. a psychotropic drug database covering individuals living in a defined catchment area and a second database with information on the outcome of interest).

Quality and appropriateness of everyday prescribing

At the local level, mental health professionals providing psychiatric care are interested in auditing their clinical practice. It is therefore of interest to develop monitoring systems able to collect drug and service use data, and to link these data with hard outcome indicators. These systems nowadays represent a basic quality requirement for psychiatric services that want to hold themselves as accountable.

In South Verona, a catchment area located in the north of Italy, a psychiatric case registry (PCR) is operating since 1978 [27]. The South Verona PCR routinely records, for all subjects in contact with the psychiatric service, socio-demographic characteristics, ICD-10 diagnoses, past psychiatric and medical history, clinical data, admissions and outpatient contacts. The PCR also records details of patients who leave the catchment area, and those who die. The PCR, however, does not routinely collect information on prescriptions of psychotropic drugs, and therefore no accurate, routinely collected data on this specific sector of clinical activity were available. A registry which includes data on every patient receiving psychotropic medications in ordinary practice was developed to monitor psychotropic drug prescriptions (psychotropic drug registry, PDR) in an innovative way [28]. The PDR was linked to the PCR in order to get data on social and demographic characteristics, clinical symptoms, diagnosis, use of services and outcomes. No exclusion criteria are allowed; anyone receiving treatment is automatically included. Information on the proportion of subjects discontinuing treatment, switching medication because of side effects, recovery or lack of efficacy, can be generated, as well as on the proportion of subjects failing to return to the physician, and the proportion of patients who improve. The innovative aspect of this approach is that this registry was developed, organised and utilised only by physicians interested in monitoring their clinical practice and in providing patients, relatives and the public with accurate information on drug use in their specific context of care.

In addition to monitoring systems, there are epidemiological studies addressing specific questions related to the appropriateness of everyday prescribing. These studies employ and develop innovative ways of tackling these questions, for example, exploring the possibility of adopting qualitative approaches to data collection, analysis and interpretation. In the field of antidepressants, it has frequently been asserted that general practitioners should increasingly recognise and treat patients with depression. However, little research has been conducted so far to measure the *coverage* of antidepressants, that is, the proportion of those receiving prescriptions of all those who might be expected to benefit from them. In the Italian general practice setting, two different cutoff scores on a screening test for depression [29] have been used to predict rates for depression and rates for depressive patients thought likely to benefit from antidepressants, according to a severity criterion [30]. This study found that individual general practitioners varied enormously in their concept of depression, but the variation between the patient populations consulting them was much less. In total, less than 40% of those who might have benefited from an antidepressant actually received such a prescription. Although this strongly suggests the need to increase the coverage of antidepressants, it seems similarly relevant to document their focusing, that is, the proportion of those receiving antidepressants who really needed them. In fact, policies aiming at increasing the coverage of antidepressants can have negative consequences in terms of focusing, that is, they can increase the proportion of those receiving antidepressants who do not need them [31].

The roads ahead

Pragmatic trials

The need for reliable evidence for medical interventions has long been recognised and the history of attempts to produce this evidence is thoroughly documented in the James Lind library (www.jameslindlibrary.org). The status of RCTs as the most reliable method for evaluating the effects of treatments is now well established. Although the basic principles of the randomised trial have a long developmental history, it is often considered that the first modern medical RCT was the UK Medical Research Council trial of streptomycin in the treatment of tuberculosis [32]. In the years following this trial, many randomised trials were conducted on a number of key questions in a number of disease areas including psychiatry and mental health. During the next decades until the early 1980s, a number of other trials were conducted investigating key issues about the newly introduced drug treatments in psychiatry. From the 1980s, the situation changed considerably, and in the area of pharmaceutical treatments public funding declined, and the vast majority of clinical trials of drug treatments in psychiatry are now sponsored and conducted by the pharmaceutical industry.

This change had a number of effects. Firstly, the number of trials increased dramatically. Secondly, trials were increasingly conducted by industry on single patented compounds and were designed to meet the requirements of regulatory bodies such as the Food and Drug Administration in the United States and the European Medicines Agency in Europe. Although the criterion for the regulatory bodies is that the drugs should be safe and effective, the design of trials that are conducted for regulatory purposes often involves clinical compromises in order not to delay the introduction of drugs onto the market. The majority of such trials are short-term, highly controlled, highly monitored and typically designed to separate between new drug and placebo as efficiently as possible. This approach to clinical trial design has been described as *explanatory* [33], in which the aim is to determine if the treatment *can* work. Patients in these trials are characteristically highly selected, follow-up is short and outcomes are essentially sensitive proxies of clinically relevant outcomes. Because the design of these trials is based on a negotiation between regulators and industry, these trials often have substantial limitations for answering clinical questions in the real world and, hence, limited clinical credibility.

Whilst the limitations of the available trials are often emphasised in the systematic reviews that are undertaken to inform the policy statement, the guideline developers understandably wish to base their recommendations on the best available evidence, and so they will often choose to use the existing randomised evidence rather than no evidence at all. The results of the available evidence often need to be extrapolated – to an unknown degree – when they are applied to the target clinical question.

The dominance of highly controlled efficacy trials has clearly had a substantial negative effect on the amount of clinically applicable randomised evidence. There are also concerns that the extensive monitoring of trial conduct required under the *International Conference on Harmonisation of Technical Requirements for Registration of Pharmaceuticals for Human Use* guidelines for Good Clinical Practice makes the cost of clinical trials prohibitive to all but the very largest drug companies. Even for pharmaceutical companies, the risk of mounting a very large expensive clinical trial on a promising compound has to be offset against the risk that such a trial will demonstrate that the investigational compound is either of limited or no efficacy, or causes serious adverse effects. Pharmaceutical companies are therefore under pressure to do everything they can to design the trial to show their product in the optimal light and to ensure that any positive results have maximum impact, leading to as rapid uptake of the new drug as possible following market authorisation.

It has been recognised for at least two decades that the effects of many treatments, although clinically worthwhile, are still only moderately sized, and that much larger trials are required to provide precise estimates of their risk and benefits [34]. The key to achieving large numbers and reasonable costs is to make the trial procedures very simple and efficient and allow widespread recruitment by practising clinicians [35]. Facilitating widespread recruitment has a further benefit: representative samples of patients can be enrolled in the trial, which means that the results will be of widespread applicability to future patients. The key design aspects of large simple trials focus on maximising internal validity and avoiding bias whilst at the same time making the trial procedures as simple as possible.

The main principles that inform the design of such trials are as follows:

- The benefits of medical treatments on important outcomes are usually only moderately sized, although they may still be clinically worthwhile. This means that the trial needs to be very large to be able to detect the effect reliably and with sufficient precision.
- Inclusion criteria are broad and as unrestrictive as possible. Unrestrictive entry criteria make it more likely that the required sample size will be achieved if a broad, heterogeneous range of patients can be recruited, thereby increasing the general applicability of the trial results. The key entry criterion is that both the patient and investigator are substantially uncertain which of the trial treatments would be most appropriate. This 'uncertainty principle' has been successfully used in other large-scale trials. It is ethical because it effectively excludes patients for whom a specific treatment is known to be most appropriate. It maximises recruitment by allowing the widest possible eligibility for trial entry.
- All trial procedures should be radically simplified. One of the key barriers to participation in trials by clinicians is time availability. Removing this barrier by keeping the trial procedures and data collection to an absolute minimum is essential to achieve widespread participation and, hence, required sample size for realising the key objectives of the trial. The trial should have adequate support materials to make sure that patients understand the reasons for the trial and have additional verbal explanation from their physician. The latter two principles have led to such trials being termed *pragmatic* [33]. In contrast to the question of '*Can* the treatment work?' answered by the explanatory trial, pragmatic – or practical – trials ask '*Does* the treatment work?' [36]. The concept of the large simple trial is beginning to be of interest in psychiatry, however, with the encouraging signs that there is once again an interest in independent clinical trials being run on important clinical questions.

Funding is likely to remain an issue. Public funding for clinical trials appears to be declining, and trial expertise in the academic sector is also limited. To date – because there is more familiarity with the explanatory trial design – many trials continue to use complex procedures that are at least as complex as most industry phase III trials. This has made these trials feasible only in specialist centres with extra staff, and there has not been the widespread participation or scalability that is the hallmark of the true large simple trial. There remains reluctance to focus on one simple hard end point, and many trials continue to involve a huge number of rating scales that require independent raters.

Pragmatic trials should not be seen as a research design that should replace explanatory trials. There is a continuum between explanatory and pragmatic trials, and, ideally, pragmatic trials should be conducted after the results of explanatory trials allow a new medicine to enter the market. Recent examples of pragmatic trials in psychopharmacology include the Clinical Antipsychotic Trials of Intervention Effectiveness (CATIE) [37], the Cost Utility of the Latest Antipsychotic Drugs in Schizophrenia Study (CUtLASS) [38] and the Clozapine plus Haloperidol or Aripiprazole Trial (CHAT) [39].

Multiple treatments meta-analysis (or network meta-analysis)

By synthesising evidence from studies with similar design which address the same research question within the frame of a systematic review, pair-wise meta-analyses (or standard meta-analyses) are one of the most effective tools in evidence-based medicine; however, one of their main drawbacks is that they can compare only two alternative treatments at a time [40]. For most clinical conditions where many treatment regimens already exist, standard meta-analysis approaches result in a plethora of pair-wise comparisons and do not inform on the comparative efficacy of all treatments simultaneously. Moreover, if no trials exist which directly compare two interventions, it is not possible to estimate their relative efficacy, and thus this specific information is missing from the overall picture. All this has led to the development of meta-analytical techniques that allow the incorporation of evidence from both direct and indirect comparisons in a network of trials and different interventions to estimate summary treatment effects as comprehensively and precisely as possible [41]. This meta-analytical technique is called *multiple treatments meta-analysis* (MTM), also known as *mixed-treatment comparison* or *network meta-analysis*. The combination of direct and indirect estimates into a single effect size not only can provide information on missing comparisons but also can increase precision of treatment estimates of already existing direct comparisons, reducing confidence intervals and strengthening inferences concerning the relative efficacy of two treatments [42, 43].

Another fruitful role of MTM technique is to facilitate simultaneous inference regarding all treatments in order to rank them according to any outcome of interest, for instance, efficacy and acceptability [44, 45]. Using MTMs within the frame of a more complex statistical procedure, it is possible to calculate the probability of each treatment to be the most effective (first-best) regimen, the second-best, the third-best and so on, and thus to rank treatments according to this hierarchical order. This is a very easy to understand and straightforward way to present MTM results, most of all for clinicians who want to know which is the best treatment to be prescribed to patients on average [46].

Recently, MTMs have become more widely employed and demanded, with the increased complexity of analyses that underpin clinical guidelines and health technology appraisals [47]. Expert statistical support, as well as subject expertise, is required for carrying out and interpreting MTM results. Several applications of the methodology have depicted the benefits of a joint analysis, but MTM approaches are far from being an established practice in the medical literature. Concerns have been expressed about the validity of MTM methods as they rely on assumptions that are difficult to test [46]. Although randomised evidence is used and MTM techniques preserve the randomisation, indirect evidence is not randomised evidence as treatments have originally been compared within but not across studies. Therefore, indirect evidence may suffer the biases of observational studies (i.e. confounding or selection bias). In this respect, direct evidence remains more robust, and in situations when both direct and indirect comparisons are available in a review, any use of MTM should be to supplement, rather than replace, the direct comparisons. Several techniques exist which can account for but not eliminate the impact of effect modifiers across studies involving different interventions [46]. However, recent empirical evidence suggests that direct and indirect evidence are in agreement in the majority of cases, and that methods based on indirect evidence (such as MTM) can address biases that cannot be addressed in a standard meta-analysis, such as sponsorship bias and optimism bias [48, 49].

Guideline implementation

According to the principles of evidence-based medicine, research findings should guide doctors when taking decisions in clinical practice. However, not all research findings are attributed equal value, as randomised evidence is considered more reliable than observational evidence, and systematic reviews of RCTs are nowadays at the pinnacle of the evidence hierarchy [50]. In such a system, a crucial issue is how the results of systematic reviews may effectively be translated into evidence-based practice, considering that access and use of systematic reviews may not be straightforward for most doctors in most countries of the world. In recent years, in order to overcome this global issue, new methodologies for aggregating, synthesising and grading the quality of evidence extracted from systematic reviews have progressively been developed, and approaches for creating clinical practice guidelines based on explicit assessments of the evidence base are nowadays commonly employed in several fields of medicine, including mental health care. The WHO, for example, is in the process of developing evidence-based recommendations to facilitate care at first- and second-level facilities by the non-specialist health-care providers in low- and middle-income countries. WHO recommendations are based on the *Grading of Recommendations Assessment, Development and Evaluation* (GRADE) methodology [51]. This system wisely considers that the development of recommendations not only involves a systematic review and assessment of quality of evidence but also explicitly considers other issues such as value judgements, resource use, local context characteristics and feasibility, which are major considerations [52].

Surprisingly, however, whilst the pathway from evidence generation to evidence synthesis and guideline development is highly developed and quite sophisticated, the pathway from evidence-based guidelines to an evidence-based practice is much less developed. The key issues are whether guidelines may have any impact on doctor/practitioner performance and so on patient outcomes, and how implementation should be conducted to maximise benefit at sustainable costs. This is particularly relevant for those involved in producing and delivering evidence-based recommendations, including international organisations such as the WHO, scientific bodies such as the World Psychiatric Association or the American Psychiatric Association, national institutes such as the UK National Institute for Health and Clinical Excellence, but also for those with responsibilities in delivering high-quality mental health care, including national and local managers of mental health-care systems, scientific organisations or even single health-care professionals.

Current knowledge on how implementation programmes should be developed is still very scant. Implementation of treatment recommendations depends on the capacity of health services, available financial, human and material resources and the community context [53]. According to the WHO, in settings where functioning mental health systems are not available, such as in some low- and middle-income countries, the prerequisite for any implementation and delivery strategies includes political commitment, in order to acquire the necessary human and financial resources; a situation analysis, in order to understand the needs related to mental health care, and help guide effective prioritisation and phasing of interventions; a supportive policy that specifies the framework to be put in place to manage and prevent priority mental health conditions; a supportive legislative infrastructure that consolidates the fundamental principles, values, aims and objectives of mental health policies and programmes; and a strong integration of mental health into primary health care, in order to enable the largest number of people to get easier and faster access to services. In settings where functioning mental health systems are available, or a new mental health system has been developed, some principles may be relevant for successful implementation programmes. First of all, *local adaption* is very important: treatment recommendations should be developed as locally as possible, or should be adapted locally, in order to take into account issues such as value judgements, resource use, local context characteristics and feasibility, which are aspects that may be widely different in different contexts. In this sense, making evidence-based recommendations is a relative concept, although explicit criteria may help increase transparency, reproducibility and internal consistency [52].

Secondly, recommendations should keep a balanced approach between care of individual patients and how work is organised (*organisational changes*). This may be particularly relevant in mental health care, where new and better interventions cannot be delivered in the absence of functioning mental health systems [54]. Another important aspect is that treatment recommendations should not be confused with decisions taken on individual patients. According to the principles of evidence-based medicine, the evidence base, summarised in the format of evidence-based treatment recommendations, represents only one of the ingredients that should inform decisions. Clinical reasoning on psychopathology and clinical phenomenology, a careful assessment of patients' needs and expectations, and the clinical team's past experience have been described as key ingredients that should always be part of any clinical decision process. In this perspective, there is no expectation of a 100% coherence between what treatment recommendations state and what professionals do. The key element is that professionals pay due consideration to the evidence base, but then, as reported by Brian Haynes and associates, 'evidence does not make decisions, people do' [55].

Implementation programmes should always be described and documented (*research*), in order to increase our knowledge on how to make the best use of available evidence to improve practice. Audit and feedback systems should be part of any implementation strategies (*monitoring*). Audit and feedback of professionals' performance is essential for fidelity reasons, that is, to check the degree of coherence between what professionals recommend and what they actually do. Audit and feedback of patient outcomes is additionally essential for internal accountability reasons, that is, to provide continuous feedback to professionals and to mental health-care planners, and for external accountability reasons, that is, to provide patients, families and the public with data that may be used for making more informed choices, and to provide feedback to science, by producing process and outcome data that may generate new research hypotheses that may be formally tested using experimental designs.

References

[1] Sox HC, Helfand M, Grimshaw J et al. (2010) Comparative effectiveness research: challenges for medical journals. *Cochrane Database Systematic Reviews* **8**: ED000003.

[2] Guyatt G, Cairns J, Churchill D et al. (1992) Evidence-based medicine. A new approach to teaching the practice of medicine. *Journal of American Medical Association* **268**: 2420–2425.

[3] Lind J. (1753) *A Treatise of the Scurvy in Three Parts. Containing an Inquiry into the Nature, Causes and Cure of That Disease, Together with a Critical and Chronological View of What Has Been Published on the Subject*. London: A. Millar.

[4] Cochrane AL. (1972) *Effectiveness and Efficiency. Random Reflections on Health Services*. London: Royal Society of Medicine Press Limited.

[5] Smith ML, Glass GV. (1977) Meta-analysis of psychotherapy outcome studies. *American Psychologist* **32**: 752–760.

[6] Mulrow CD. (1994) Rationale for systematic reviews. *BMJ* **309**: 597–599.

[7] Stroup DF, Berlin JA, Morton SC et al. (2000) Meta-analysis of observational studies in epidemiology: a proposal for reporting. Meta-analysis Of Observational Studies in Epidemiology (MOOSE) group. *Journal of Amercian Medical Association* **283**: 2008–2012.

[8] Sterling TD. (1959) Publication decisions and their possible effects on inferences drawn from tests of significance – or vice-versa. *Journal of the American Statistical Association* **54**: 30–34.

[9] Egger M, Davey Smith G, Schneider M et al. (1997) Bias in meta-analysis detected by a simple, graphical test. *BMJ* **315**: 629–634.

[10] Cook DJ, Guyatt GH, Ryan G et al. (1993) Should unpublished data be included in meta-analyses? Current convictions and controversies. *Journal of American Medical Association* **269**: 2749–2753.

[11] Peto R, Collins R, Gray R. (1993) Large-scale randomized evidence: large, simple trials and overviews of trials. *Annals of the New York Academy of Sciences* **703**: 314–340.

[12] Juni P, Witschi A, Bloch R et al. (1999) The hazards of scoring the quality of clinical trials for meta-analysis. *Journal of American Medical Association* **282**: 1054–1060.

[13] Higgins JPT, Green S (eds.). (2011) *Cochrane Handbook for Systematic Reviews of Interventions* Version 5.1.0. Cochrane Collaboration. Available from: www.cochrane-handbook.org. Accessed on 2 January 2013.

[14] Grasela T. (1996) Pharmacoepidemiology: a scientific basis for outcome research. *Annals of Pharmacotherapy* **30**: 188–190.

[15] WHO Collaborating Centre for Drug Statistic Methodology. (2003) *Guidelines for ATC Classification and DDD Assignment.* Oslo: WHO Collaborating Centre for Drug Statistic Methodology.

[16] Tansella M, De Salvia D, Williams P. (1987) The Italian psychiatric reform: some quantitative evidence. *Social Psychiatry* **22**: 37–48.

[17] Williams P, Bellantuono C, Fiorio R et al. (1986) Psychotropic drug use in Italy: national trends and regional differences. *Psychological Medicine* **16**: 841–850.

[18] Andretta M, Ciuna A, Corbari L et al. (2005) Impact of regulatory changes on first- and second-generation antipsychotic drug consumption and expenditure in Italy. *Social Psychiatry and Psychiatric Epidemiology* **40**: 72–77.

[19] Percudani M, Barbui C. (2003) Cost and outcome implications of using typical and atypical antipsychotics in ordinary practice in Italy. *Journal of Clinical Psychiatry* **64**: 1293–1299.

[20] Ciuna A, Andretta M, Corbari L et al. (2004) Are we going to increase the use of antidepressants up to that of benzodiazepines? *European Journal of Clinical Pharmacology* **60**: 629–634.

[21] Robinson WS. (1950) Ecological correlations and the behaviour of individuals. *American Sociological Review* **15**: 351–357.

[22] Raschetti R, Spila-Alegiani S, Diana G. (1993) Antipsychotic drug prescription in general practice in Italy *Acta Psychiatrica Scandinavica* **87**: 317–321.

[23] Percudani M, Barbui C, Fortino I et al. (2004) Antipsychotics drug use in the elderly is cause for concern. *International Clinical Psychopharmacology* **19**: 347–350.

[24] Kaye JA, Bradbury BD, Jick H. (2003) Changes in antipsychotic drug prescribing by general practitioners in the United Kingdom from 1991 to 2000: a population-based observational study. *British Journal of Clinical Pharmacology* **56**: 569–575.

[25] Percudani M, Barbui C, Fortino I et al. (2004) Antidepressant drug use in Lombardy Italy: a population-based study. *Journal of Affective Disorders* **83**: 169–175.

[26] Posternak MA, Zimmerman M, Keitner GI. (2002) A re-evaluation of the exclusion criteria used in antidepressant efficacy trials. *American Journal of Psychiatry* **159**: 191–200.

[27] Amaddeo F, Beecham J, Bonizzato P et al. (1997) The use of a case register to evaluate the costs of psychiatric care. *Acta Psychiatrica Scandinavica* **95**: 159–198.

[28] Barbui C, Nosè M, Rambaldelli G et al. (2005) Development of a registry for monitoring psychotropic drug prescriptions: aims, methods and implications for ordinary practice and research. *International Journal of Methods in Psychiatric Research* **14**: 151–157.

[29] Rizzo R, Piccinelli M, Mazzi MA et al. (2000) The Personal Health Questionnaire: a new screening instrument for detection of ICD-10 depressive disorders in primary care. *Psychological Medicine* **30**: 831–840.

[30] Bellantuono C, Mazzi MA, Tansella M et al. (2002) The identification of depression and the coverage of antidepressant drug prescriptions in Italian general practice. *Journal of Affective Disorders* **72**: 53–59.

[31] Pariante C, Tansella M. (2005) Editorial. *Epidemiologia e Psichiatria Sociale* **14**: 51–54.

[32] Medical Research Council. (1948) Streptomycin treatment of pulmonary tuberculosis. *British Medical Journal* **2**: 769–773.

[33] Schwartz D, Lellouch J. (1967) Explanatory and pragmatic attitudes in therapeutical trials. *Journal of Chronic Diseases* **20**: 637–648.

[34] Yusuf S, Collins R, Peto R. (1984) Why do we need some large, simple randomized trials? *Statistics in Medicine* **3**: 409–422.

[35] Geddes JR. (2005) Large simple trials in psychiatry: providing reliable answers to important clinical questions. *Epidemiologia e Psichiatria Sociale* **14**: 122–126.

[36] Haynes B. (1999) Can it work? Does it work? Is it worth it? *BMJ* **319**: 652–653.

[37] Lieberman JA, Stroup TS, McEvoy JP et al. (2005) Effectiveness of antipsychotic drugs in patients with chronic schizophrenia. *New England Journal of Medicine* **353**: 1209–1223.

[38] Jones PB, Barnes TR, Davies L et al. (2006) Randomized controlled trial of the effect on quality of life of second- vs first-generation antipsychotic drugs in schizophrenia: cost utility of the latest antipsychotic drugs in schizophrenia study (cutlass 1). *Archives of General Psychiatry* **63**: 1079–1087.

[39] Barbui C, Accordini S, Nosè M et al. (2011) Aripiprazole versus haloperidol in combination with clozapine for treatment-resistant schizophrenia in routine clinical care: a randomized, controlled trial. *Journal of Clinical Psychopharmacology* **31**: 266–273.

[40] Cipriani A, Furukawa TA, Barbui C. (2011) What is a Cochrane review? *Epidemiology and Psychiatric Sciences* **20**: 231–233.

[41] Caldwell DM, Ades AE, Higgins JPT. (2005) Simultaneous comparison of multiple treatments: combining direct and indirect evidence. *BMJ* **331**: 897–900.

[42] Lu G, Ades AE. (2004) Combination of direct and indirect evidence in mixed treatment comparisons. *Statistics in Medicine* **23**: 3105–3124.

[43] Salanti G, Higgins JP, Ades AE et al. (2008) Evaluation of networks of randomized trials. *Statistical Methods in Medical Research* **17**: 279–301.

[44] Salanti G, Ades AE, Ioannidis JP. (2011) Graphical methods and numerical summaries for presenting results from multiple-treatment meta-analysis: an overview and tutorial. *Journal of Clinical Epidemiology* **64**: 163–171.

[45] Cipriani A, Barbui C, Salanti G et al. (2011) Comparative efficacy and acceptability of antimanic drugs in acute mania: a multiple-treatments meta-analysis. *Lancet* **378**: 1306–1315.

[46] Salanti G, Marinho V, Higgins JP. (2009) A case study of multiple-treatments meta-analysis demonstrates that covariates should be considered. *Journal of Clinical Epidemiology* **62**: 857–864.

[47] Barbui C, Cipriani A. (2011) What are evidence-based treatment recommendations? *Epidemiology and Psychiatric Sciences* **20**: 29–31.

[48] Song F, Harvey I, Lilford R. (2008) Adjusted indirect comparison may be less biased than direct comparison for evaluating new pharmaceutical interventions. *Journal of Clinical Epidemiology* **61**: 455–463.

[49] Salanti G, Dias S, Welton NJ et al. (2010) Evaluating novel agent effects in multiple-treatments meta-regression. *Statistics in Medicine* **29**: 2369–2383.

[50] Tyrer P. (2008) So careless of the single trial. *Evidence-Based Mental Health* **11**: 65–66.

[51] Guyatt GH, Oxman AD, Vist GE et al. (2008) GRADE: an emerging consensus on rating quality of evidence and strength of recommendations. *BMJ* **336**: 924–926.

[52] Barbui C, Dua T, van Ommeren M et al. (2010) Challenges in developing evidence-based recommendations using the GRADE approach: the case of mental, neurological, and substance use disorders. *PLoS Medicine* **7**: e1000322.

[53] Jacob KS, Sharan P, Mirza I et al. (2007) Mental health systems in countries: where are we now? *Lancet* **370**: 1061–1077.

[54] Thornicroft G, Tansella M, Law A. (2008) Steps, challenges and lessons in developing community mental health care. *World Psychiatry* **7**: 87–92.

[55] Haynes RB, Devereaux PJ, Guyatt GH. (2002) Physicians' and patients' choices in evidence based practice. *BMJ* **324**: 1350.

CHAPTER 22

Services for people with severe mental disorders in high-income countries: From efficacy to effectiveness

Paul Bebbington¹, Elizabeth Kuipers² and David Fowler³

¹ Mental Health Sciences Unit, Faculty of Brain Sciences, UCL, London, UK
² Department of Psychology, Institute of Psychiatry, King's College London, London, UK
³ Division of Health Policy and Practice, School of Medicine, University of East Anglia, Norwich, UK

Introduction

The human costs of schizophrenia and related disorders include a decrease in life expectancy of up to 15 years, prolonged disability, a greatly increased risk of suicide and major impacts on informal carers. Medication helps to prevent relapse, and speeds the process of discharge from hospital, and its more effective deployment would help matters. Nevertheless, these disorders retain an unexplained heterogeneity of outcome [1]. The cost and suffering would be considerably reduced if we were able to bring the worst outcomes appreciably closer to the best.

However, while outcomes have improved over the past half century, this progress appears to have stalled. Across industrialised economies, psychiatric services for the severely mentally ill have gone through various iterations. Nevertheless, as we will demonstrate, the service innovations of the last two decades have not been effective in reducing the prognostic variance of psychosis: they do not ameliorate social and clinical outcomes. This is despite affluence, heavy investment and a commitment to the provision of effective care based as much as possible in community settings. There is a clear gap between the efficacy of treatment and its effectiveness.

In this chapter, we will review the limitations of current systems of care in the developed world, using British services and policies as exemplars of the wider problem. We will argue that the key issues are the delivery of treatment and the demonstration that delivered treatment is effective in the community setting. If the situation is to be improved, services must do more than engage clients and

Improving Mental Health Care: The Global Challenge, First Edition.
Edited by Graham Thornicroft, Mirella Ruggeri and David Goldberg.
© 2013 John Wiley & Sons, Ltd. Published 2013 by John Wiley & Sons, Ltd.

exhort them to take medication. We think the remedy lies to a large extent in the introduction of a range of novel, evidence-based treatments into the process of service delivery. Some of these treatments are specialised, and probably need to be deployed selectively, but others could be made available more widely. Broadly speaking, the treatments we will describe are research-based psychological and social interventions developed around cognitive models, both of psychosis itself and of the process of informal care. While they have important direct effects, they also encourage a benign context for optimising the use of medication.

The variation in outcome of schizophrenia parallels a comparable variety in the phenomena experienced and reported by individual clients at various phases of the disorder. We contend that in order to improve outcome, we must analyse the antecedents and mechanisms of these phenomena. We also need to study people's responses to the fact and experience of having psychosis – metacognitions such as illness perceptions, awareness of stigma and self-stigmatisation, all of which have an impact on outcome. This knowledge is needed in order to continue the development of specific treatments. We must then assess the needs of individual clients in terms of the phenomena they experience, and their response to them, using this to identify the treatments and combinations of treatment that will be appropriate. Finally we need to include their carers or significant others (where they exist) in treatment plans, and to offer them help for themselves where appropriate.

The effect of specific treatments in the individual case is itself very variable, ranging from failure to occasionally spectacular success, and we are still unable to predict precisely who will respond. Treatments therefore have to be deployed flexibly, abandoning approaches that seem unproductive, but always attempting to identify promising alternatives.

Community psychiatric services: Fit for purpose? Which purpose?

Community psychiatric services have a number of functions. They monitor people who may be socially disruptive. They deliver care, which is the unambitious cousin of treatment. Most would agree, however, that community services should also be mechanisms for delivering treatment. This immediately raises a number of questions. What attributes of disorder should be targeted? Are treatments offered and delivered? Are the treatments delivered as intended? Can the intended treatments be delivered in the setting of a community team? If delivered as intended, are the treatments effective? In order to justify the provision of a service, these questions must all be answered.

The first provision of systematic psychiatric care in the late eighteenth and nineteenth centuries involved the building of local mental hospitals. Initially, they had two purposes: the segregation of mentally disturbed people and their humane and effective treatment [2]. Unfortunately, only the first purpose survived the gradual overcrowding of the hospitals. The effect was an ever-increasing psychiatric inpatient population, which in Britain and the United States peaked in the mid-1950s [3]. The development of a policy of community psychiatry was contemporaneous with, and benefited from, the introduction of neuroleptic medication, but was not dependent upon it [4]. The purpose of the policy was the decarceration of people with severe mental illness. It was developed from the bottom up by well-motivated psychiatric professionals, who felt that the well-being of discharged patients would be increased by properly supported residence in the community. However, in hindsight, perhaps inevitably, an inadvertent and unholy alliance with fiscal conservatism emerged, such that the decarceration proceeded without adequate provision of alternative community services [3].

Community psychiatric provision was not properly funded and implemented in the United Kingdom until the 1990s. By then, the programme of mental hospital closure was well-advanced, and the care of people with severe mental illness was managed by generic CMHTs with characteristics borrowed from US and Italian models. These offered continuity of care based on an accepted responsibility for a stipulated caseload. Responsibility was made clear by having a defined client group (those with severe mental illness), a defined catchment area and the key worker system. The teams included staff from a range of disciplines, which could include community nurses, social workers, psychologists, psychiatrists and community occupational therapists. They adopted a multidisciplinary approach that encouraged flexible client management underwritten by the availability of a range of resources. Teams were not necessarily medically led, and tended to have a flat management hierarchy, with sharing and rotation of management tasks. Key workers had access to backup from other team members. These teams were designed to provide long-term support to clients in the community, some of which involved assistance with the various responsibilities of community living, such as housing needs, self-care and help with benefits and budgeting. There was some, albeit limited, access to structured activity, and much of the focus was on the encouragement of compliance with medication. However, the pharmacological treatment of positive symptoms of psychosis is only moderately successful [5], and part of this lack of success arises from discontinuation, sometimes due to side effects, sometimes not [6, 7]. Thus, medication may be ineffective for purely pharmacological reasons, or it may be ineffective because it is difficult to persuade people that they should take it, or, having taken it, that it is important enough to persist with. The management of people with severe mental disorders in the community may end up looking like the failed management of medication.

Beyond the generic community mental health team

The effectiveness of these generic CMHTs was reviewed by Tyrer and colleagues [8], who concluded that they were associated with increased patient satisfaction, increased acceptance of treatment and less suicide. However, there was no clear advantage in relation to time spent in hospital or to overall clinical and social outcomes. This failure to achieve clinical and social improvement is a refrain we will hear again in relation to other sorts of community treatment. While the teams did, as intended, target people with severe mental illness, they were relatively ineffective in dealing with their clients in times of crisis, and had problems in helping those who were reluctant to engage, or suffered from dual diagnosis. There was, therefore, concern that generic CMHTs between them did not provide a sufficiently comprehensive service to maintain the health of all people with severe mental illness in the community. In the United Kingdom, this led to the augmentation of generic teams by more specific teams. In particular, these included assertive outreach teams (AOTs) and crisis resolution teams (CRTs).

Both these specialist teams owe their origins to the development of assertive community treatment (ACT) in the American Midwest in the 1970s. This was designed as an alternative provision for people who would otherwise be kept in hospital [9]. It was used variously to facilitate the discharge of inpatients, as an alternative to admission and as a mechanism for keeping vulnerable patients in the community. The effectiveness of ACT was systematically reviewed by Marshall and Lockwood [10]. They analysed 14 randomised controlled trials (RCTs) and concluded that on average the provision of ACT saved one admission for ten people treated, and resulted in a 42% reduction in hospital bed use. However, it did not reduce costs. It prevented disengagement, but there was no improvement in clinical outcome or social functioning. The results were better from the earlier studies.

There were, however, particular problems with the importation of ACT into the British mental health service environment. Five RCTs, ostensibly of ACT, were carried out in the United Kingdom in the 1990s. The results were disappointing. ACT led to improved contact with patients, but there was no consistent improvement in clinical or social outcomes, and costs actually increased.

This led to a quasi-theological argument about whether it was possible to distinguish between true ACT and intensive case management (ICM). (Theological, because there was no empirical evidence regarding the effective elements of ACT.) Marshall and Creed [11] made a distinction between ACT and ICM, arguing that an ICM team was merely a CMHT with fewer clients, and thus quite different from ACT. They also argued that ACT was well enough specified for fidelity to be evaluated, and pointed out that fidelity scales were available [12]. The components of true ACT included a maximum caseload of 10–12 per full-time worker, extended hours of operation, 'in vivo' contact, assertive engagement and a 'no dropouts' policy. In addition, there was a team-based approach, with regular and frequent team meetings, and the daily provision of plans. The team was to liaise with carers to support them, it was to rely on the skills of team members rather than outside agencies, and it would have its own beds, being responsible for admissions and discharges.

Marshall and Creed [11] argued that the poor results in the United Kingdom were the consequence of inadequate implementation of teams along these lines. However, ACT is a social treatment, likely to vary in its effects with the social context. The importation of ACT into the British (and European) service context was not straightforward. For instance, in the United Kingdom, in contrast to the United States, home visits were part of normal CMHT contacts with service users. This removed a key difference between ACT and CMHT models. The move into UK systems may also have been limited by other problems. Staff were often uncomfortable with a model which they saw as coercive and intrusive. Moreover, the comparison services, in the form of CMHTs, were not always very different, and might have been somewhat effective anyway. Finally, the expedient nature of the introduction of AOTs may have distorted the model.

Nevertheless, the provision of ACT by dedicated AOTs became government policy, and they were introduced across the country without adequate evidence. Thus, the National Service Framework for Mental Health [13, 14] announced that 220 AOTs and 335 CRTs would be implemented across England by 2003.

Data accrued somewhat later: the first RCT in the UK service setting to compare well-defined ACT with usual care from CMHTs was REACT [15, 16]. This involved 2 AOTs and 13 CMHTs in an inner London catchment area. After referral, data were collected from participants before randomisation. Follow-up data were collected at 9, 18 and 36 months. The primary outcome was the reduction of time spent in hospital, and the sample size of 250 was based on reducing mean bed use by one-third. The AOTs involved were rated independently as being of moderate-to-high model fidelity [17].

In the event, there were no differences between the teams in the total number of days in hospital, nor on any other measure of inpatient service use. The clients of the AOTs did show better engagement, and were less likely to be lost to follow-up. They also reported consistently greater satisfaction with the ACT service. There were no effects on other secondary outcomes, including symptoms, quality of life, the number of clients' needs that were met, adherence to medication or any other measure of clinical and social functioning. It should be noted that the CMHTs in any case had four of the seven defining characteristics of ACT. This study emphasises that it is hard to demonstrate advantages from ACT when CMHTs are functioning reasonably effectively. Moreover, the setting in inner London probably did not help: it is difficult to reduce admission in places where the admission threshold is already high.

Crisis resolution

It was demonstrated long ago that long-stay psychiatric inpatient beds can largely be replaced by community resources [18]. However, until recently it was not clear whether this was also the case for acute inpatient treatment. Despite this, there was a policy in the 1990s in the United Kingdom of progressive reduction in the availability of inpatient beds. This had untoward effects, which Tyrer [19] described as the 'profligate service', characterised by the use of beds outside the normal catchment area, the loss of continuity of care and progressive rise in admission rates. This policy was based on the assumption that CMHTs can provide adequate care in substitution for inpatient treatment. It was clear that, at that point, bed closures, certainly in inner-city areas, had gone too far.

This led to the introduction of dedicated CRTs [14, 20]. The argument for doing this was reasonable. Given the high levels of violence and the frequent necessity for compulsory detention, inpatient treatment is unpopular with both clients and their relatives. However, few CMHTs have resources for the urgent and intensive visiting required to obviate the need for admission in crisis. Perhaps a more focused and intensive community-based service could take on this function. Early examples of this approach included the work in Wisconsin [18], which, as we have already seen, also served as a model for assertive outreach. Hoult et al. [21] reported positive results from the introduction of a crisis resolution team in Sydney. These services involved 24 hour access, or at least extended hours. Treatment was generally home-based, with visits more than once a day if needed. There was also access to team professionals by phone. It was claimed that this type of intervention had the capacity to reduce bed use, and therefore costs, while increasing patient and carer satisfaction.

Early studies of intensive home treatment initiated in emergencies [18, 21, 22] provide only limited support for the current CRT model, as the experimental teams continued to provide care once the crisis had resolved, and control services did not include routine home visits by multidisciplinary teams. Nevertheless, policy again ran ahead of empirical research into effectiveness [13, 14]. There had been virtually no RCTs or even natural experiments with appropriate controls in Britain. Up to a point, this is understandable: it is extremely difficult to overcome the logistic problems of researching the impact of interventions designed to resolve crises. Early studies relied on temporal or geographical comparisons. Reynolds et al. [23] reported results from a small survey following the introduction of a crisis resolution team, based on historical controls. There appeared to be a small reduction in bed use, and both service users and carers expressed satisfaction with the change. Minghella et al. [24] took advantage of a natural experiment in Birmingham, in which a crisis resolution team was introduced in one area but not in a comparison area. Although there was no diminution in psychiatric symptoms, the authors reported reduced admission rates, lower costs and increased satisfaction in the CRT arm. However, they made no adjustment for baseline differences between the groups, and the response rate was very poor.

Thus, it became apparent, even as CRTs were being introduced, that the research base was insufficient. The only evidence involved comparison with services that had identifiable inadequacies. It was not clear that CRTs reduced admission rates in areas with high thresholds for admission, nor was it possible to calculate how many beds might be closed as a result of their introduction. Finally, CRTs appeared incapable of improving clinical or social functioning, social networks or quality of life. For this reason, Johnson and her colleagues [25, 26] set up a pair of linked controlled trials in a deprived catchment area in inner London. The first was a before and after comparison trial in South Islington, while the second was an RCT in North Islington. This tandem design maximises inferential validity and generalisability through a process of triangulation. Before and after trials lack the benefits of randomisation, but are likely to include a wider range of participants, and their results may thereby imply more general application.

The South Islington CRT study involved the estimation of costs and outcomes relating to the introduction of CRTs. One of the central methodological problems of this design is the identification of crises. Once the crisis resolution team has been set up, the clients accepted by the team can be identified as being in crisis. However, before that, the definition of a crisis is much more problematic. One of the advantages of the South Islington study was the development and use of an operational definition of a crisis [25]. Using this, an independent clinical panel decided whether the criteria for a crisis had been met. Data were then collected at baseline, and at six weeks and six months afterwards. The baseline assessment was detailed and wide-ranging, in order to allow for a large number of potential confounders.

The North Islington CRT study was based on randomisation. Clearly, this is difficult to carry out at a time of crisis. The procedure depended on using a 24 hour telephone randomisation service once referrals had been accepted as appropriate by team staff members. There are also ethical issues that require to be resolved, as clients in crisis might not be capable of valid consent. There was an arrangement whereby clients already known to the service could opt into the study before they were in crisis, and in other cases consent was obtained from next of kin. No other clients who lacked capacity took part. All in all, 260 subjects were randomised. Data were collected at baseline, and eight weeks and six months after the crisis, using information from staff and clinical files. Participants were themselves interviewed at the eight-week stage (response rate 87%).

In both studies, there was a substantial reduction in admissions during the crisis. Before the existence of the CRT in South Islington, 70% of people in crisis had been admitted in the following six weeks. This was reduced to 48% following the introduction of the CRT. This was reflected in an average reduction from 19 to 13 days in hospital. After adjustment for baseline differences, these results remained highly significant. There was also significantly greater satisfaction on the part of clients with the CRT-based service. The eight-week results from the RCT were similar, and again highly significant: of the participants in the experimental group, 21% had been admitted, compared with 59% of the controls. The reduction in bed days was considerable, from 17.8 to 6.6. These differences were maintained: in the six months after the crisis, 29% of the experimental group had been admitted, in contrast to 67% of the control group. The equivalent bed days in hospital were 16 and 35. However, there was relatively little difference in the number of participants who required to be admitted *compulsorily*. This indicates that the benefits were greatest for the less severe crises; the introduction of CRTs might, therefore, have untoward effects on the atmosphere in inpatient units. One difference between the before and after comparison and the RCT was that there was no improvement in client satisfaction in the latter.

Taken together, these studies suggest that CRT had an impact on bed use, mainly on voluntary admissions. There may be an effect on satisfaction, but this is not definite. However, there was no short-term impact on other variables of interest: social functioning, symptoms or quality of life.

Problems in identifying cost-effectiveness

The trials of assertive outreach and crisis resolution described here suggest strongly that CRTs have an effect on bed occupancy, while AOTS do not. This has been made particularly clear by an elegant study carried out by Glover and his colleagues [27]. This demonstrated that over a number of years, bed use was declining generally. AOTs had no effect on this decline, whereas it was accelerated by the introduction of CRTs (see Figure 22.1).

What to make of these results? Assertive outreach and crisis intervention both have the explicit intention of keeping people out of hospital if at all possible. This was assumed, with some justice, to be laudable. However, in the case of assertive outreach, the *primary* goal was the engagement of people reluctant to accept services. Again, this is based on an implicit assumption, to wit, that the mere fact of engagement will encourage acceptance of, and benefit from, treatment. Assessing the cost-effectiveness of assertive outreach is problematic. This is because increased engagement with services inevitably increases costs. Costs would only be reduced if there was indeed a reduction in bed use, given the very high cost of inpatient care. Thus, the ideal outcome for an assertive outreach intervention is that the increased costs of engagement would be more than compensated for by the reduction in hospital bed use. However, there is a danger that closer contact with clients experiencing difficult problems may actually increase bed use, as the full extent of their problems is recognised and monitored, particularly if they seem incapable of resolution. In the event, AOTs might be either more or less expensive than ordinary CMHTs. These costs will be reflected in a range of outcomes. Ideally, these would include social and clinical improvements. However, these have generally been unchanged by ACT, and this was so in the REACT trial described earlier. Other outcomes include effective engagement and the satisfaction of the client, which are likely to go hand in hand. In their economic study of the REACT trial, McCrone and his colleagues [28] opted to assess cost-effectiveness in terms of client satisfaction. They found that the total follow-up costs over 18 months were marginally *higher* for the ACT

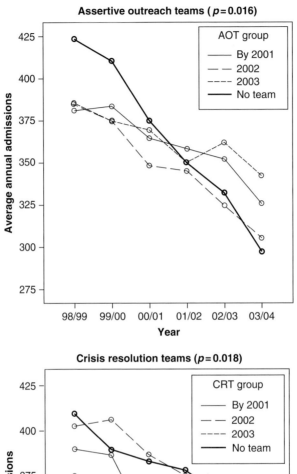

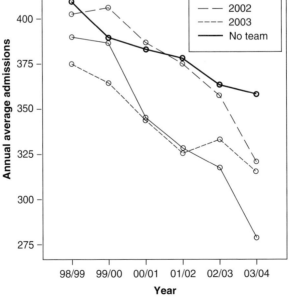

Figure 22.1 The effect of introducing crisis resolution teams and assertive outreach team on bed occupancy in the United Kingdom. Taken from Glover et al. [27].

group, partly because they had spent a little more time in hospital. However, this was not statistically significant. They calculated that a one-unit improvement in satisfaction scores in the ACT group was associated with extra costs of nearly £500. While client satisfaction is an intrinsic good, most professionals and most clients would, quite reasonably, prefer outcomes that included social and clinical improvement.

The clue to the primary aim of crisis resolution lies in the name, although its effectiveness is very closely tied up with the prevention of hospital admission, which has therefore been used consistently in trials as a proxy measure of outcome. It is nevertheless possible to conceive of crises being unpleasantly prolonged as a result of the drive to prevent admission, and the objective of crisis resolution, there-fore, does not map perfectly onto admission rates. In an ideal world, the actions of a crisis resolution team would be to shorten the crisis and reduce its impact on client and carers, with reduced admission to hospital as a benign side effect. However, it is also possible to effect a reduction in admissions merely by fiercer gate-keeping. The advantage of the service so closely targeting the process of emergency admission is that there would be sizeable cost reductions if it were effective.

Economic analyses were carried out in both the South Islington and North Islington trials of crisis intervention [29, 30]. At follow-up in South Islington, mean costs for the post-CRT patients were appreciably less, albeit not significantly so. However, when patients with any CRT contact were compared with those with none, the cost reduction per patient became significant, at £2189. The RCT of crisis intervention in North Islington provided quantitatively similar results. The primary outcome measure in the economic analysis was inpatient days over a six-month follow-up period. Patients receiving care from the CRT had *non-inpatient* costs nearly £800 higher than patients receiving standard care, reflecting the greater degree of involvement by the team. However, after the inclusion of inpatient costs, the CRT group cost about £2500 less than standard care. This gave a 99.5% likelihood of the CRT being cost-effective.

CRTs can be justified because they provide similar clinical and social outcomes for less cost than standard care, and perhaps increase client satisfaction. Assertive outreach, on the other hand, provides equivalent outcomes, but with no reduction in cost, and possibly a slight increase. The only identifiable justifi-cation is therefore in terms of client satisfaction, but without improved social and clinical outcomes, this is far from persuasive.

Social and psychological interventions in psychosis

Family intervention for psychosis
Research on informal carers dates back to the 1950s, following the decline in bed numbers in asylums in the United Kingdom and the United States. As a result, informal (unpaid) carers (usually relatives) found themselves increasingly

involved in the day-to-day care of people with serious mental health problems. Such caring has always been demanding and stressful, and is often prolonged [31–34]. Up to a third of carers of people with psychosis meet criteria for post-traumatic stress disorder (PTSD) [35] and depression [36]. The sense of grief and loss is comparable to levels recorded in bereavement [37].

The first empirical research linking family atmosphere and the outcome of psychosis dates back to the 1960s [38–40]. This made it clear that, although family involvement could be helpful, some reactions – particularly if critical or overinvolved – were associated with subsequent relapse of the service user. These reactions were encapsulated in the concept of expressed emotion (EE) [39]. High levels of EE in key relatives reliably predict patient outcomes in schizophrenia: overall, the relapse rate for those returning to low EE families was 21% compared with a 50% relapse rate in families with high EE [41].

The earliest RCTs of family intervention in psychosis (FI-p) date back to the early 1980s [42, 43], and the treatment is well-established. There is robust evidence from a large number of clinical trials that it reduces the rate of relapse in psychosis by around 20% [44–49]. While this effect appears to be independent of the amount of pharmaceutical treatment, the best outcomes occur when family intervention is accompanied by regular adherence to anti-psychotic medication [41]. However, in routine service settings, the implementation of family intervention has tended to be poor, and it is inapplicable for the many patients in inner cities without close carers. The reason may be that the treatment is complex, requires training and supervision and does not enter the job description of most care staff [50, 51]. While there are successful training initiatives in some British locations, such as Meriden in the Midlands [52], the effectiveness of such training in increasing access to FI-p or in improving outcomes as a result has not yet been well-demonstrated.

The first attempts to modify outcome by family intervention resulted from the EE research into the effects of poor relationships on outcome in schizophrenia [42, 43]. These early interventions were developed from evidence about the problems carers faced and from behaviour therapy approaches to modifying unproductive patterns of problem solving in families. However, these early approaches lacked a detailed understanding of the particular cognitive and affective problems associated with caring roles in psychosis. We now know much more about this [53, 54]. For instance, it is clear that high EE relates to attributions and appraisal of the problems, rather than to the problems per se [55–57]. This contributes to the sense of burden, stress and distress experienced by carers [58], to other poor outcomes such as low self-esteem, and to less effective, avoidant coping, even at first episode [36, 59, 60].

High levels of negative EE, such as criticism from carers, seem to have their effects on patients via mood: critical and intrusive relationships increase anxiety and depression [61, 62]. In contrast, supportive relationships are likely to reduce negative affect. This is seen in some trials of psychological therapy in which the control 'befriending' or supportive therapy resulted in improvements in affect and positive symptoms [63], and may explain the better response to psychological treatments in those patients with carers than in those without [64]. More recent evidence suggests a mechanism for this: service users are able to perceive criticism from their carers accurately, and perceptions of carer criticism have in turn been linked to poorer service user functioning [65–67].

We proposed that individuals' appraisal of their illness also influences their own mood and engagement with treatment, influencing longer-term outcomes [68]. Recent research has indeed confirmed that the illness perception of people with psychosis has a strong relationship to negative affect, both anxiety and depression [69, 70], although a longer-term impact on outcomes has yet to be demonstrated.

Thus, carers' appraisals of their circumstances and of the resources they have to cope with them are crucial to both carer and service user outcomes, much more so than the apparent severity or scope of the problems faced [31]. Such appraisals contribute to the well-being of service users as well as of carers, and it has been argued more recently that carers merit targeting in treatment in their own right [50].

In physical ill health, carers' illness perceptions and their resultant decisions are more important than illness severity in determining outcomes [71]. This is equally true in psychosis [72, 73]. Carers experience more stress and depression, and have more negative views of the impact of care, if they feel they are not in control of their relative's illness, and that it will last a long time. When, as commonly happens, these illness perceptions run counter to those of service users, carers are more likely to experience low mood and self-esteem [74]. Such disagreements are observed more frequently in high-EE relationships [72].

Recently, more attention has been given to positive aspects of caregiving relationships and their links with carer and service user outcomes [57, 75]. Many carers report positive caregiving experiences, with associated feelings of satisfaction and improved self-esteem [76, 77]. Moreover, carer warmth can serve as a protective factor against relapse [10, 78, 79].

There is firm evidence about the coping responses most advantageous to carers of people with psychosis [80–82]. Coping is dependent on accurate appraisal of situations, on the individual's resources and on how these are deployed [83]. In psychosis, avoidant coping (characterised by 'hoping problems will go away') may be useful for temporary problems that resolve naturally, but not for more enduring or worsening problems. Active and proactive strategies seem more capable of reducing carer burden, even early in the illness [31, 81, 84]. Such strategies are usually shaped and encouraged as part of family interventions [85, 86]. The stigma and shame associated with mental ill health can lead to a significant reduction in social networks, even for carers [87, 88]. The importance of social support, particularly access to a confidante, in reducing distress and encouraging more proactive coping in carers has been confirmed [87, 89].

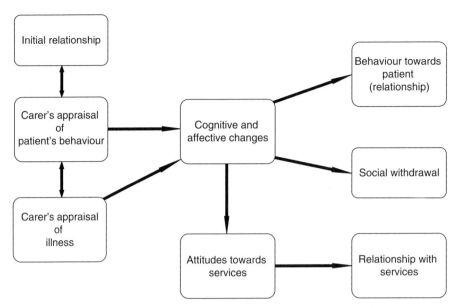

Figure 22.2 Cognitive model of carer responses in psychosis after Kuipers et al. [54].

This information has now been integrated into a cognitive model of family intervention (see Figure 22.2) [54]. The model uses information from empirical research to shape the degree, complexity and content of treatment. Treatment is described in terms of different carer responses: positive, emotionally over involved or hostile and critical. This is an example of how detailed assessment of individual cases can indicate the appropriate elements of an intervention.

Cognitive behaviour therapy for psychosis

Cognitive behaviour therapy for psychosis (CBT-p) has consistently been shown to reduce psychotic symptoms in people with medication-resistant symptoms [46, 47, 90, 91]. Although there were early indications that it may also reduce relapse [92] and emotional distress [93], the evidence for effectiveness is most robust in patients with enduring, medication-resistant and distressing positive symptoms. However, even for positive symptom reduction, effect sizes remain moderate, at only 0.35 and 0.37 in recent meta-analyses [91, 94, 95]. It should be noted that this is based on an *additional* effect in people already benefiting from medication. It thus compares reasonably well with the effect sizes of 0.48 for second-generation antipsychotics compared with placebo [96].

However, Tarrier and Wykes [94] and Wykes et al. [95] have queried the methodological standards used in CBT studies, showing that smaller effect sizes were seen in trials with blind raters. The most recent Cochrane meta-analysis of 30 trials [97] concluded that 'no overall effectiveness was found between CBT and other talking therapies...although there might be some longer term advantage in CBT for dealing with emotions and distressing feelings'. However, one of the perennial issues in meta-analysis concerns which trials are included and which excluded, and the rationale for these decisions. A further issue is that the more recent trials have focused on unselected samples. Thus, reduced effect sizes over time might have more than one cause.

Recent guidelines, which have their own strict methodology and trial quality standards, have looked at the evidence independently, and both the UK National Institute for Health and Clinical Excellence (NICE) [98, 99] and the US Patient Outcomes Research Team (PORT) guidelines [100] recommend that CBT-p and FI-p should be made more widely available. Additional support for CBT-p comes from the recent POSITIVE trial in Germany, a methodologically sophisticated multisite RCT with blind ratings of 330 patients with persistent symptoms of psychosis [101]. Participants were randomised to receive 20 sessions of CBT-p or supportive therapy (another manualised talking treatment). Outcomes were assessed over a two-year follow-up. Participants had symptoms of medium severity, and some degree of social impairment, and 92% were adherent to medication. Around 10% of sessions were assessed for therapist competence, and demonstrated high levels of skill for both therapy conditions. At nine-month follow-up, the CBT-p group showed significantly greater improvement, with an effect size of 0.33 over and above the effect of supportive therapy (Prof. Stefan Klingberg, personal communication). The formal publication of the results of this important trial is expected in 2013.

Preventing relapse with CBT-p

The 2003 NICE guideline identified a need for research on the effectiveness of CBT in preventing relapse. This led to the Psychological Prevention of Relapse in Psychosis (PRP) trial [64, 102]. This large, multicentre trial was designed specifically to evaluate the effect of CBT-p in reducing future relapses and improving symptoms in patients recovering from a recent psychotic relapse. It comprised two pathways. In the first, patients who had carers were allocated to one of three alternatives: treatment as usual (TAU), CBT-p plus TAU or FI-p plus TAU. In the second, patients without carers were allocated to TAU or to CBT-p plus TAU. The treatments were focused on preventing further relapse, in up to 20 sessions spread over nine months. In all, 301 patients and 83 carers took part, and primary outcome data were available on 96% of the total sample. The CBT and family intervention had no effect on rates of remission and relapse or on days in hospital at 12 or 24 months. The ineffectiveness of family intervention on relapse was particularly surprising, given the strong contrary evidence in the existing literature: it might be attributable to the low overall relapse rate in clients with carers in this study, who were also primarily low in EE. CBT-p showed a beneficial effect on depression at 24 months, but family intervention did not. In people with carers, CBT-p significantly improved delusional distress and social functioning. In the light of these results, we concluded that generic CBT-p should be reserved for the original target group: people with distressing medication-resistant positive symptoms. We saw no grounds for using it routinely to forestall relapse in people recovering from recent episodes of psychosis.

These negative findings might have arisen because the participants were a medication-sensitive group, having in many cases relapsed precisely because they had stopped taking medication. When this was reinstated, many recovered, and were then reluctant to engage with CBT-p. Thus, positive results might have been restricted to the subgroup of participants who had received CBT-p as per protocol.

However, the analysis of subgroups in randomised trials is usually a methodological solecism: it is carried out in a way that removes the advantages of randomisation and opens the door to false inference (see Dunn, Chapter 19). Nevertheless, we thought it important to assess the delivery of the different elements of treatment and their effect on outcome. This was because CBT-p involves a range of interventions, the deployment and timing of which is determined by discussion between therapist and client. The treatment is manualised, and therapy sessions were routinely taped, allowing detailed evaluations of therapy delivery and of client engagement during the study (something no previous study of CBT-p had attempted). In a pre-planned analysis, we therefore applied novel statistical methods to assess the differential effect of the type of treatment delivered on the effectiveness of CBT-p [102]. This involved the use of principal stratification (based on structural equation modelling with finite mixtures) to estimate intention-to-treat (ITT) effects for subgroups of participants. These were defined by qualitative and quantitative differences in the receipt of therapy. This technique allowed us effectively to maintain the constraints and inferential benefits of randomisation.

The findings were interesting. The consistent delivery of *full therapy*, defined *a priori* by specific cognitive and behavioural interventions, led to clinically and statistically significant increases in months in remission, and diminution of psychotic and affective symptoms. Delivery of *partial therapy* (which involved assessment and engagement by highly skilled clinicians) was not effective. These analyses suggest that CBT-p is of clinically significant benefit in patients able to engage in the full range of therapy procedures. In this group, CBT-p had a significant impact on relapse prevention, paralleled by symptomatic improvements.

The findings do raise the question of the prior identification of patients likely to benefit. We were, however, unable to predict from the individual characteristics of participants in the PRP trial which patients would engage in the sometimes difficult process of full therapy. However, a subsequent study showed that aspects of illness perception were predictive of engagement in full therapy – essentially those who saw psychological therapy as relevant and likely to help them gain 'control' over their problems [103]. This kind of screening measure may be of use in the future. Other predictors of good outcome in CBT-p show that those with good memory and planning do better [104], and those with a 'chink of insight', that is, who have some doubt about their delusions before therapy starts, improve more quickly [105]. Finally, it now seems clear that therapists should not persist in trying to deliver full therapy if it becomes apparent that clients are unable to meet its demands.

Treatment innovations and the attributes of psychosis

FI-p and CBT-p are both treatments of considerable complexity. This is understandable, as they were developed in response to theoretically based evidence of the processes and mechanisms involved in the generation of psychotic symptoms. Treating people with these techniques has in turn increased our knowledge of process. Freeman et al. [106] argue that attempts to improve CBT should use this knowledge to develop more specific interventions. This carries the possibility of the individual tailoring of treatment. It may also identify specific, relatively brief, interventions that could be delivered following brief protocol-based training to a wider range of patients by staff such as care coordinators or support workers. A recent pilot study has shown this can reduce symptoms, improve affect and help participants to reach their goals [107].

Psychosis is clearly a complex condition, with complex origins in the interaction of biological, psychological and social factors. Likewise, it has a complex course, and the appropriateness of treatment almost certainly varies with the phase of illness. A number of cognitive models of positive psychotic symptoms have been published. Although these recognise and accept the importance of biological processes, they emphasise the contribution of psychological mechanisms to the development and persistence of psychosis, particularly those involving emotional and reasoning processes [68, 108–112]. They also include a significant role for a social aetiology, as they propose that the emotional disturbance occurs in the context of a conducive social-cognitive background [59, 68]. Models like this provide a powerful impetus for investigating mechanisms, and have stimulated a major research effort over the last decade or so. Their significance for the present chapter is that they feed into the elaboration of techniques suitable for consideration in the process of CBT-p and FI-p. One of the earlier examples of these cognitive models [68, 109] is illustrated in Figure 22.3.

The continuum of psychotic experience

Cognitive models postulate that symptoms of psychosis lie on a continuum from subclinical to clinical. However, psychotic experiences are in themselves insufficient to ensure passage across the threshold of diagnosable disorder. Since the late 1980s, there have been reports that experiences similar to those of psychotic patients are identifiable in the general population [113]. Large-scale population studies have confirmed this, although prevalence varies with the instruments used, the phenomena covered and the population surveyed [114]. Thus, 5.5% of participants in the 2000 British National Psychiatric Morbidity Survey reported some kind of psychotic experience [115], compared with 17.5% in the Dutch NEMESIS

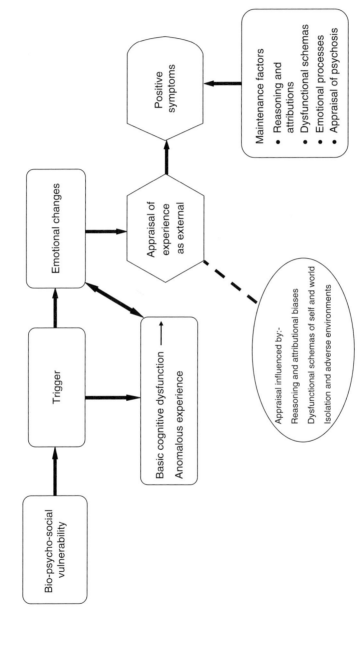

Figure 22.3 Cognitive model of positive symptoms of psychosis after Garety et al. [68].

survey [116]. Up to 30% of a young adult internet sample had some level of paranoid ideation [117]. van Os et al. [118] argued that the psychosis phenotype is expressed as a continuous distribution of experiences, and that it may be 50 times more common than the medical concept. The substantial literature supporting this idea has been summarised by Hanssen et al. [118] and Linscott and van Os [119].

Are subclinical psychotic experiences really made of the same cloth as their counterparts seen in the clinic? The characteristics of auditory hallucinations in non-clinical samples have been reviewed by Larøi et al. [120]. The classical phenomenological attributes seem similar in clinical and non-clinical groups. However, in the former, the experience is usually infrequent and brief, and often occurs in unusual circumstances such as sleep deprivation and stress. While voices may be accompanied by subclinical delusions, they are rarely associated with negative symptoms. Non-clinical voice-hearers generally feel more in control of their voices, which tend to be more mundane and less self-referential. Voices with negative content are more characteristic of clinical groups. Interestingly, non-clinical voice hearers seem more likely to attribute them to spiritual experiences than to real people. Finally, clinical and subclinical experiences demonstrate similar associations with demographic attributes and environmental risk factors [121–123]. While psychotic-like experiences in the general population are rarely elicited in the rigorous manner of a detailed clinical interview, the similarities therefore appear to be considerable. Finally and importantly, it is clear that transitions occur over time from the subclinical to the clinical [124–126]. This begs for an explanation of why transitions occur and an exposition of the consequent implications for treatment.

Emotion and psychotic experience

Cognitive models propose that the emergence of clinical disorder is encouraged by both cognitive and emotional factors. The emphasis on emotional processes is novel. It is held that they act alone or in combination with cognitive biases in vulnerable individuals to increase the risk of positive symptom formation through the resulting appraisal patterns [68, 110, 111, 127, 128]. Thus, distress is a key factor distinguishing clinical from non-clinical populations [126, 129–132]. Baseline and follow-up data from the 2000 British National Psychiatric Morbidity Survey showed neurotic symptoms were associated with both current and future paranoia and other psychotic symptoms [103, 106, 133]. The function of affective symptoms in maintaining paranoid ideation in people with psychosis was recently confirmed in a longitudinal clinical study [134]. These results emphasise the importance in therapy of specific techniques designed to ameliorate the emotional component of psychosis.

Worry and psychosis

Some cognitive theorists have emphasised the role of 'meta-cognitive' processes in the development of delusions, for instance, ways of thinking, such as a ruminative style [111, 128]. Worry is repetitive ruminative thinking about experiences.

It inevitably has an affective quality, and is seen as important in emotional disorders, particularly because it involves catastrophisation, whereby the negative significance of personal circumstances becomes exaggerated. In line with the well-established affective component in psychosis, worry may also have a role in maintaining delusions of negative content, such as persecutory delusions [110]. It correlates with the severity of delusional distress [135]. In one longitudinal study of patients with acute psychosis and persecutory delusions, worry processes contributed to delusional conviction and persistence at follow-up [136]. It predicts emerging paranoia in general population samples [103]. Pilot work using brief cognitive interventions to deal with worry has shown reductions in persecutory delusions [137, 138].

Insomnia and psychosis

Insomnia is common in people with psychosis [139], and does not appear to be the result of neuroleptic medication [140]. As well as impairing quality of life [141], increasing insomnia is often associated with the emergence or re-emergence of psychotic symptoms. Even in the mentally well, insomnia has the capacity to distort thinking, particularly in the small hours, and it is conceivable that in psychosis this distortion builds and persists. Insomnia is clearly a correlate and a predictor of paranoia in general population samples [103, 106]. Some of its effect is mediated through anxiety and depression. If insomnia is a mediator of delusional thinking rather than the product or concomitant of it, it should be possible to modify delusions by the effective treatment of insomnia. A pilot study has suggested that this is so, using a four-session cognitive approach [142].

Recent epidemiological findings

The last 15 years or so have seen an increasing volume of research into the social correlates of psychosis, adding greatly to the plausibility of a major social component in its aetiology. Much of this work has implications for social and psychological treatment, some very direct, some less so.

A number of environmental factors are now accepted as influencing the development of schizophrenia: these include urban birth and rearing, migrant status and membership of ethnic minorities [143–148]. The understanding of these environmental factors has relied strongly on hypotheses about individual social class and social capital, indices of neighbourhood deprivation, racial discrimination and life events such as childhood parental separation [148, 149]. They are certainly consistent with cognitive models, which postulate psychological mechanisms for the action of environmental factors, such as an increased vulnerability to anxiety, depression and low self-esteem and an enduring cognitive bias affecting the processing of events and experiences. The latter emerges from the consequences of adversity on expectations, and includes schematic beliefs about self and others, and distortions in attributional style, such as a tendency to attribute power and control to others [68, 150, 151].

However, these epidemiological correlates are merely suggestive of psychological approaches to treatment. This is not the case with the effects of trauma, which feeds directly into treatment options. There is now strong evidence that psychosis is often preceded by childhood trauma, including sexual abuse and victimisation [152–157]. Cognitive models have provided differing accounts for the mechanism of the effects of trauma on psychosis. Hallucinations are particularly common in people with psychosis who have experienced traumas [158, 159]. One hypothesis is that intrusive memories of traumatic experiences are the re-experiencing symptoms seen in PTSD. However, in psychosis they are not recognised as such and are thus misinterpreted [160]. Such direct and intrusive PTSD-like re-experiencing is relatively uncommon. Traumatic experiences more typically facilitate the emergence of psychosis by creating emotional disturbance and negative schematic beliefs about the self and others, and by increasing anomalous experiences [68, 161]. Hardy et al. [158] found that hallucinations could be considered a form of re-experienced traumatic memories in only 12.5% of people with psychosis and a history of traumas. In nearly half, the links between the traumas experienced and the psychotic symptoms were solely schematic, and in around 40%, no interpretable links could be identified. Bullying and childhood sexual abuse were the types of trauma most often associated with hallucinations.

It may be possible to adapt some of the ideas underlying the successful treatment of trauma to benefit people with psychosis who have a traumatic history. Pilot work on this has shown that up to three-quarters of those with persistent delusions or hallucinations have intrusive images and memories associated with their beliefs [162, 163]. Other work at a preliminary stage suggests that, for some people, rescripting of these upsetting images can be helpful.

Negative schematic beliefs and psychosis

Although low self-esteem and depressed mood are correlated, it has been found that negative schematic beliefs – relatively enduring beliefs about the self and others – contribute to the development and persistence of psychosis, over and above the effects of depressed or anxious mood [55, 164]. Mood and schemas are independently associated with psychotic and psychotic-like symptoms in clinical and non-clinical populations [164, 165]. A combination of very negative extreme self (as weak, vulnerable, inadequate) and extreme negative other (devious, threatening, bad) schemas, in association with anxiety, was found to be specifically associated with paranoia. The schema patterns associated with hallucinations and grandiose delusions were quite distinct [166].

Appraisals and reasoning processes

A key component of the cognitive model is bias in probabilistic reasoning, thought to contribute to the development of delusions by influencing the appraisal of disturbing anomalous experiences and adverse events. There is strong evidence that people with psychosis 'jump to conclusions' (JTC); that is, they gather less data than controls in reaching a decision [167]. JTC appears to be specifically related to delusions [168, 169], and it is present, in attenuated form, in people defined in various ways as 'at risk' for psychosis [170–172]. It is also identifiable in people who have recovered from delusions [169, 173]. These results suggest that JTC is a trait representing liability to psychosis, particularly if the psychosis phenotype is characterised by delusions [171]. It is also exacerbated in acute psychosis, thus showing state as well as trait characteristics [173].

There have been some attempts to examine the mechanisms underlying JTC. It is negatively associated with 'belief flexibility', the metacognitive ability to generate alternative hypotheses for one's beliefs, and to reflect on the evidence [168, 174]. JTC does not seem related to cognitive impairment, but is related to poor belief flexibility [175]. Because of the link with delusions, attempts are in progress to modify JTC and belief flexibility in clinical populations.

In summary, there is now strong evidence that depressed and anxious mood states, worry, insomnia and negative schematic beliefs contribute to the symptoms of psychosis. Longitudinal data suggest that these emotion-related variables play a causal role in the development and maintenance of psychotic symptoms, facilitating transition to psychosis and contributing to symptom persistence and severity. Reasoning bias and belief flexibility can also maintain symptoms. Thus, these features can act as targets for individualised treatment.

Negative symptoms

Negative symptoms are another important feature of schizophrenia: blunted affect and emotion, poverty of speech, anhedonia, lack of sociability and lack of motivation. Their effect on quality of life, functional disability and the burden on others is greater than that of positive symptoms. Perhaps one-third of patients with schizophrenia in the community have prominent negative symptoms [176]. Antipsychotic medication may improve them through its effect on positive symptoms, but there is always the risk that their extrapyramidal side effects may accentuate negative symptoms [177, 178]. Overall, medication has little effect in improving social functioning [96].

Poor social outcome is widely acknowledged as a major impediment to a full and rewarding life for people who have psychosis. The barriers to improving psychosocial recovery in psychosis are complex. They include the presence of residual psychotic symptoms, underlying neurocognitive deficits, sensitivity to stress, and self-restriction due to affective symptoms and consciousness of impairment, stigma and discrimination. Neurocognitive deficits affect attention, social cognition, working memory, verbal learning, psychomotor speed and executive functions. There is an Atlantic divide over these issues, with American authorities placing more weight on them than their European counterparts. The European view, to which we adhere, acknowledges the role of such deficits, but within the constellation of other factors.

Cognitive remediation is a direct attempt at improving cognitive performance, using a range of techniques such as compensation strategies, environmental aids and exercises to improve executive function and cognition. In the short term, it improves performance on neuropsychological tests, but it is harder to demonstrate effects on functional outcome. The techniques are not yet capable of delivering prolonged effects once treatment has finished; follow-up data are typically short term [179, 180].

A number of studies have provided suggestive evidence for the efficacy of CBT-p in improving negative symptoms [63, 92, 95, 181, 182]. Although these were only assessed as secondary outcomes, they suggested the possibility of combining CBT-p and CRT with vocational case management, as we shall see later.

Towards personalised treatment

There is much discussion of personalised medicine in many conditions including severe psychiatric disorders. When there is great heterogeneity in the form and course of a disorder, there is a clear requirement for personalising treatments. Only in this way is overall outcome likely to be improved. However, a lack of information may restrict our ability to design specific treatment plans. At the moment, this is true of drug treatment in psychosis [96], although with psychological and social treatments even now there may be more scope. Personalisation may be completely individual, by choosing elements of treatment (such as the ones described earlier) in accordance with particular symptoms and problems. Alternatively, it may take the form of identifying subgroups of patients defined in terms of the phase or characteristics of their disorder. Examples of the latter include treatments targeted at the prodromal or initial stages of disorder, or at particular life stages.

Combining interventions

Early intervention services
The onset of psychosis is a particularly critical time, made more so by the fact that treatment may be delayed by the patient and by dilatory service responses. A prolonged duration of untreated psychosis (DUP) causes suffering, but may

also have a malign effect on the subsequent course. Early intervention services (EISs) were developed to address this problem, in the hope that reducing DUP would improve prognosis [183, 184]. They were introduced in Australia, the United States, Canada, New Zealand and elsewhere even though at the time there was little evidence for effectiveness. The National Service Framework for Mental Health [13] and NICE [98] recommended the widespread deployment of such services, since when the provision of EISs has steadily increased, with around 150 EISs currently operating in the United Kingdom [185].

A particularly interesting feature of EISs is that they now usually consist of community-based multidisciplinary mental health teams providing pharmacotherapy, FI-p, CBT-p, problem-solving skills training, vocational help, crisis management and case management [186, 187], in other words, an individually tailored combination of evidence-based psychological interventions. The widespread dissemination of this approach, together with an integral evaluation, characterises the hopeful development of the GETUP project in northern Italy (Prof. Mirella Ruggeri, personal communication; see also Chapter 5 of this volume).

Bird et al. [185] recently carried out a systematic review of EISs for people with a first or early episode of psychosis. They also evaluated the separate use of CBT-p and FI-p in the context of early psychosis. Four EISs, four studies of CBT-p and three studies of FI-p met their quality criteria. They found that EISs reduced hospital admission, relapse rates and symptom severity, and improved access to and engagement with treatment. Used alone, FI-p reduced relapse and hospital admission rates, whereas CBT-p reduced the severity of symptoms, but with little impact on relapse or hospital admission.

Combining CBT-p and vocational case management

The poor social outcome of schizophrenia is most clearly demonstrated in barriers to competitive employment [188–190]. For example, in the tri-national European study carried out by Marwaha et al. [190], the overall employment rate of participants was 22%. This did vary somewhat between countries and sites, with rates of 13% in the United Kingdom, 12% in France and 30% in Germany. The proportion of people in each country who were supporting themselves entirely through working without receiving welfare benefits was much less variable: 9% in the United Kingdom, 8% in France and 12% in Germany. Long-term follow-up studies agree that poor social outcomes become established early in the course of disorder [191, 192].

Fowler et al. [193] developed a form of CBT specifically focused on improving constructive social behaviour while managing sensitivity to stress, social anxiety and psychotic symptoms in early psychosis. This was combined with vocational case management typified by individual placement and support working practices. The intervention formed the basis of an RCT [193]. As social recovery is a complex construct with several domains, the primary measure of outcome in this trial comprised time spent engaged in structured social and constructive economic activity. Seventy-seven participants with affective and non-affective psychosis were randomised after recruitment from secondary mental health teams. They had presented with a history of unemployment and poor social outcome. The treatment was delivered over a nine-month period, in a mean of 12 sessions. The cognitive work, delivered in three stages, included negotiating a formulation with the client, promoting a sense of agency, and addressing hopelessness, feelings of stigma and negative beliefs about self and others. Social activity, work, education and leisure were actively promoted by linking them to meaningful goals in the third stage. ITT analysis showed no significant impact on primary or secondary outcomes. However, a pre-planned analysis with diagnostic subgroups showed important benefits of CBT specifically in people with non-affective psychosis who had problems with social recovery. There was some evidence that the beneficial effects might be mediated by reducing hopelessness and improving positive beliefs about self and others, particularly in participants with non-affective psychosis [194]. These results are sufficiently promising to justify a larger RCT of this approach. It is an interesting combination of social and psychological interventions, and with refinement may be capable, at any rate in some individuals, of mitigating one of the central problems in the management of psychosis: how to improve meaningful activity and employment after an episode.

Conclusions

As Tandon et al. [96] point out, it is clear that in the last 25 years our understanding of treatments for schizophrenia has changed remarkably little. No single treatment, whether pharmacological or psychological, produces improvement that is reliable at the individual level, despite moderately good group effects. Group effects in ordinary clinical practice are, however, vitiated by the availability and implementation of treatment. In principle, the prime responsibility of community psychiatric services is the delivery of treatments whose efficacy is established, at least at the group level. Team structures do not in themselves improve outcomes unless the teams deliver effective evidence-based treatments and interventions. Hence, the team structures that do well are those that do this – notably early intervention teams [185].

However, the differential responses of individual patients to particular treatments are such that it is very difficult to predict who will respond to what. This means that the delivery of treatment should be flexible in the light of a continuing process of assessment. Treatments should be negotiated between clinicians and clients in the light of preference, vulnerability and need, and renegotiations in the light of new information should be the norm, in an essentially iterative process. The timing of treatment is likely to be important too – sometimes patients will consider a treatment two or three years into their illness that they would not have countenanced at its beginning.

The key to improvements in treatment is knowledge: increased knowledge of the disorder, its attributes and mechanisms and increased knowledge of the detailed effects of treatments, whether psychological, social or pharmacological. This research knowledge must then be disseminated and supported effectively at team level. Only then will we be able to narrow the gap between efficacy and effectiveness.

References

[1] van Os J, Kapur S. (2009) Schizophrenia. *Lancet* **374**: 635–645.

[2] Prichard JC. (1833) *A Treatise on Insanity*. London: Marchant.

[3] Thornicroft G, Bebbington PE. (1989) Deinstitutionalisation: from hospital closure to service development. *British Journal of Psychiatry* **155**: 739–753.

[4] Grad J, Sainsbury P. (1966) Evaluating community psychiatric service in Chichester – results. *Milbank Memorial Fund Quarterly* **44**: 279–287.

[5] Leucht S, Arbter D, Engel RR et al. (2009) How effective are second generation antipsychotic drugs? A meta-analysis of placebo-controlled trials. *Molecular Psychiatry* **14**: 429–447.

[6] Lieberman JA, Stroup TS, McEvoy JP et al. (2005) Effectiveness of antipsychotic drugs in patients with chronic schizophrenia. *New England Journal of Medicine* **353**: 1209–1223.

[7] Jones PB, Barnes TRE, Davies L et al. (2006) Randomized controlled trial of the effect on quality of life of second- vs first-generation antipsychotic drugs in schizophrenia – Cost Utility of the Latest Antipsychotic Drugs in Schizophrenia Study (CUtLASS 1). *Archives of General Psychiatry* **63**: 1079–1087.

[8] Tyrer P, Coid J, Simmonds S et al. (2000) Community Mental Health Teams (CMHTs) for people with severe mental illnesses and disordered personality. *Cochrane Database of Systematic Reviews* **2**: CD000270.

[9] Marx AJ, Test MA, Stein LI. (1973) Extra-hospital management of severe mental illness – feasibility and effects of social functioning. *Archives of General Psychiatry* **29**: 505–511.

[10] Marshall M, Lockwood A. (1998) Assertive community treatment for people with severe mental disorders (Cochrane Review). *Cochrane Library* **4**: CD001089.

[11] Marshall M, Creed F. (2000) Assertive community treatment – is it the future of community care in the UK? *International Review of Psychiatry* **12**: 191–196.

[12] Teague GP, Bond GR, Drake RE. (1998) Programme fidelity in community treatment: development and views of measure. *American Journal of Orthopsychiatry* **68**: 216–231.

[13] Department of Health. (1999) *National Service Framework for Mental Health*. Available from: http://www.dh.gov.uk/en/publicationsandstatistics/Lettersandcirculars/index.htm. Accessed on 31 December 2012.

[14] Department of Health. (2001) *Mental Health Policy Implementation Guide*. Available from: http://www.dh.gov.uk/en/Publicationsandstatistics/Publications/PublicationsPolicy AndGuidance/DH_4009350. Accessed on 31 December 2012.

[15] Killaspy H, Bebbington PE, Blizard R et al. (2006) The REACT study: a randomised evaluation of assertive community treatment in north London. *BMJ* **332**: 815–820.

[16] Killaspy H, Kingett S, Bebbington PE et al. (2009) Three year outcomes of participants in the REACT (Randomised Evaluation of Assertive Community Treatment in North London) study. *British Journal of Psychiatry* **195**: 81–82.

[17] Wright C, Burns T, James P et al. (2003) Assertive outreach teams in London: models of operation – Pan-London Assertive Outreach Study Part I. *British Journal of Psychiatry* **183**: 132–138.

[18] Stein PLI, Test MA. (1980) Alternative to mental hospital treatment. I. Conceptual model treatment program, and clinical evaluation. *Archives of General Psychiatry* **37**: 392–397.

[19] Tyrer P. (1988) Cost-effective or profligate community psychiatry? *British Journal of Psychiatry* **172**: 1–3.

[20] Johnson S. (2004) Crisis resolution and intensive home treatment teams. *Psychiatry* **3**: 22–25.

[21] Hoult J, Reynolds I, Charbonneaupowis M et al. (1983) Psychiatric hospital versus community treatment – the results of a randomised trial. *Australian and New Zealand Journal of Psychiatry* **17**: 160–167.

[22] Marks IM,Connolly J, Muijen M et al. (1994) Home-based versus hospital-based care for people with seriousmental illness. *British Journal of Psychiatry* **165**: 179–194.

[23] Reynolds I, Jones JE, Berry DW et al. (1990) A crisis team for the mentally ill: the effect on patients, relatives and admissions. *Medical Journal of Australia* **152**: 646–652.

[24] Minghella E, Ford R, Freeman T et al. (1998) *Open All Hours: 24 Hour Response for People with Mental Health Emergencies*. London: Sainsbury Centre for Mental Health.

[25] Johnson S, Nolan F, Hoult J et al. (2005) Outcomes of crises before and after introduction of a crisis resolution team: Islington Crisis Studies 1. *British Journal of Psychiatry* **187**: 68–75.

[26] Johnson S, Nolan F, Pilling S et al. (2005) Randomised controlled trial of care by a crisis resolution team: the North Islington Crisis Study. *BMJ* **331**: 599–602.

[27] Glover G, Arts G, Babu KS. (2006) Crisis resolution/home treatment teams and psychiatric admission rates in England. *British Journal of Psychiatry* **189**: 441–445.

[28] McCrone P, Johnson S, Nolan F et al. (2009) Impact of a crisis resolution team on service costs in the UK. *Psychiatric Bulletin* **33**: 17–19.

[29] McCrone P, Killaspy H, Bebbington P et al. (2009) The REACT study: cost-effectiveness of assertive community treatment in north London. *Psychiatric Services* **60**: 908–913.

[30] McCrone P, Pilling S, Sandor A et al. (2009) Economic evaluation of a crisis resolution service: the north Islington crisis study. *Epidemiologia e Psichiatria Sociale* **18**: 54–58.

[31] Scazufca M, Kuipers E. (1996) Links between expressed emotion and burden of care in relatives of patients with schizophrenia. *British Journal of Psychiatry* **168**: 580–587.

[32] Brown S, Birtwistle J. (1998) People with schizophrenia and their families. Fifteen-year outcome. *British Journal of Psychiatry* **173**: 139–144.

[33] Kuipers E, Bebbington PE. (2005) Research on burden and coping strategies in families of people with mental disorders; problems and perspectives. In: Leff J, Sartorius N, Maj M (eds.), *Families and Mental Disorders: From Burden to Empowerment*. Chichester: John Wiley & Sons, Ltd, pp. 217–234.

[34] Roick C, Heider D, Bebbington PE et al. (2007) Burden on caregivers of schizophrenia patients: a comparison between Germany and Great Britain. *British Journal of Psychiatry* **190**: 333–338.

[35] Barton K, Jackson C. (2008) Reducing symptoms of trauma among carers of people with psychosis: pilot study examining the impact of writing about caregiving experiences. *Australian and New Zealand Journal of Psychiatry* **42**: 693–701.

[36] Raune D, Kuipers E, Bebbington PE. (2004) Expressed emotion at first episode psychosis: investigating a carer appraisal model. *British Journal of Psychiatry* **184**: 321–326.

[37] Patterson P, Birchwood M, Cochrane R. (2005) Expressed emotion as an adaptation to loss: prospective study in first-episode psychosis. *British Journal of Psychiatry* **187** (Suppl. 48): s59–s64.

[38] Brown GW, Monck EM, Carstairs GM et al. (1962) Influence of family life on the course of schizophrenic illness. *British Journal of Preventive and Social Medicine* **16**: 55–68.

[39] Rutter M, Brown GW. (1966) Reliability and validity of measures of family life and relationships in families containing a psychiatric patient. *Social Psychiatry* **1**: 38–53.

[40] Brown GW, Birley JLT, Wing JK. (1972) Influence of family life on the course of schizophrenic disorders: a replication. *British Journal of Psychiatry* **121**: 241–258.

[41] Bebbington PE, Kuipers L. (1994) The predictive utility of expressed emotion in schizophrenia: an aggregate analysis. *Psychological Medicine* **24**: 707–718.

[42] Falloon IRH, Boyd JL, McGill CW et al. (1982) Family management in the prevention of exacerbations of schizophrenia: a controlled study. *New England Journal of Medicine* **306**: 1437–1440.

[43] Leff J, Kuipers L, Berkowitz R et al. (1982) A controlled trial of social intervention in the families of schizophrenic patients. *British Journal of Psychiatry* **141**: 121–134.

[44] Bustillo JR, Lauriello J, Horan WP et al. (2001) The psychosocial treatment of schizophrenia: an update. *American Journal of Psychiatry* **158**: 163–175.

[45] Pitschel-Walz G, Leucht S, Bäuml J et al. (2001) The effect of family interventions on relapse and rehospitalization in schizophrenia: a metaanalysis. *Schizophrenia Bulletin* **27**: 73–92.

[46] Pilling S, Bebbington P, Kuipers E et al. (2002) Psychological treatments in schizophrenia. I: meta-analysis of family intervention and cognitive behaviour therapy. *Psychological Medicine* **32**: 763–782.

[47] Pfammatter M, Junghan UM, Brenner HD. (2006) Efficacy of psychological therapy in schizophrenia: conclusions from meta-analyses. *Schizophrenia Bulletin* **32** (Suppl. 1): S64–S80.

[48] Pharoah F, Mari J, Rathbone J et al. (2006) Family intervention for schizophrenia. *Cochrane Database of Systematic Review* **18** (4): CD000088.

[49] Pharoah F, Mari J, Rathbone J et al. (2010) Family intervention for schizophrenia. *Cochrane Database of Systematic Reviews* **12**: CD000088.

[50] Kuipers E. (2010) Time for a separate psychosis caregiver service? *Journal of Mental Health* **19**: 401–404.

[51] Prytys M, Garety PA, Jolley S et al. (2011) Implementating the NICE Guideline for schizophrenia recommendations for psychological therapies: a qualitative analysis of the attitudes of CMHT staff. *Clinical Psychology and Psychotherapy* **18**: 48–59.

[52] Fadden G, Heelis R. (2011) The Meriden family programme: lessons learnt over 10 years. *Journal of Mental Health* **20**: 79–88.

[53] Askey R, Holmshaw J, Gamble C et al. (2009) What do carers of people with psychosis need from mental health services? Exploring the views of carers, service users and professionals. *Journal of Family Therapy* **31**: 310–331.

[54] Kuipers E, Onwumere J, Bebbington P. (2010) Cognitive model of care-giving in psychosis. *British Journal of Psychiatry* **196**: 259–264.

[55] Barrowclough C, Tarrier N, Humphreys L et al. (2003) Self-esteem in schizophrenia: relationships between self-evaluation, family attitudes, and symptomatology. *Journal of Abnormal Psychology* **112**: 92–99.

[56] Barrowclough C, Hooley JM. (2003) Attributions and EE: a review. *Clinical Psychology Review* **23**: 849–888.

[57] Grice SJ, Kuipers E, Bebbington PE et al. (2009) Carers' attributions about positive events in psychosis relate to expressed emotion. *Behaviour Research and Therapy* **47**: 783–789.

[58] Scazufca M, Kuipers E. (1998) Stability of expressed emotion in relatives of those with schizophrenia and its relationship with burden of care and perception of patients' social functioning. *Psychological Medicine* **28**: 453–461.

[59] Kuipers E, Garety P, Fowler D et al. (2006) Cognitive, emotional, and social processes in psychosis: refining cognitive behavioral therapy for persistent positive symptoms. *Schizophrenia Bulletin* **32** (Suppl. 1): S24–S31.

[60] Onwumere J, Kuipers E, Bebbington P et al. (2011) Coping styles in carers of people with recent and long-term psychosis. *Journal of Nervous and Mental Disease* **199**: 423–424.

[61] Tarrier N, Vaughn C, Lader M et al. (1979) Bodily reactions to people and events in schizophrenia. *Archives of General Psychiatry* **36**: 311–315.

[62] Kuipers E, Bebbington P, Dunn G et al. (2006) Influence of carer expressed emotion and affect on relapse in non-affective psychosis. *British Journal of Psychiatry* **188**: 173–179.

[63] Sensky T, Turkington D, Kingdon D et al. (2000) A randomized controlled trial of cognitive-behavioral therapy for persistent symptoms in schizophrenia resistant to medication. *Archives of General Psychiatry* **57**: 165–172.

[64] Garety PA, Fowler DG, Freeman D et al. (2008) A randomised controlled trial of cognitive behavioural therapy and family intervention for the prevention of relapse and reduction of symptoms in psychosis. *British Journal of Psychiatry* **192**: 412–423.

[65] Bachmann S, Bottmer C, Jacob S et al. (2006) Perceived criticism in schizophrenia: a comparison of instruments for the assessment of the patient's perspective and its relation to relatives' expressed emotion. *Psychiatry Research* **142**: 167–175.

[66] Cutting LP, Aakre J, Docherty NM. (2006) Schizophrenia patients' perceptions of stress, expressed emotion attitudes, and sensitivity to criticism. *Schizophrenia Bulletin* **32**: 743–750.

[67] Onwumere J, Kuipers E, Bebbington PE et al. (2009) Patient perceptions of caregiver criticism in pychosis: links with patient and caregiver functioning. *Journal of Nervous and Mental Disease* **197**: 85–91.

[68] Garety PA, Kuipers E, Fowler D et al. (2001) A cognitive model of the positive symptoms of psychosis. *Psychological Medicine* **31**: 189–195.

[69] Lobban F, Barrowclough C, Jones S. (2004) The impact of beliefs about mental health problems and coping on outcome in schizophrenia. *Psychological Medicine* **34**: 1165–1176.

[70] Watson PW, Garety PA, Weinman J et al. (2006) Emotional dysfunction in schizophrenia spectrum psychosis: the role of illness perceptions. *Psychological Medicine* **36**: 761–770.

[71] Hagger MS, Orbell S. (2003) A meta-analytic review of the common-sense model of illness representations. *Psychology & Health* **18**: 141–184.

[72] Lobban F, Barrowclough C, Jones S. (2005) Assessing cognitive representations of mental health problems. II. The illness perception questionnaire for schizophrenia: relatives' version. *British Journal of Clinical Psychology* **44**: 163–179.

[73] Onwumere J, Kuipers E, Bebbington P et al. (2008) Care-giving and illness beliefs in the course of psychotic illness. *Canadian Journal of Psychiatry* **53**: 460–468.

[74] Kuipers E, Watson P, Onwumere J et al. (2007) Discrepant illness perceptions affect and expressed emotion in people with psychosis and their carers. *Social Psychiatry and Psychiatric Epidemiology* **42**: 277–283.

[75] O'Brien MP, Gordon JL, Bearden CE et al. (2006) Positive family environment predicts improvement in symptoms and social functioning among adolescents at imminent risk for onset of psychosis. *Schizophrenia Research* **81**: 269–275.

[76] Veltman A, Cameron JI, Stewart DE. (2002) The experience of providing care to relatives with chronic mental illness. *Journal of Nervous and Mental Disease* **190**: 108–114.

[77] Chen FP, Greenberg JS. (2004) A positive aspect of caregiving: the influence of social support on caregiving gains for family members of relatives with schizophrenia. *Community Mental Health Journal* **40**: 423–435.

[78] Bertrando P, Beltz J, Bressi C et al. (1992) Expressed emotion and schizophrenia in Italy. A study of an urban population. *British Journal of Psychiatry* **161**: 223–229.

[79] Ivanović M, Vuletić Z, Bebbington P. (1994) Expressed emotion in the families of patients with schizophrenia and its influence on the course of illness. *Social Psychiatry and Psychiatric Epidemiology* **29**: 61–65.

[80] Birchwood M, Cochrane R. (1990) Families coping with schizophrenia – coping styles, their origins and correlates. *Psychological Medicine* **20**: 857–865.

[81] Scazufca M, Kuipers E. (1999) Coping strategies in relatives of people with schizophrenia before and after psychiatric admission. *British Journal of Psychiatry* **174**: 154–158.

[82] Barrowclough C, Parle M. (1997) Appraisal, psychological adjustment and expressed emotion in relatives of patients suffering from schizophrenia. *British Journal of Psychiatry* **171**: 26–30.

[83] Lazarus RS, Folkman S. (1984) *Stress Appraisal and Coping.* New York: Springer.

[84] Magliano L, Fadden G, Economou M et al. (2000) Family burden and coping strategies in schizophrenia: 1-year follow-up data from the BIOMED I study. *Social Psychiatry and Psychiatric Epidemiology* **35**: 109–115.

[85] Barrowclough C, Tarrier N. (1992) *Families of Schizophrenic Patients: Cognitive Behavioural Intervention.* London: Chapman & Hall.

[86] Leff J, Kuipers E, Lam D. (2002) *Family Work for Schizophrenia: A Practical Guide*, 2nd edn. London: Gaskell.

[87] Magliano L, Fiorillo A, Malangone C et al. (2003) The effect of social network on burden and pessimism in relatives of patients with schizophrenia. *American Journal of Orthopsychiatry* **73**: 302–309.

[88] Gutiérrez-Maldonado J, Caqueo-Urízar A, Kavanagh D. (2005) Burden of care and general health in families of patients with schizophrenia. *Social Psychiatry and Psychiatric Epidemiology* **40**: 899–904.

[89] Joyce J, Leese M, Kuipers E et al. (2003) Evaluating a model of caregiving for people with psychosis. *Social Psychiatry and Psychiatric Epidemiology* **38**: 189–195.

[90] Jones C, Cormac I, Silveira Da Mota Neto JI et al. (2004) Cognitive behaviour therapy for schizophrenia. *Cochrane Database of Systematic Review* **18** (4): CD000524.

[91] Zimmermann G, Favrod J, Trieu VH et al. (2005) The effect of cognitive behavioral treatment on the positive symptoms of schizophrenia spectrum disorders: a meta-analysis. *Schizophrenia Research* **77**: 1–9.

[92] Gumley A, O'Grady M, McNay L et al. (2003) Early intervention for relapse in schizophrenia: results of a 12-month randomized controlled trial of cognitive behavioural therapy. *Psychological Medicine* **33**: 419–431.

[93] Trower P, Birchwood M, Meaden A et al. (2004) Cognitive therapy for command hallucinations: randomised controlled trial. *British Journal of Psychiatry* **184**: 312–320.

[94] Tarrier N, Wykes T. (2004) Is there evidence that CBT is an effective treatment for schizophrenia? A cautious or cautionary tale. *Behaviour Research and Therapy* **42**: 1371–1401.

[95] Wykes T, Steel C, Everitt B et al. (2008) Cognitive behavior therapy for schizophrenia: effect sizes, clinical models, and methodological rigor. *Schizophrenia Bulletin* **34**: 523–537.

[96] Tandon R, Nasrallah HA, Keshavan MS. (2010) Schizophrenia, "just the facts" 5. Treatment and prevention past, present, and future. *Schizophrenia Research* **122**: 1–23.

[97] Jones C, Hacker D, Cormac I et al. (2012) Cognitive behaviour therapy versus other psychosocial treatments for schizophrenia. *Cochrane Database of Systematic Reviews* **4**: CD008712.

[98] National Institute for Health and Clinical Excellence. (2003) *Schizophrenia: Core Interventions in the Treatment and Management of Schizophrenia in Primary and Secondary Care (Full Guideline).* London: Gaskell & British Psychological Society.

[99] National Institute for Health and Clinical Excellence. (2009) *Schizophrenia: Core Interventions in the Treatment and Management of Schizophrenia in Primary and Secondary Care (Update).* London: National Institute of Clinical and Health Excellence.

[100] Kreyenbuhl J, Buchanan RW, Dickerson FB et al. (2010) The Schizophrenia Patient Outcomes Research Team (PORT): updated treatment recommendations 2009. *Schizophrenia Bulletin* **36**: 94–103.

[101] Klingberg S, Wittorf A, Meisner C et al. (2010) Cognitive behavioural therapy versus supportive therapy for persistent positive symptoms in psychotic disorders: the POSITIVE Study, a multicenter, prospective, single-blind, randomised controlled clinical trial. *Trials* **11**: 123.

[102] Dunn G, Fowler D, Rollinson R et al. (2012) Effective elements of cognitive behaviour therapy for psychosis: results of a novel type of subgroup analysis based on principal stratification. *Psychological Medicine* **42**: 1057–1068.

[103] Freeman D, Stahl D, McManus S et al. (2012) Insomnia, worry, anxiety and depression as predictors of the occurrence and of the persistence of persecutory ideation: a longitudinal analysis from the British National Psychiatric Morbidity Survey Programme. *Social Psychiatry and Psychiatric Epidemiology* **47**: 1195–1203.

[104] Kumari V, Peters ER, Fannon D et al. (2009) Dorsolateral prefrontal cortex activity predicts responsiveness to cognitive-behavioral therapy in schizophrenia. *Biological Psychiatry* **66**: 594–602.

[105] Garety P, Fowler D, Kuipers E et al. (1997) The London-East Anglia randomised controlled trial of cognitive behaviour therapy for psychosis. II: predictors of outcome. *British Journal of Psychiatry* **171**: 420–426.

[106] Freeman D, McManus S, Brugha T et al. (2011) Concomitants of paranoia in the general population. *Psychological Medicine* **41**: 923–936.

[107] Waller H, Freeman D, Jolley S et al. (2011) Targeting reasoning biases in delusions: a pilot study of the Maudsley Review Training Programme for individuals with persistent, high conviction delusions. *Journal of Behavior Therapy and Experimental Psychiatry* **42**: 414–421.

[108] Bentall RP, Corcoran R, Howard R et al. (2001) Persecutory delusions: a review and theoretical integration. *Clinical Psychology Review* **21**: 1143–1192.

[109] Garety PA, Bebbington P, Fowler D et al. (2007) Implications for neurobiological research of cognitive models of psychosis: a theoretical paper. *Psychological Medicine* **37**: 1377–1391.

[110] Freeman D, Garety PA, Kuipers E et al. (2002) A cognitive model of persecutory delusions. *British Journal of Clinical Psychology* **41**: 331–347.

[111] Morrison AP. (2001) The interpretation of intrusions in psychosis: an integrative cognitive approach to hallucinations and delusions. *Behavioral and Cognitive Psychotherapy* **29**: 257–276.

[112] Bentall RP, Rowse G, Shryane N et al. (2009) The cognitive and affective structure of paranoid delusions: a transdiagnostic investigation of patients with schizophrenia spectrum disorders and depression. *Archives of General Psychiatry* **66**: 236–247.

[113] Bentall RP, Claridge GS, Slade PD. (1989) The multidimensional nature of schizotypal traits: a factor analytic study with normal subjects. *British Journal of Clinical Psychology* **28**: 363–375.

[114] Beavan V, Read J, Cartwright C. (2011) The prevalence of voice-hearing in the general population: a literature review. *Journal of Mental Health* **20**: 281–292.

[115] Johns LC, Cannon M, Singleton N et al. (2004) Prevalence and correlates of self-reported psychotic symptoms in the British population. *British Journal of Psychiatry* **185**: 298–305.

[116] van Os J, Hanssen M, Bijl RV et al. (2000) Strauss (1969) revisited: a psychosis continuum in the general population? *Schizophrenia Research* **45**: 11–20.

[117] Freeman D, Garety PA, Bebbington PE et al. (2005) Psychological investigation of the structure of paranoia in a non-clinical population. *British Journal of Psychiatry* **186**: 427–435.

[118] Hanssen M, Krabbendam L, Vollema M et al. (2006) Evidence for instrument and family-specific variation of subclinical psychosis dimensions in the general population. *Journal of Abnormal Psychology* **115**: 5–14.

[119] Linscott RJ, van Os J. (2010) Systematic reviews of categorical versus continuum models in psychosis: evidence for discontinuous subpopulations underlying a psychometric continuum. Implications for DSM-V, DSM-VI, and DSM-VII. *Annual Review of Clinical Psychology* **6**: 391–419.

[120] Larøi F, Sommer IE, Blom JD et al. (2012) The characteristic features of auditory verbal hallucinations in clinical and nonclinical groups: state-of-the-art overview and future directions. *Schizophrenia Bulletin* **38**(4): 724–733.

[121] Peters E, Day S, McKenna J et al. (1999) Delusional ideation in religious and psychotic populations. *British Journal of Clinical Psychology* **38**: 83–96.

[122] Johns LC, van Os J. (2001) The continuity of psychotic experiences in the general population. *Clinical Psychology Review* **21**: 1125–1141.

[123] Arseneault L, Cannon M, Poulton R et al. (2002) Cannabis use in adolescence and risk for adult psychosis: longitudinal prospective study. *BMJ* **325**: 1212–1213.

[124] Chapman LJ, Chapman JP, Kwapil TR et al. (1994) Putatively psychosis-prone subjects 10 years later. *Journal of Abnormal Psychology* **103**: 171–183.

[125] Poulton R, Caspi A, Moffitt TE et al. (2000) Children's self-reported psychotic symptoms and adult schizophreniform disorder: a 15-year longitudinal study. *Archives of General Psychiatry* **57**: 1053–1058.

[126] Hanssen M, Krabbendam L, de Graaf R et al. (2005) Role of distress in delusion formation. *British Journal of Psychiatry* **48** (Suppl.): s55–s58.

[127] Birchwood M. (2003) Pathways to emotional dysfunction in first episode psychosis. *British Journal of Psychiatry* **182**: 373–375.

[128] Freeman D, Garety PA. (2003) Connecting neurosis and psychosis: the direct influence of emotion on delusions and hallucinations. *Behaviour Research and Therapy* **41**: 923–947.

[129] Peters ER, Joseph SA, Garety PA. (1999) Measurement of delusional ideation in the normal population: introducing the PDI (Peters et al. Delusions Inventory). *Schizophrenia Bulletin* **25**: 553–576.

[130] Krabbendam L, Myin-Germeys I, Hanssen M et al. (2004) Hallucinatory experiences and onset of psychotic disorder: evidence that the risk is mediated by delusion formation. *Acta Psychiatrica Scandinavica* **110**: 264–272.

[131] Krabbendam L, Myin-Germeys I, Hanssen M et al. (2005) Development of depressed mood predicts onset of psychotic disorder in individuals who report hallucinatory experiences. *British Journal of Clinical Psychology* **44**: 113–125.

[132] Krabbendam L, van Os J. (2005) Affective processes in the onset and persistence of psychosis. *European Archives of Psychiatry and Clinical Neuroscience* **255**: 185–189.

[133] Wiles NJ, Zammit S, Bebbington P et al. (2006) Self-reported psychotic symptoms in the general population: results from the longitudinal study of the British National Psychiatric Morbidity Survey. *British Journal of Psychiatry* **188**: 519–526.

[134] Fowler D, Hodgekins J, Garety P et al. (2012) Negative cognition, depressed mood and paranoia: a longitudinal pathway analysis using structural equation modelling. *Schizophrenia Bulletin* **38**(5): 1063–1073.

[135] Freeman D, Garety PA. (1999) Comments on the content of persecutory delusions: does the definition need clarification? *British Journal of Clinical Psychology* **39**: 407–414.

[136] Startup H, Freeman D, Garety PA. (2007) Persecutory delusions and catastrophic worry in psychosis: developing the understanding of delusion distress and persistence. *Behaviour Research and Therapy* **45**: 523–537.

[137] Foster C, Startup H, Potts L et al. (2010) A randomised controlled trial of a worry intervention for individuals with persistent persecutory delusions. *Journal of Behavior Therapy and Experimental Psychiatry* **41**: 45–51.

[138] Hepworth C, Startup H, Freeman D. (2011) Developing treatments of persistent persecutory delusions the impact of an emotional processing and metacognitive awareness intervention. *Journal of Nervous and Mental Disease* **199**: 653–658.

[139] Freeman D, Pugh K, Vorontsova N et al. (2009) Insomnia and paranoia. *Schizophrenia Research* **108**: 280–284.

[140] Chouinard S, Poulin J, Stip E et al. (2004) Sleep in untreated patients with schizophrenia: a meta-analysis. *Schizophrenia Bulletin* **30**: 957–967.

[141] Ritsner M, Kurs R, Ponizovsky A et al. (2004) Perceived quality of life in schizophrenia: Relationships to sleep quality. *Qualilty of Life Research* **13**: 783–791.

[142] Myers E, Startup H, Freeman D. (2011) Cognitive behavioural treatment of insomnia in individuals with persistent persecutory delusions: a pilot trial. *Journal of Behavior Therapy and Experimental Psychiatry* **42**: 330–336.

[143] Arseneault L, Cannon M, Witton J et al. (2004) Causal association between cannabis and psychosis: examination of the evidence. *British Journal of Psychiatry* **184**: 110–117.

[144] van Os J, Krabbendam L, Myin-Germeys I et al. (2005) The schizophrenia envirome. *Current Opinion in Psychiatry* **58**: 141–145.

[145] Cantor-Graae E, Selten JP. (2005) Schizophrenia and migration: a meta-analysis and review. *American Journal of Psychiatry* **162**: 12–24.

[146] McGrath JJ. (2006) Variations in the incidence of schizophrenia: data versus dogma. *Schizophrenia Bulletin* **32**: 195–197.

[147] Fearon P, Kirkbride JB, Morgan C et al. (2006) Incidence of schizophrenia and other psychoses in ethnic minority groups: results from the MRC AESOP Study. *Psychological Medicine* **36**: 1–10.

[148] Kirkbride JB, Fearon P, Morgan C et al. (2006) Heterogeneity in incidence rates of schizophrenia and other psychotic syndromes: findings from the 3-center AeSOP study. *Archives of General Psychiatry* **63**: 250–258.

[149] Fearon P, Morgan C. (2006) Environmental factors in schizophrenia: the role of migrant studies. *Schizophrenia Bulletin* **32**: 405–408.

[150] Birchwood M, Gilbert P, Gilbert J et al. (2004) Interpersonal and rolerelated schema influence the relationship with the dominant 'voice' in schizophrenia: a comparison of three models. *Psychological Medicine* **34**: 1571–1580.

[151] Cooper C, Morgan C, Byrne M et al. (2008) Perceptions of social disadvantage, ethnicity and psychosis: results from the AESOP study. *British Journal of Psychiatry* **192**: 185–190.

[152] Mueser KT, Goodman LB, Trumbetta SL et al. (1998) Trauma and post traumatic stress disorder in severe mental illness. *Journal of Consulting and Clinical Psychology* **66**: 493–499.

[153] Bebbington PE, Bhugra D, Brugha T et al. (2004) Psychosis, victimisation and childhood disadvantage: evidence from the second British National Survey of psychiatric morbidity. *British Journal of Psychiatry* **185**: 220–226.

[154] Bebbington PE, Jonas S, Kuipers E et al. (2011) Sexual abuse and psychosis: data from an English National Survey. *British Journal of Psychiatry* **199**: 29–37.

[155] Janssen I, Krabbendam L, Bak M et al. (2004) Childhood abuse as a risk factor for psychotic xperiences. *Acta Psychiatrica Scandinavica* **109**: 38–45.

[156] Read J, van Os J, Morrison AP et al. (2005) Childhood trauma, psychosis and schizophrenia: a literature review with theoretical and clinical implications. *Acta Psychiatrica Scandinavica* **112**: 330–350.

[157] Spauwen J, Krabbendam L, Lieb R et al. (2006) Impact of psychological trauma on the development of psychotic symptoms: relationship with psychosis proneness. *British Journal of Psychiatry* **188**: 527–533.

[158] Hardy A, Fowler D, Freeman D et al. (2005) Trauma and hallucinatory experience in psychosis. *Journal of Nervous and Mental Disease* **193**: 501–507.

[159] Gracie A, Freeman D, Green S et al. (2007) The association between traumatic experience, paranoia and hallucinations: a test of psychological models. *Acta Psychiatrica Scandinavica* **116**: 280–289.

[160] Morrison AP, Frame L, Larkin W. (2003) Relationships between trauma and psychosis: a review and integration. *British Journal of Clinical Psychology* **42**: 331–353.

[161] Fowler D. (2000) Psychological formulation of early episodes of psychosis: a cognitive model. In: Birchwood M, Fowler D, Jackson C (eds.), *Early Intervention in Psychosis: A Guide to Concepts, Evidence and Interventions*. Chichester: John Wiley & Sons, Ltd, pp. 101–127.

[162] Schulze K, Freeman D, Kuipers E. (2013) Intrusive mental imagery in people with persecutory delusions. *Behaviour Research and Therapy* **51**: 7–14.

[163] Ison R, Medoro L, Keen N et al. (in press) Image rescripting for people with psychosis who hear voices. *Behavioural and Cognitive Psychotherapy*.

[164] Fowler D, Freeman D, Smith B et al. (2006) The Brief Core Schema Scales (BCSS): psychometric properties and associations with paranoia and grandiosity in non-clinical and psychosis samples. *Psychological Medicine* **36**: 749–759.

[165] Smith B, Fowler DG, Freeman D et al. (2006) Emotion and psychosis: links between depression, self-esteem, negative schematic beliefs and delusions and hallucinations. *Schizophrenia Research* **86**: 181–188.

[166] Garety P, Gittins M, Jolley S et al. (2012) Differences in cognitive and emotional processes between persecutory and grandiose delusions. *Schizophrenia Bulletin*. April 12 [Epub ahead of print].

[167] Garety P, Freeman D. (1999) Cognitive approaches to delusions: a critical review of theories and evidence. *British Journal of Clinical Psychology* **38**: 113–154.

[168] Garety PA, Freeman D, Jolley S et al. (2005) Reasoning, emotions, and delusional conviction in psychosis. *Journal of Abnormal Psychology* **114**: 373–384.

[169] Moritz S, Woodward TS. (2005) Jumping to conclusions in delusional and non-delusional schizophrenic patients. *British Journal of Clinical Psychology* **44**: 193–207.

[170] Colbert SM, Peters ER. (2002) Need for closure and jumping to conclusions in delusion-prone individuals. *Journal of Nervous and Mental Disease* **190**: 27–31.

[171] van Dael F, Versmissen D, Janssen I et al. (2006) Data gathering: biased in psychosis? *Schizophrenia Bulletin* **32**: 341–351.

[172] Broome MR, Johns LC, Valli I et al. (2007) Delusion formation and reasoning biases in those at clinical high risk for psychosis. *British Journal of Psychiatry* **191** (Suppl. 51): S38–S42.

[173] Peters E, Garety P. (2006) Cognitive functioning in delusions: a longitudinal analysis. *Behaviour Research and Therapy* **44**: 481–514.

[174] Freeman D, Garety PA, Fowler D et al. (2004) Why do people with delusions fail to choose more realistic explanations for their experiences? An empirical investigation. *Journal of Consulting and Clinical Psychology* **72**: 671–680.

[175] So SH, Freeman D, Dunn G et al. (2012) Jumping to conclusions, a lack of belief inflexibility and delusion conviction in psychosis: a longitudinal investigation of the structure, frequency and relatedness of reasoning biases. *Journal of Abnormal Psychology* **121**: 129–139.

[176] Bebbington PE, Angermeyer M, Azorin J-M et al. (2005) The European Schizophrenia Cohort (EuroSC): a naturalistic prognostic and economic study. *Social Psychiatry and Psychiatric Epidemiology* **40**: 707–717.

[177] Tandon R, Ribeiro SCM, DeQuardo JR et al. (1993) Covariance of positive and negative symptoms during neuroleptic treatment in schizophrenia: a replication. *Biological Psychiatry* **34**: 495–497.

[178] Stahl SM, Buckley PF. (2007) Negative symptoms of schizophrenia: a problem that will not go away. *Acta Psychiatrica Scandinavica* **115**: 4–11.

[179] Wykes T, Huddy V. (2009) Cognitive remediation for schizophrenia: it is even more complicated. *Current Opinion in Psychiatry* **22**: 161–167.

[180] Wykes T, Huddy V, Cellard C et al. (2011) A meta-analysis of cognitive remediation for schizophrenia: methodology and effect sizes. *American Journal of Psychiatry* **168**: 472–485.

[181] Turkington D, Kingdon D, Turer T. (2002) Effectiveness of a brief cognitive-behavioural therapy intervention in the treatment of schizophrenia. *British Journal of Psychiatry* **180**: 523–527.

[182] Durham RC, Guthrie M, Morton RV et al. (2003) Tayside-Fife clinical trial of cognitive-behavioural therapy for medication-resistant psychotic symptoms – results to 3-month follow-up. *British Journal of Psychiatry* **182**: 303–311.

[183] Harrigan S, McGorry P, Krstev H. (2003) Does treatment delay in first-episode psychosis really matter? *Psychological Medicine* **33**: 97–110.

[184] Bottlender R, Sato T, Jager M. (2009) The impact of the duration of untreated psychosis prior to first psychiatric admission on the 15-year outcome in schizophrenia. *Schizophrenia Research* **62**: 37–44.

[185] Bird V, Premkumar P, Kendall T et al. (2010) Early intervention services, cognitive-behavioural therapy and family intervention in early psychosis: systematic review. *British Journal of Psychiatry* **197**: 350–356.

[186] Craig T, Garety P, Power P et al. (2004) The Lambeth Early Onset (LEO) team: randomised controlled trial of the effectiveness of specialised care for early psychosis. *BMJ* **329**: 1067–1071.

[187] Grawe RW, Falloon IR, Widen JH et al. (2006) Two years of continued early treatment for recent-onset schizophrenia: a randomised controlled study. *Acta Psychiatrica Scandinavica* **114**: 328–336.

[188] Harrison G, Croudace T, Mason P et al. (1996) Predicting the long-term outcome of schizophrenia. *Psychological Medicine* **26**: 697–705.

[189] Marwaha S, Johnson S. (2004) Schizophrenia and employment: a review. *Social Psychiatry and Psychiatric Epidemiology* **39**: 337–349.

[190] Marwaha S, Johnson S, Bebbington P et al. (2007) Rates and correlates of employment in people with schizophrenia in the UK, France and Germany. *British Journal of Psychiatry* **191**: 30–37.

[191] Strauss JS, Carpenter WT. (1977) Prediction of outcome in schizophrenia. III. Five-year outcome and its predictors. *Archives of General Psychiatry* **34**: 159–163.

[192] Carpenter WT, Strauss JS. (1991) The prediction of outcome in schizophrenia. IV. 11 year follow-up of the Washington IPSS cohort. *Journal of Nervous and Mental Disease* **179**: 517–525.

[193] Fowler D, Hodgekins J, Painter M et al. (2009) Cognitive behaviour therapy for improving social recovery in psychosis: a report from the ISREP MRC trial pplatform study (Improving Social Recovery in Early Psychosis). *Psychological Medicine* **39**: 1627–1636.

[194] Hodgekins J, Fowler D. (2010) CBT and recovery from psychosis in the ISREP trial: mediating effects of hope and positive beliefs on activity. *Psychiatric Services* **61**: 321–324.

CHAPTER 23

The management of mental disorders in the primary care setting

Matteo Balestrieri

Department of Experimental and Clinical Medical Sciences, University of Udine, Udine, Italy

Introduction

A large number of surveys have documented that a significant proportion of primary care patients are affected by affective and/or anxiety disorders [1–6]. If we consider the last decades, the interest for the study in this field has grown dramatically: Figure 23.1 shows that using the keywords 'primary care' and 'mental health' in Pubmed only 65 papers in 1985 but 985 in 2011 were found, while using the words 'primary care' and 'psychotropic drugs' the respective numbers were 21 and 227. Many of these papers tried to shed light on critical issues, such as the best kind of primary services' organisation for mental health, the intervention to improve the detection of depression and anxiety by primary care physicians (PCPs) and the efficacy of psychotropic drug and psychosocial treatments. This chapter tries to put together the information available on several of these issues, using a selection of papers, reviews and meta-analyses which propose sound data.

Organisation of primary care services

In 2008, the World Organization of Family Doctors (WONCA) in collaboration with the World Health Organization (WHO) stated that by providing mental health services in primary health care, more people will be able to receive the mental health care needed because of *better physical accessibility* (primary health care is the easiest level of contact with the national health system to access), *better financial accessibility* (if mental health services are integrated into primary health care, health-care costs are greatly reduced) and *better acceptability* (linked to reduced

Improving Mental Health Care: The Global Challenge, First Edition.
Edited by Graham Thornicroft, Mirella Ruggeri and David Goldberg.
© 2013 John Wiley & Sons, Ltd. Published 2013 by John Wiley & Sons, Ltd.

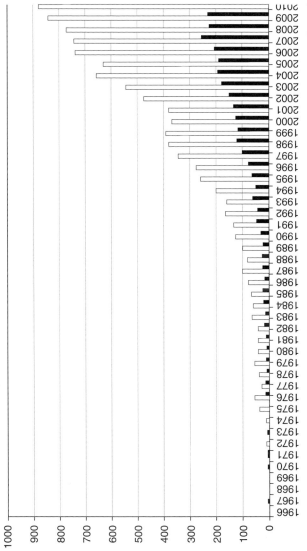

Figure 23.1 Number of papers found in Pubmed using the keywords 'Primary care' plus, respectively, 'Mental Health' (□) and 'Psychotropic drugs' (■).

stigma and easier communication with health-care providers) [7]. To reach these goals, consistently with the international standards of good practices, countries must strengthen existing networks of services, including those in primary health care, to provide mental health services. Funds must therefore be shifted or redistributed from tertiary/secondary to primary levels of care, and eventually new funds must be made available. It remains to be established which type of organisation of care would be better to achieve the goals indicated by the WONCA.

Competence of care

How far can PCPs be considered competent in mental health care? The 'pathways to care' model by Goldberg and Huxley [8] can be used to define such competence. This model produces similar proportion of morbidity at the various levels in Europe [9, 10], while in the United States, it has been observed what has been called 'the American bypass', that is, the direct referral of patients to mental health professionals.

According to the 'pathway to care' model, accessing mental health care involves passing through five levels and four filters. The first level is that of the general population with whatsoever mental health disorder. In countries where primary care services are widely and easily accessible to the population, the subsequent level (level 2), composed by all adults who seek help from a PCP, includes a reduced proportion of people, corresponding to about 80% of the population at level 1. The difference between the two levels derives from an attitude called 'illness behaviour' (filter 1), which describes the propensity to seek help from a PCP for a physical and/or mental disease, and depends on both personal factors and characteristics of the organisation of mental health services. Where PCPs are freely and easily accessible, the first filter is widely permeable. On the other hand, when specialist care is widely available, the patients can refer directly to mental health professionals (level 4).

Level 3 is represented by all adults who are considered mentally disordered by their PCPs, whether or not they satisfy research criteria. This is also called 'conspicuous morbidity' (50–60% of the population at level 2). The referral of a patient to mental health services represents filter 3, which gives access to the morbidity present in the mental health services (level 4), and – after a further filter – to the mentally ill persons admitted to hospital (level 5). This model highlights the importance of the PCPs, whose ability to detect a disorder (filter 2) and propensity to refer (filter 3) represents key barriers to care.

Bearing in mind the 'pathway to care' model, we must consider that the characteristics of the patients present at the various filter levels are different. Mental health disorders are not all the same; they have dissimilar severity, carry on different gradients of burden on people and families, determine distinct and specific limitations in the capacities and social participation and require treatments of different complexities. PCP can reasonably manage only a proportion of the general mental health morbidity.

Bower and Gilbody [11] proposed the following categorisation:

1 Severe mental disorders, like schizophrenia, organic disorders and bipolar disorder: they involve both primary and secondary care.

2 Other disorders for which there are effective pharmacological and psychological treatments, like anxious depression, pure depression, generalised anxiety, panic disorder, obsessive–compulsive disorder: they can usually be managed entirely within primary care.

3 Disorders in which psychotropic drugs have a more limited role, while psychological therapies are effective, like phobias, distress-related somatoform disorders, eating disorders, chronic fatigue: they are rarely treated within primary care, and only a small proportion of cases are treated by specialist services.

4 Disorders that tend to resolve spontaneously, like bereavement and adjustment disorders: they need supportive help, rather than a specific mental health skill.

In my opinion, some annotations are necessary to this categorisation. At level 1, we must agree on the fact that the primacy is for the specialist services, which must coordinate the management with the ancillary, although essential, help of the PCP. At level 2, I would introduce a gradient of severity, since all these disorders are responsive to the therapies addressed by the PCPs only until resistances to the treatment occur or severity is high. At level 3, it is true that these disorders are rarely treated in primary care, but is less true that pharmacologic treatment has a minor role. Moreover, there are numerous examples of specialist services equipped to manage these disorders specifically. Finally, at level 4, adjustment disorders (with the exception of bereavement) often need to be treated by a skilled physician or psychotherapist [12, 13].

These differing opinions are more substantial for the last two levels. I believe that public health services should be able to manage a broad range of mental health problems, that is, belonging to all four categories, whereas the list of Bower and Gilbody implies a small involvement of specialist services, a high level of competence of primary care, but above all an involvement of health services only in the first two categories. In a period of reduction of resources such as the one we are witnessing, the categorisation by Bower and Gilbody might be more adherent to the reality, and indeed nowadays differences do exist between the United Kingdom and Italy, in terms of a more pronounced emphasis on privatisation in the United Kingdom [14]. Is that the solution in times of reduction of resources?

Recently, Thornicroft and Tansella [15] proposed another model, which differentiates the mental health service development according to availability of resources worldwide. This 'balanced care model', was framed in three sequential steps relevant to settings with different levels of resources: (a) low-resource settings, which need to focus on improving the recognition and treatment of people with mental illnesses in primary care; (b) medium-resource settings, which in addition can develop general adult mental health services, namely, outpatient clinics, community mental health teams, acute inpatient services, community residential care and work/occupation; (c) high-resource settings, which can also provide specialised services in areas such as eating disorders and treatment-resistant affective disorders and for people with comorbid psychotic and substance misuse/dependence disorders or for mentally ill mothers.

Models of primary care involvement in the frame of mental health-care organisation

We can imagine different models of mental health-care organisation which involve primary care.

Replacement

The psychiatrists and other specialists take the principal responsibility for the management of mental health problems, with little or no participation of the PCP. Replacement is also associated with psychological or drug therapy provided by private professionals. In South Verona, we reported that in 1991, the one-month prevalence of patients seen by private psychiatrists was about one-third of the prevalence of the community mental health centre (CMHC), and that the vast majority of these patients did not have contacts with psychiatric services in the previous year [16]. In any case, it was quite self-evident that private psychiatrists were replacing PCPs in the management of mental health problems.

Referral

The PCP is the first-contact physician, but the subsequent referral of the patient to the psychiatric services is encouraged. The referral to specialist care depends on the skills available in the primary care team and the accessibility to mental health care [17]. The referral to psychiatrists is often motivated by a request of diagnostic assessment. In a trial by Burton et al. [18], about half of patients referred to secondary care with a diagnosis of 'unexplained medical symptoms' met the criteria for current depression, anxiety or panic disorders.

Consultation-liaison

Mental health specialists enter into an ongoing educational relationship with PCPs, to support them in caring for individual patients. Sometimes it includes a systematic training of primary care staff aimed at improving prescribing or providing skills in psychological therapy. Training can also imply a widespread dissemination of information and guidelines or more intensive practice-based education seminars. Recently, two meta-analyses have been performed on consultation-liaison (C-L) in primary care, with contrasting results. In the five trials selected by Cape et al. [19], there was no significant effect of C-L on antidepressant (AD) use or depression outcomes in the short or long term. On the contrary, in the ten trials selected by van der Feltz-Cornelis et al. [20], the assessment of illness burden was significantly superior as compared with usual care. This produced a reduction of utilisation of health-care services.

Collaborative care

'Case managers' who work with patients and coordinate with PCPs and specialists are involved in order to improve quality of care. This model is based on the principles of chronic disease management. A recent meta-analysis on randomised controlled trials comparing collaborative care models (i.e. including at least three of six fundamental components: patient self-management support, delivery system redesign, use of clinical information systems, provider decision support, linkage to community resources and health-care organisation support) with other care conditions indicated significant effects across disorders and care settings for depression as well as for mental and physical quality of life and social role function [21].

Stepped care

This model was proposed in the National Institute for Health and Clinical Excellence (NICE) guidelines for depression and anxiety [22] and consists of treatments of differing intensity graded to the patient's needs, so that the least intrusive or restrictive intervention is first provided. For the management of common mental disorders, five steps were devised: (a) PCP treatment, (b) PCP treatment supervised by CMHCs, (c) consultation with CMHCs, (d) shared care between PCPs and CMHCs and (e) treatment at the CMHC. These steps are ordered along a dimension of increasing CMHC involvement and decreasing PCP responsibility; referral of patients to CMHC is expected from the third step upwards. In Italy, a stepped care model implemented in Bologna showed that about 58% of patients were referred by PCPs [23]. As to the pattern of care, patients living in the urban area were more likely to receive shared care – that is, step (d) – compared with those living in a non-urban area, while the reverse was true for the consultation intervention – that is, step (c) . Also Franx et al. [24] proved that with a stepped care approach, PCPs report improvements in the management of different levels of care, in the prescription of ADs and in the working relationships with patients and colleagues.

The prevalence of mental health disorders in primary care

The prevalence of mental disorders in primary care is subject to different confounding factors. One is the intrinsic weakness of the diagnostic criteria in psychiatry even at the specialist level. This difficulty is amplified by the uncertainty to translate those criteria at the primary care level, where the disorders can be different in terms of symptom presentation and severity. Another factor is the difference between level 2 and level 3 of Goldberg and Huxley's model, that is, the ability of PCPs in recognising and correctly identifying the mental disorders of their patients (filter 2).

Diagnostic issues

In a country with a widespread access to primary care, the prevalence at this level should not be much different from the one existing in the population. A popular concept is the so-called 'one in four', which sustains the notion that one in four people will have a mental health problem at some point in their lives, but this assumption is still debated [25, 26]. For example, a 2005 meta-analysis estimated a yearly prevalence of 27% for the European Union [27], but a 2010 update of this work revised this to 38% a year [28], as a result of including more disorders such as insomnia and attention-deficit hyperactivity disorder.

A further problem is that PCPs are uneasy with the psychiatric diagnoses also because these are still very much a work in progress. The WHO is currently revising the Primary Health Care version of the International Classification of Disease (ICD11-PHC) [29]. Ad hoc symptom scales can help in detecting common mental disorders such as anxiety and depression, while more complex disorders need to be detected and referred to the mental health specialists.

Detection of mental disorders in primary care

Although in primary care settings patients with depressive disorders are common and report high levels of personal suffering and disability resulting in high medical and social costs, about half of them are undetected and untreated. Inadequate detection of psychiatric disorders can occur as a result of either underestimation or overestimation. Some studies have documented that PCPs fail to detect from 10% to 50% of patients suffering from clinically relevant psychiatric disorders [6, 30, 31]. Other studies have focused on the proportion of patients who are labelled as depressed by PCPs, but who do not satisfy international diagnostic criteria for major depressive episodes [32, 33].

PCPs recognise depression poorly due to their more physical and demand-led orientation [34–36]. Moreover, the rates of non-detection of depressed patients are high when somatic symptoms are present [37] and when depression is of mild severity [38]. In a recent paper, Piek et al. [39] reported that patients who did not consult their PCPs for mental problems and were without comorbid anxiety disorders were less often recognised. On the contrary, an Italian primary care survey showed that PCPs over-detect depression in subjects who are divorced, separated or widowed and in individuals with a moderate to poor quality of life [6].

How to improve the ability of PCPs to recognise mild mental health disorders (e.g. anxiety and depression) is still a debated question. The use of screening questionnaires in primary care has become the most commonly used quality improvement strategy for depression care. Even if this solution appeared to respond positively to this problem, methodological sound analyses did not confirm the success of this strategy [40]. In a comprehensive review, Barbui and Tansella [41] showed that screening alone does not improve the recognition, management and outcome of depression, management strategies are supported by insufficient evidence, while strong evidence exists to encourage PCPs to prescribe effective doses of ADs in patients with moderate to severe depression. More recently, these results were confirmed by a systematic review conducted by Gilbody et al. [42]. Figure 23.2 shows that in high-risk patients (four studies), screening and case-finding instruments had a borderline positive impact on the rate of recognition of depression by clinicians, while in unselected patients (seven studies), screening and case-finding instruments had no effect on depression. The conclusion is that, if used alone, case-finding or screening questionnaires for depression appear to have little or no impact on the detection and management of depression by PCPs.

Psychotropic drug treatment

So far, literature findings have not been able to draw firm conclusions on the cost-effectiveness of psychotherapies in comparison with usual care or psychotropic drug treatment. Even the cost-effectiveness of counselling in comparison with usual care and psychotropic drug treatment is yet to be established. Meta-analyses show that psychotherapy is significantly more expensive than usual care, but not significantly more expensive than AD treatment [43, 44]. In the next paragraphs, ADs are taken as reference drugs for psychotropic drug treatments, since most of the literature is focused on these drugs. Other drugs such as benzodiazepines are equally important but would introduce a discussion on different aspects of prescription [45, 46], while antipsychotic drugs and mood stabilisers are less prescribed in primary care.

Communication

A recent review identified 17 studies which addressed the perception of depression by PCPs [47]. The results indicated that PCPs are unsure about the exact nature of the relationship between mood and social problems and of their role in managing it. Ambivalent attitudes to working with depressed people, a lack of confidence, the use of a limited number of management options and a belief that a diagnosis of depression is stigmatising interfere negatively with the management of depression by PCP and might result in the fact that PCPs commonly consider AD treatment their only option.

But is it that what the patients want? A systematic review shed light on the patients' preferences regarding psychotherapy and AD medication in the primary care setting [48]. The majority of patients preferred psychotherapy in all available studies, while ADs were often regarded only as an addictive option. A further literature review by Deledda et al. [49] on 27 studies focusing on primary care patients' perspective showed that most of the expectations were related to the function 'fostering the relationship'. The authors' conclusion was that patients do have concrete expectations regarding each of the goals to be met

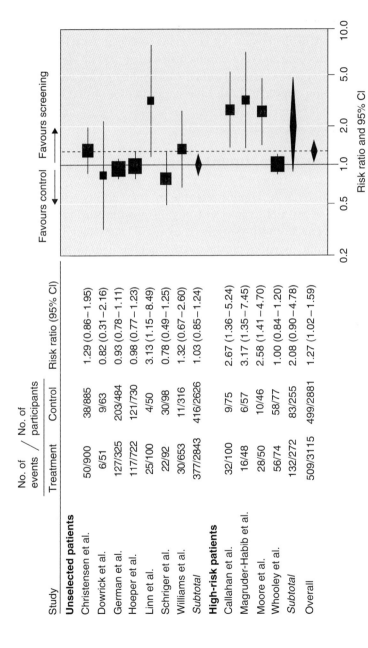

Study	No. of events / No. of participants		Risk ratio (95% CI)
	Treatment	Control	
Unselected patients			
Christensen et al.	50/900	38/885	1.29 (0.86–1.95)
Dowrick et al.	6/51	9/63	0.82 (0.31–2.16)
German et al.	127/325	203/484	0.93 (0.78–1.11)
Hoeper et al.	117/722	121/730	0.98 (0.77–1.23)
Linn et al.	25/100	4/50	3.13 (1.15–8.49)
Schriger et al.	22/92	30/98	0.78 (0.49–1.25)
Williams et al.	30/653	11/316	1.32 (0.67–2.60)
Subtotal	377/2843	416/2626	1.03 (0.85–1.24)
High-risk patients			
Callahan et al.	32/100	9/75	2.67 (1.36–5.24)
Magruder-Habib et al.	16/48	6/57	3.17 (1.35–7.45)
Moore et al.	28/50	10/46	2.58 (1.41–4.70)
Whooley et al.	56/74	58/77	1.00 (0.84–1.20)
Subtotal	132/272	83/255	2.08 (0.90–4.78)
Overall	509/3115	499/2881	1.27 (1.02–1.59)

Figure 23.2 Effect of screening and case-finding instruments on the recognition of depression by clinicians, by method of patient selection (Gilbody et al. [42], reprinted with permission).

in the medical encounters, and the physicians should perform each of their tasks according to the patients' perspective.

Trends in prescription

As a matter of fact, the AD drug prescriptions are increasing all over the world. In Italy, the use of tricyclic ADs (TADs) remained substantially stable from 1983 to 2000, while the use of selective serotonin reuptake inhibitor (SSRI) and newer agents dramatically increased. Overall, the use of ADs increased about fourfold in that period [50]. Surveys conducted both at national level [51] and regional levels confirmed a substantial increase of AD prescription [52, 53].

In England, AD prescribing increased by 10% per year on average from 1998 to 2010 [54]. An analysis of 170 UK practices between 1993 and 2005 showed that ADs prescribing nearly doubled during the study period – the average number of prescriptions issued per patient increased from 2.8 in 1993 to 5.6 in 2004 [55]. An analysis of PCP AD prescription in Scotland showed that the total drug volume increased threefold between 1995/1996 and 2006/2007, largely driven by increases in SSRI [56].

In the United States, the rate of AD prescription increased from about 6% in 1996 to about 10% in 2005 [57]. Among ADs users, the percentage of patients treated for depression did not significantly change, while those undergoing psychotherapy declined. Data from the National Health and Nutrition Examination Surveys showed that from 1988–1994 through 2005–2008, the rate of ADs used in the United States increased nearly fourfold, so that nowadays about one in ten Americans aged 12 and over takes an AD medication [58].

Even examining the literature on pattern of AD prescription in other geographical areas, there is no doubt that ADs have taken an important place in the pharmacological armamentarium of the PCPs. Some of the quoted papers do not seem to indicate that an increase of recognition of depression is the main reason. Other possibilities are that ADs have broadened their indication, or that there is an increase in the duration of treatment [56].

Clinical appropriateness

ADs are by far no more prescribed just for depression, but have a wide indication for several anxiety disorders. Despite that, off-label prescription is still widespread. Radley et al. [59] used US nationally representative data to define prescribing patterns by diagnosis for 160 commonly prescribed drugs. According to their analysis, off-label use of psychotropic drugs was 31%, with gabapentin (83%) and amitriptyline hydrochloride (81%) having the greatest proportion of off-label use (with over 60% of little/no scientific support). A recent analysis of the Quebec database of prescriptions in the primary care confirmed that off-label prescribing is common and varies by drug, patient and physician characteristics [60]. Off-label use was highest for central nervous system drugs (26.3%), including anticonvulsants (66.6%), antipsychotics (43.8%) and ADs (33.4%).

To note, physicians with evidence-based orientation were less likely to prescribe 'off-label'.

Until a decade ago, the doses of AD drugs prescribed for patients identified as depressed were often inadequate, falling below the recommended therapeutic range [61–63]. More recently, probably as a consequence of the simplification of administration (once a day administration, single tablet corresponding to the daily dosage) largely driven by increases in SSRI prescribing, higher mean daily dose prescription has been reported [56, 64].

A further point is the duration of treatment, which in primary care is, in general, quite short. A primary care cohort study from a database of 237 Scottish practices showed that among patients who started an AD treatment during one year (2.2% of all patients), only 75% continued beyond 30 days, 56% beyond 90 days and 40% beyond 180 days. Treatment was less likely to be continued in patients living in areas with high socioeconomic deprivation, in patients under 35 years and in those for whom the PCPs recorded no relevant diagnostic code [65].

Piek et al. [66] reviewed 13 guideline recommendations for long-term treatment with ADs in primary care, concluding that no randomised clinical trials addressing the efficacy of maintenance treatment with ADs as compared to placebo were performed in primary care. Thus, recommendations on maintenance treatment with ADs in primary care cannot be considered evidence-based.

Comparison with instruments measuring depression severity or adequacy of treatment

According to studies by Paykel [67] and Elkin et al. [68], only patients scoring 13 or more on the Hamilton Rating Scale for Depression 17 items (HRSD high scorers) are likely to respond significantly better than placebo to an AD and should, therefore, be considered for drug treatment [69]. In one of our surveys, we took in consideration two parameters [38]: (a) the *decision to start a treatment*, analysed in patients who were HRSD high scorers and not on drug and (b) the *coverage* (i.e. the proportion of patients who would benefit from an AD and who were actually receiving such drugs). Our results showed that only 13% of HRSD high scorers started a new drug treatment, and only about 21% of patients potentially beneficiary of an AD treatment were effectively treated.

A quite recent survey conducted in 38 general practices in the United Kingdom used as reference instruments the 9-item Patient Health Questionnaire (PHQ-9) and the Hospital Anxiety and Depression Scale (HADS) [70]. Overall, 79.1% of depressed patients assessed with either PHQ-9 or HADS received a prescription for an AD, and 22.8% were referred to specialist services. Prescriptions and referrals were significantly associated with higher severity scores at both instruments, while rates of treatment were lower for older patients and for patients with comorbid physical illness. The authors concluded that PCPs did not decide on drug treatment or referral for depression on the basis of questionnaire scores alone, but also took account of other factors such as age and physical illness.

Another observational study of adults attending four PCP practices in Scotland showed that the proportion of participants rated as depressed by PCPs and that of participants receiving ADs differed significantly by HADS depression scores [71]. PCPs recognised 52% participants with HADS 'probable' depression as having a clinically significant depression. There was little evidence of prescribing without relevant indication, but around half of patients with significant symptoms were not identified by their PCPs as suffering from a depressive disorder. In conclusion, these PCPs were initiating AD treatments quite conservatively.

Finally, a very recent retrospective cohort study using routine primary care records conducted in 13 UK general practices examined the association between the severity scores obtained with the PHQ-9 at initial diagnosis and a subsequent PHQ-9 within six months [72]. Patients who showed an inadequate response in score change at the time of second assessment were nearly five times as likely to experience a subsequent change to treatment in comparison with those who showed an adequate response. Thus, PCPs' decisions to change treatment following a second PHQ-9 appear to be in line with NICE guidelines for the monitoring of depression in primary care.

The adequacy of treatment can be assessed with instruments created ad hoc. One of these is the Antidepressant Treatment and History Form (ATHF), a validated instrument rating the adequacy of AD treatment [73]. Using this instrument, Joo et al. [74] assessed the adequacy of overall physician depression management, basing their assessment on severity of depression, adequate AD dosage as determined by the ATHF rating, adequate duration of medication trial and physician-reported next step in depression management. About 75% of the 389 patients treated by PCPs included in this study were judged to receive adequate depression management; a lower rate of adequacy was associated with mild to moderate depressive symptoms (as opposed to remitted or severe symptoms) and specific medications. This is an interesting method to explore the adequacy of treatment, since it allows a comparison between primary care practice and a well-defined standard of good practice. However, while other studies using ATHF have been published [75], no other study was conducted in the primary care.

Comparison with specialist treatment

In general, psychiatrists treat mild depression more aggressively than PCPs, as demonstrated by Lawrence et al. [76] in a US survey where they showed a vignette of an old man with depressive symptoms to psychiatrists and PCPs. Compared with PCPs, psychiatrists were more likely to recommend an AD (70% vs 56%), counselling (86% vs 54%) or the combination of medication and counselling (61% vs 30%).

Fernández et al. [77] analysed the data derived from the Spanish sample of the European Study of the Epidemiology of Mental Disorders (ESEMeD), a

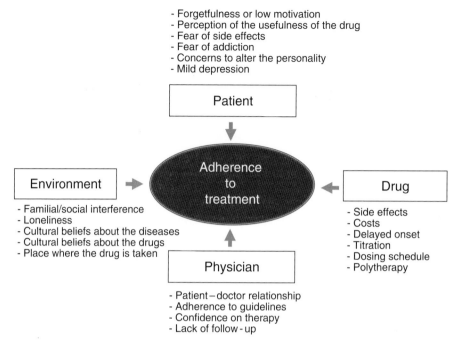

Figure 23.3 Factors involved in adherence to psychotropic drug treatment.

cross-sectional study in a representative sample of adults. Their results showed that similar proportions (only about 30%) of patients in specialty and general medical treatment received a minimally adequate treatment.

Adherence to treatment

A very recent review on AD adherence identified 5 studies conducted in psychiatric populations over the past ten years, while the literature search in primary care populations provided 13 studies [78]. The overall non-adherence rates for AD prescriptions in primary care ranged from 5.4% to 87.6%, with an average rate of AD non-adherence during a six-month period of 46.2%. For comparison, the overall non-adherence rates for AD prescriptions in psychiatric populations ranged from 13% to 55.7%. The conclusions are that about 50% of patients discontinue AD therapy prematurely, without meaningful differences between psychiatric and primary care populations.

Figure 23.3 shows that the reasons for non-adherence can be classified as patient-, clinician-, drug- and environment-related. An important issue regards the beliefs of patients about the treatment. Aikens et al. [79] tried to identify the medication beliefs that could predict the adherence during the maintenance phase of AD treatment. They identified four patient attitudes towards ADs: scepticism, indifference, ambivalence and acceptance. They concluded that adherence is lowest when perceived harm exceeds perceived needs, and highest when perceived needs exceed perceived harm.

Non-adherence has been dealt with several methods, but there is a wide consensus on the necessity to provide multifaceted interventions consisting of collaborative management by the PCPs and a consulting psychiatrist [80]. According to the review by Vergouwen et al. [81], educational interventions alone fail to demonstrate a clear benefit on adherence, while collaborative care interventions tested in primary care demonstrated significant improvements in adherence during the acute and continuation phase of treatment and were associated with clinical benefit, especially in patients suffering from major depression who had been prescribed adequate dosages of ADs.

A very recent review by Chong et al. [82] on effectiveness of interventions for improving adherence provided similar results. Among the 28 interventions tested, about 57% showed significant effects on AD adherence outcomes. The interventions which showed significant improvement in outcomes were primarily multifaceted and complex, with proactive care management and involvement of mental health specialists. The most commonly used elements of multifaceted interventions included patient educational strategies, telephone follow-up to monitor patients' progress as well as providing medication support and feedback to primary care providers. On the contrary, educational interventions alone were ineffective.

Effectiveness of AD treatment

There is no a priori reason to think that trials conducted in primary care are different from those conducted at the specialist level, provided that we control for all variables involved. One of these variables is, for example, the severity of depression, which is usually lower in primary care. If we accept that ADs are effective in acute depressive episodes moderate to severe, we also know that ADs are not effective in mild depression. In a study on the effectiveness of mental health interventions for patients with common somatic conditions, Raine et al. [83] demonstrated that treatments were more effective in patients in secondary care than in primary care, and this happened because secondary care patients had more severe disease, they received a different treatment regimen and the intervention was more closely supervised.

As a consequence, we would be more comfortable if we could have evidence of studies conducted in primary care–based samples. Arroll et al. [84] took stock of the available knowledge with a Cochrane meta-analysis on the efficacy of ADs in primary care. There were 14 studies included in their review, of which 10 studies examined TAD, 2 examined SSRI and 2 included both classes, all compared with placebo. Pooled estimates of efficacy data showed that both TAD and SSRI were effective for depression treated in primary care. Thus, even if we need further data, so far we can consider this meta-analysis as a milestone for the confirmation of the efficacy of ADs even at the primary care level.

Conclusions

In 1985, I co-authored an Italian book edited by Michele Tansella on the epidemiological approach to psychiatry [1]. After about 30 years from the publication of that book, can we say that we have more information and competency in the management of mental health in primary care? Probably the response is 'yes', but with some caveats. For example, following the 'pathway to care' model, several proposals of organisation of primary care services for mental health have been put forward and tested in Italy as well and in other countries. The good news is that most of them (e.g. C-L, collaborative care, stepped care) seem to work well.

On the other hand, less information is available about the methods that might be implemented to improve the ability of PCPs in detecting anxiety and depressive disorders. If used alone, case-finding and screening questionnaires have demonstrated little or no impact on the probability of detection. Yet, even if it is recognised that training primary care staff is necessary, few analyses have been carried out on continuing education of PCPs in the mental health field.

Psychotropic drug prescription increased in the last decades, but undoubtedly this cannot be the sole response to mental health disease. Patients want more communication with their PCPs and would like some kind of non-drug intervention. Counselling is a potential treatment for these patients, but there is still a lack of consensus over its effectiveness in primary care. The appropriateness of prescriptions is less than optimal, but the psychotropic drugs – at least the ADs – seem to be efficacious and thus represent a useful tool for PCPs. The critical point is the adherence of the patients to the treatment. This again involves the necessity to provide multifaceted interventions consisting of collaborative management by the PCPs and the consulting psychiatrists, since only these interventions have demonstrated significant improvements in adherence during the acute and continuation phase of treatment.

In conclusion, the key message to be put forward is that PCPs must improve their medical competence in the management of mental health disorders, but in so doing they have to know how to balance this personal competence with the ability to collaborate with specialist services. Mental health is often not just a question of symptoms but also of perceived quality of life and social participation. This implies the necessity of complex interventions where PCPs and mental health specialists can cooperate.

References

[1]   Tansella M (ed.). (1985) *L'Approccio Epidemiologico in Psichiatria*. Milano: Boringhieri.
[2]   Goldberg DP, Lecrubier Y. (1995) Form and frequency of mental disorders across centres. In: Ustun TB, Sartorius N (eds.), *Mental Illness in General Health Care: An International Study*. Chichester: John Wiley & Sons, Ltd on behalf of WHO, pp. 323–334.

[3] Lepine JP, Gastpar M, Mendlewicz J et al. (1997) Depression in the community: the first pan-European study DEPRES (Depression Research in European Society). *International Clinical Psychopharmacology* **12**: 19–29.

[4] Rucci P, Gherardi S, Tansella M et al. (2003) Subthreshold psychiatric disorders in primary care: prevalence and associated characteristics. *Journal of Affective Disorders* **76**: 171–181.

[5] Ansseau M, Dierick M, Buntinkx F et al. (2004) High prevalence of mental disorders in primary care. *Journal of Affective Disorders* **78**: 49–55.

[6] Balestrieri M, Baldacci S, Bellomo A et al. (2007) Clinical vs. structured interview on anxiety and affective disorders by primary care physicians. Understanding diagnostic discordance. *Epidemiologia e Psichiatria Sociale* **16**: 144–151.

[7] WONCA. (2008) What is primary care mental health? WHO and WONCA Working Party on Mental Health. *Mental Health in Family Medicine* **5**: 9–13.

[8] Goldberg D, Huxley P. (1980) *Mental Illness in the Community: The Pathway to Psychiatric Care.* London: Tavistock Publications.

[9] Goldberg D. (1995) Epidemiology of mental disorders in primary care settings. *Epidemiologic Reviews* **17**: 182–190.

[10] Tansella M, Williams P. (1989) The spectrum of psychiatric morbidity in a defined geographical area. *Psychological Medicine* **19**: 765–770.

[11] Bower P, Gilbody S. (2005) Managing common mental health disorders in primary care: conceptual models and evidence base. *BMJ* **330**: 839–842.

[12] Carta MG, Balestrieri M, Murru A et al. (2009) Adjustment disorder: epidemiology, diagnosis and treatment. *Clinical Practice and Epidemiology in Mental Health* **26**: 5–15.

[13] Fernández A, Mendive JM, Salvador-Carulla L et al. (2012) Adjustment disorders in primary care: prevalence, recognition and use of services. *British Journal of Psychiatry* **201**: 137–142.

[14] Peedell C. (2011) Further privatisation is inevitable under the proposed NHS reforms. *BMJ* **342**: d2996.

[15] Thornicroft G, Tansella M. (2012) The balanced care model for global mental health. *Psychological Medicine* **11**: 1–15.

[16] Balestrieri M, Bon MG, Rodriguez-Sacristan A et al. (1994) Pathways to psychiatric care in south-Verona, Italy. *Psychological Medicine* **24**: 641–649.

[17] Goldberg D. (1999) The management of anxious depression in primary care. *Journal of Clinical Psychiatry* **60** (Suppl. 7): 39–42.

[18] Burton C, McGorm K, Weller D et al. (2011) Depression and anxiety in patients repeatedly referred to secondary care with medically unexplained symptoms: a case-control study. *Psychological Medicine* **41**: 555–563.

[19] Cape J, Whittington C, Bower P. (2010) What is the role of consultation-liaison psychiatry in the management of depression in primary care? A systematic review and meta-analysis. *General Hospital Psychiatry* **32**: 246–254.

[20] van der Feltz-Cornelis CM, Van Os TW, Van Marwijk HW et al. (2010) Effect of psychiatric consultation models in primary care. A systematic review and meta-analysis of randomized clinical trials. *Journal of Psychosomatic Research* **68**: 521–533.

[21] Woltmann E, Grogan-Kaylor A, Perron B et al. (2012) Comparative effectiveness of collaborative chronic care models for mental health conditions across primary, specialty, and behavioral health care settings: systematic review and meta-analysis. *American Journal of Psychiatry* **169**: 790–804.

[22] National Collaborating Centre for Mental Health. (2009) *Depression: The Treatment and Management of Depression in Adults: NICE Clinical Guideline 90.* London: National Institute for Health and Clinical Excellence.

[23] Rucci P, Piazza A, Menchetti M et al. (2012) Integration between primary care and mental health services in Italy: determinants of referral and stepped care. *International Journal of Family Medicine* **2012**: 507464.

[24] Franx G, Oud M, de Lange J et al. (2012) Implementing a stepped-care approach in primary care: results of a qualitative study. *Implementation Science* **7**: 8.

[25] Goldberg D, Huxley P. (2012) At least 25% with a mental health problem is a conservative estimate. *BMJ* **344**: e1776.

[26] Ginn S, Horder J. (2012) "One in four" with a mental health problem: the anatomy of a statistic. *BMJ* **344**: e1302.

[27] Wittchen HU, Jacobi F. (2005) Size and burden of mental disorders in Europe: a critical review and appraisal of 27 studies. *European Neuropsychopharmacology* **15**: 357–376.

[28] Wittchen HU, Jacobi F, Rehm J et al. (2011) The size and burden of mental disorders and other disorders of the brain in Europe 2010. *European Neuropsychopharmacology* **21**: 655–679.

[29] Goldberg DP, Prisciandaro JJ, Williams P. (2012) The primary health care version of ICD-11: the detection of common mental disorders in general medical settings. *General Hospital Psychiatry* **34**: 665–670.

[30] Coyne JC, Schwenk TL, Fechner-Bates S. (1995) Non-detection of depression by primary care physicians reconsidered. *General Hospital Psychiatry* **17**: 3–12.

[31] Tiemens BG, Ormel J, Simon GE. (1996) Occurrence, recognition, and outcome of psychological disorders in primary care. *American Journal of Psychiatry* **153**: 636–644.

[32] Tiemens BG, Von Korff M, Lin EH. (1999) Diagnosis of depression by primary care physicians versus a structured diagnostic interview. Understanding discordance. *General Hospital Psychiatry* **21**: 87–96.

[33] Bellantuono C, Rizzo R, Mazzi M et al. (2002) The identification of depression and the coverage of AD drug prescriptions in Italian general practice. *Journal of Affective Disorders* **72**: 53–59.

[34] Berardi D, Menchetti M, Cevenini N et al. (2005) Increased recognition of depression in primary care. Comparison between primary-care physician and ICD-10 diagnosis of depression. *Psychotherapy and Psychosomatics* **74**: 225–230.

[35] Wittchen HU, Höfler M, Meister W. (2001) Prevalence and recognition of depressive syndromes in German primary care settings: poorly recognized and treated? *International Clinical Psychopharmacology* **16**: 121–135.

[36] Cepoiu M, McCusker J, Cole MG et al. (2008) Recognition of depression by non-psychiatric physicians – a systematic literature review and meta-analysis. *Journal of General Internal Medicine* **23**: 25–36.

[37] Bridges K, Goldberg D. (1992) Somatic presentation of depressive illness in primary care. *Journal of Royal College of General Practitioners* **36**: 9–11.

[38] Balestrieri M, Carta MG, Leonetti S et al. (2004) Recognition of depression and appropriateness of AD treatment in Italian primary care. *Social Psychiatry and Psychiatric Epidemiology* **39**: 171–176.

[39] Piek E, Nolen WA, van der Meer K et al. (2012) Determinants of (non-)recognition of depression by general practitioners: results of the Netherlands Study of Depression and Anxiety. *Journal of Affective Disorders* **138**: 397–404.

[40] Tylee A, Walters P. (2007) Underrecognition of anxiety and mood disorders in primary care: why does the problem exist and what can be done? *Journal of Clinical Psychiatry* **68** (Suppl. 2): 27–30.

[41] Barbui C, Tansella M. (2006) Identification and management of depression in primary care settings. A meta-review of evidence. *Epidemiologia e Psichiatria Sociale* **15**: 276–283.

[42] Gilbody S, Sheldon T, House A. (2008) Screening and case-finding instruments for depression: a meta-analysis. *Canadian Medical Association Journal* **178**: 997–1003.

[43] Wolf NJ, Hopko DR. (2008) Psychosocial and pharmacological interventions for depressed adults in primary care: a critical review. *Clinical Psychological Review* **28**: 131–161.

[44] Bosmans JE, van Schaik DJ, de Bruijne MC et al. (2008) Are psychological treatments for depression in primary care cost-effective? *Journal of Mental Health Policy and Economics* **11**: 3–15.

[45] Balestrieri M, Bortolomasi M, Galletta M et al. (1997) Patterns of hypnotic drug prescription in Italy. A two-week community survey. *British Journal of Psychiatry* **170**: 176–180.

[46] Balestrieri M, Marcon G, Samani F et al. (2005) Mental disorders associated with benzodiazepine use among older primary care attenders. A regional survey. *Social Psychiatry and Psychiatric Epidemiology* **40**: 308–315.

[47] Barley EA, Murray J, Walters P et al. (2011) Managing depression in primary care: a meta-synthesis of qualitative and quantitative research from the UK to identify barriers and facilitators. *BMC Family Practice* **12**: 47.

[48] van Schaik DJ, Klijn AF, van Hout HP et al. (2004) Patients' preferences in the treatment of depressive disorder in primary care. *General Hospital Psychiatry* **26**: 184–189.

[49] Deledda G, Moretti F, Rimondini M et al. (2012) How patients want their doctor to communicate. A literature review on primary care patients' perspective. *Patient Education Counseling*. Available from: http://dx.doi.org/10.1016/j.pec.2012.05.005. Accessed on 3 January 2013.

[50] Guaiana G, Andretta M, Corbari L et al. (2005) Antidepressant drug consumption and public health indicators in Italy, 1955 to 2000. *Journal of Clinical Psychiatry* **66**: 750–755.

[51] Trifirò G, Tillati S, Spina E et al. (2013) A nationwide prospective study on prescribing pattern of antidepressant drugs in Italian primary care. *European Journal of Clinical Pharmacology* **69** (2): 227–236.

[52] Percudani M, Barbui C, Fortino I et al. (2004) Antidepressant drug use in Lombardy, Italy: a population-based study. *Journal of Affective Disorders* **83**: 169–175.

[53] Guaiana G, Andretta M, Griez E et al. (2011) Sales of antidepressants, suicides and hospital admissions for depression in Veneto Region, Italy, from 2000 to 2005: an ecological study. *Annals of General Psychiatry* **10**: 24.

[54] Ilyas S, Moncrieff J. (2012) Trends in prescriptions and costs of drugs for mental disorders in England, 1998–2010. *British Journal of Psychiatry* **200**: 393–398.

[55] Moore M, Yuen HM, Dunn N et al. (2009) Explaining the rise in antidepressant prescribing: a descriptive study using the general practice research database. *BMJ* **339**: b3999.

[56] Lockhart P, Guthrie B. (2011) Trends in primary care antidepressant prescribing 1995–2007: a longitudinal population database analysis. *British Journal of General Practice* **61**: e565–e572.

[57] Olfson M, Marcus SC. (2009) National patterns in antidepressant medication treatment. *Archives of General Psychiatry* **66**: 848–856.

[58] Pratt LA, Brody DJ, Gu Q. (2008) *Antidepressant Use in Persons Aged 12 and Over: United States, 2005–2008*. NCHS Data Brief no. 76. Hyattsville: National Center for Health Statistics, pp. 1–8.

[59] Radley DC, Finkelstein SN, Stafford RS. (2006) Off-label prescribing among office-based physicians. *Archives of Internal Medicine* **166**: 1021–1026.

[60] Eguale T, Buckeridge DL, Winslade NE et al. (2012) Drug, patient, and physician characteristics associated with off-label prescribing in primary care. *Archives of Internal Medicine* **172**: 781–788.

[61] Katon W, Von Korff M, Lin E et al. (1992) Adequacy and duration of AD treatment in primary care. *Medical Care* **30**: 67–76.

[62] Isometsa E, Seppala I, Henriksson M et al. (1998) Inadequate dosaging in general practice of tricyclic vs. other ADs for depression. *Acta Psychiatrica Scandinavica* **98**: 451–454.

[63] Davidson J, Meltzer-Brody S. (1999) The underrecognition and undertreatment of depression: what is the breadth and depth of the problem? *Journal of Clinical Psychiatry* **60** (Suppl. 7): 4–9.

[64] Weilburg JB, O'Leary KM, Meigs JB et al. (2003) Evaluation of the adequacy of outpatient antidepressant treatment. *Psychiatric Services* **54**: 1233–1239.

[65] Burton C, Anderson N, Wilde K et al. (2012) Factors associated with new antidepressant treatment. Analysis of a large primary care database. *British Journal of General Practice* **62**: e104–e112.

[66] Piek E, van der Meer K, Nolen WA. (2010) Guideline recommendations for long-term treatment of depression with antidepressants in primary care – a critical review. *European Journal of General Practice* **16**: 106–112.

[67] Paykel ES. (1988) Antidepressants: their efficacy and place in therapy. *Journal of Psychopharmacology* **2**: 105–118.

[68] Elkin I, Shea MT, Watkins JT et al. (1989) National Institute of Mental Health Treatment of Depression Collaborative Research Program. General effectiveness of treatments. *Archives of General Psychiatry* **46**: 971–982.

[69] Paykel ES, Priest RG. (1992) Recognition and management of depression in general practice: consensus statement. *BMJ* **305** (6863): 1198–1202.

[70] Kendrick T, Dowrick C, McBride A et al. (2009) Management of depression in UK general practice in relation to scores on depression severity questionnaires: analysis of medical record data. *BMJ* **338**: b750.

[71] Cameron IM, Lawton K, Reid IC. (2009) Appropriateness of antidepressant prescribing: an observational study in a Scottish primary-care setting. *British Journal of General Practice* **59**: 644–649.

[72] Moore M, Ali S, Stuart B et al. (2012) Depression management in primary care: an observational study of management changes related to PHQ-9 score for depression monitoring. *British Journal of General Practice* **62**: 451–457.

[73] Oquendo MA, Baca-Garcia E, Kartachov A et al. (2003) A computer algorithm for calculating the adequacy of AD treatment in unipolar and bipolar depression. *Journal of Clinical Psychiatry* **64**: 825–833.

[74] Joo JH, Solano FX, Mulsant BH et al. (2005) Predictors of adequacy of depression management in the primary care setting. *Psychiatric Services* **56**: 1524–1528.

[75] Kocsis JH, Gelenberg AJ, Rothbaum B et al. (2008) Chronic forms of major depression are still undertreated in the 21st century: systematic assessment of 801 patients presenting for treatment. *Journal of Affective Disorders* **110**: 55–61.

[76] Lawrence RE, Rasinski KA, Yoon JD et al. (2012) Primary care physicians' and psychiatrists' approaches to treating mild depression. *Acta Psychiatrica Scandinavica* **126** (5): 385–392.

[77] Fernández A, Haro JM, Codony M et al. (2006) Treatment adequacy of anxiety and depressive disorders: primary versus specialised care in Spain. *Journal of Affective Disorders* **96**: 9–20.

[78] Sansone RA, Sansone LA. (2012) Antidepressant adherence: are patients taking their medications? *Innovations in Clinical Neuroscience* **9**: 41–46.

[79] Aikens JE, Nease DE Jr, Nau DP et al. (2005) Adherence to maintenance-phase antidepressant medication as a function of patient beliefs about medication. *Annals of Family Medicine* **3**: 23–30.

[80] Katon W, Von Korff M, Lin E et al. (1995) Collaborative management to achieve treatment guidelines. Impact on depression in primary care. *Journal of American Medical Association* **273**: 1026–1031.

[81] Vergouwen AC, Bakker A, Katon WJ et al. (2003) Improving adherence to antidepressants: a systematic review of interventions. *Journal of Clinical Psychiatry* **64**: 1415–1420.

[82] Chong WW, Aslani P, Chen TF. (2011) Effectiveness of interventions to improve AD medication adherence: a systematic review. *International Journal of Clinical Practice* **65**: 954–975.

[83] Raine R, Haines A, Sensky T et al. (2002) Systematic review of mental health interventions for patients with common somatic symptoms: can research evidence from secondary care be extrapolated to primary care? *BMJ* **325** (7372): 1082.

[84] Arroll B, Elley CR, Fishman T et al. (2009) Antidepressants versus placebo for depression in primary care. *Cochrane Database of Systematic Reviews* **3**: CD007954.

CHAPTER 24

Some wobbly planks in the platform of mental health care

Norman Sartorius

Association for the Improvement of Mental Health Programmes, Geneva, Switzerland

Introduction

Mental disorders are a major public health problem. They are highly prevalent. Most of them can have severe consequences unless appropriately treated. It is probable that the extended life expectancy, the neglect of the prevention of brain diseases, the epidemic of anomie linked to rampant urbanisation and the enhanced environmental stresses will make the prevalence of mental disorders grow even further in the future. It is thus to be expected that governments will formulate policies and programmes that can deal with the problems that mental disorders can produce for individuals and societies.

Many governments produced mental health policies; 74 countries did not do so [1]. Not all of the countries that have formulated a policy also have a programme that would serve to implement the policy. Some have both a policy and a programme but do not pay much attention to either when it comes to budgeting for health care or organising it. Yet, even those that have formulated a programme and are implementing it often admit that there are areas of neglect and failure parallel to successful implementation of their plans built on their mental health policies and programmes.

A possible explanation of this failure is that the premises of our policies and programmes are faulty. This paper will examine the validity of some of these premises to see whether they are still valid and make it easier for people with mental illness and their families to receive the care that they need. Other premises, not discussed in this chapter, should also be carefully examined; to do so in this chapter will not be possible in view of the limited space allowed for each of the chapters.

Estimating mental health needs

One of the premises of current mental health programming is that the prevalence of mental disorders is a necessary determinant of plans for mental health service.

Improving Mental Health Care: The Global Challenge, First Edition.
Edited by Graham Thornicroft, Mirella Ruggeri and David Goldberg.
© 2013 John Wiley & Sons, Ltd. Published 2013 by John Wiley & Sons, Ltd.

The prevalence of mental disorders, the argument goes, tells us how many people need mental health care. What mental health plans have to do, this premise says, is to match the numbers of facilities, staff as well as other resources, and ingredients of care accepted as valid at the point of making plans for services (e.g. that a person with an acute psychotic state will usually require two to three weeks of inpatient care), with the care of people with mental disorders. Staff and facilities that are included in this calculation are not necessarily mental health professionals; thus, the members of general practitioners and other staff in the community, for example, midwives and home-visiting nurses who are or can be given the necessary training, should be included in these considerations.

This premise is, however, wrong. First, there are people with mental disorders who do not want to receive mental health care and manage to live with their mental health problems without any contact to health services. The reasons for this may be different, but an important consideration is that the stigma of mental disorder has sometimes worse consequences than the disease itself. Often, the stigma – not the diseases or impairment – prevents people who have a stigmatised disease from getting a job, finding a house, getting married or obtaining a driving licence. Sometimes people with mental illness can manage relying on advice from practitioners of alternative medicine; sometimes they find solace in their religion; and sometimes they develop their own ways of coping with problems.

Second, depending on the circumstances and the image of the mental health service, people who do not have a well-defined mental disorder may seek help from the mental health-care workers. The demand for care may increase after a report about the great efficacy of a new treatment method is published in the media. Demand for health care will vary depending on the environmental circumstances. In times of financial crises, for example, the numbers of those who contact health (and mental health) services will increase. People who care for seriously disabled individuals for a long time contact services (including mental health services) more often than the general population demanding help, looking for a sympathetic listener or seeking advice about problems that could be symptoms of mental disorders.

Third, the need for mental health care depends on whether there is an intervention effective in the resolution of a problem that the health service can offer. When the health service has no effective intervention that can help in resolving a particular problem, the problem should not be counted among the needs for that service. Thus, people with dementia and their family might well need significant support and help from social services: for the time being, they should not be counted among needs for mental health services.

Thus, the need for the service is not equal to the prevalence of mental disorders, although to an extent it depends on it. Needs for service equal the demands for help by people (or their families) with a recognisable mental disorder for which the service has an effective answer. It is also important to remember that demands which are not related to an existing mental disorder (for which the service has a treatment) have to be taken into account in planning services because they will take time of the health practitioners who have to examine the persons requesting help and refer them to the agency that can help or discourage them from seeking support from the service. How much time will be taken dealing with demands will depend on the skills of the health professionals and on environmental factors. It is difficult to predict how the demands will vary, although it can be expected that the continuous increase of knowledge of those who demand help as well as a clearer definition of what a service can do are likely to reduce the variation. The demands by themselves are, however, also not equal to needs for mental health services.

Providing community care

Although the first mental hospitals in Europe were built in the fifteenth century, it was in the nineteenth century that the notion that people with mental disorders have to be given protection, support and treatment gained strength. Mentally ill people were no longer to be sent down the rivers in the ships of fools nor exposed to the mockery and violence in the streets. It appeared logical that this could best be done by building sufficient numbers of hospitals to protect the patients from the community and to offer them inpatient care. The wish to remove the mentally ill from the public places might have also played a role as a motivating factor to construct asylums. Some of the leading psychiatrists – for example, Griesinger – suggested that it might be better to provide care in the community with an outreach service than in a hospital. Geel, a small town in the Duchy of Brabant, maintained, for nearly a thousand years, a system of health care for the mentally ill that could or should have been a model of helping patients in the community by entrusting the care for them to foster families [2]. The proposals of Griesinger and the example of Geel (and possibly other isolated examples which were not described) did not attract many followers. As countries of Europe became richer, they built hospitals for the mentally ill, sometimes using the spoils of war like it happened in the instance of Germany's victory over France in the 1870 war when the reparations received by Germany were to a large extent used to build hospitals for the mentally ill. With a slight delay, European powers built hospitals similar in structure to those in Europe in their colonies at the beginning of the twentieth century.

While serving some of their purposes (e.g. removing the mentally ill from the public places and protecting those ill from the crowds), the mental hospitals large in size and often short of staff did not provide appropriate care to those who were admitted for treatment. The long stay in the overcrowded institutions contributed to the disability and impairments of the mentally ill. Stay in hospitals contributed to the interruption of social links and connections with the family and the home community. Mental hospitals often had a bad name, and this influenced the quality of staff who applied to work there. Quality control of services in the hospital was often missing, and there was little concern about the rights of the mentally ill. In the absence of demonstrably effective treatment and in the absence of external control of the service, psychiatrists tried out a variety of treatments. The horrifying mutilations in the search for foci of infection (foci that, according to the theory, were producing the toxins leading to mental disorders) by Dr Cotton in the Trenton hospital [3] exemplify the worst of active interventions: most often, however, patients received no treatment, and patients and their needs were neglected by all.

The alternative to a stay in a mental hospital was to receive treatment while living in the community. Some of the psychiatrists were for this option but many were opposed. The families who were to provide care were ambivalent. Other members of the community were usually reluctant to have mentally ill people living among them. Eventually, the work of pioneers of community psychiatry provided evidence that treatment in the community is possible, that it can be effective, that it prevents the effects of institutionalisation and that patients who have been offered community treatment instead of hospital care report improved quality of life. The belief that treatment can be provided in the community led governments to reduce the numbers of hospital beds and close many of the mental hospitals. The notion of treatment in the community was also attractive to Governments because it was seen as a way of saving money: the idea that the savings should be used to facilitate community care did not seem to find much acceptance. In some instances, for example, in the United States and in Italy, the reduction was very rapid, and thousands of patients found themselves suddenly without any support or treatment. Some of them ended in prisons (initiating the currently massive trend of trans-institutionalisation), others became the homeless mentally ill. Some died a violent death, and some perished because of physical illness for which they received no treatment. In other countries in which the deinstitutionalisation was slower and has been organised in parallel with an investment into community-based services, the outcome was positive.

Over time, it became possible to assemble the evidence about the requirements for a successful provision of community psychiatric care. These include the existence of a community in which the patient can live; staff of mental health services who are willing to provide care; resources that will enable the staff to do their work (e.g. regular supply of medications, means of transportation necessary to visit patients at home); support – material, moral and informational to the carers (family or others) who will be helping the person with the mental illness; a legal structure that will ensure that the patients' and health workers' safety and rights are protected; a system of quality control; and access to inpatient treatment without delays if this becomes necessary.

Mental health policies as well as most of the authorities in psychiatry today agree that community care as defined and developed in the middle and late twentieth century is the best way to organise mental health services. Yet, there are very few places in which the requirements mentioned earlier are fulfilled. First, the geographically defined communities that figure so prominently in the organisation of community mental health care are rapidly disappearing. Urbanisation happens faster than ever expected. In Argentina, for example, 85% of the population is now living in urban settings to which they moved recently and in which they have few if any contacts with the rest of the inhabitants. There are still countries or parts of countries in which communities are well composed, have social coherence, identifiable leaders and a recognisable structure: but their numbers are diminishing very fast.

Mental health professionals who spent years working in an institution are often reluctant to work in a community. Most of the education of doctors and nurses about psychiatry – at undergraduate and postgraduate level – never includes a visit to a patient's home. Health workers are often reluctant to go to poorer parts of the city and afraid of what might happen to them if they were to visit their clients in the urban slums. In many settings, the mental health service does not provide means of transportation to staff nor any incentive for work in the community.

Nor are there provisions for support to the family. In some countries, families or other carers receive a financial compensation if they are looking after a patient at home. The sums which they are receiving are ridiculously small, often equal to the value of food for the patient, for a day or two. In the past, families were often very large and could distribute the tasks of looking after a mentally ill or disabled member without difficulty. In modern times, families have become very small, nuclear, containing two partners and possibly one or two children. Providing care for the mentally ill will take most of the energy and time of at least one family member, an expenditure of time and energy that is incompatible with that person's job and other obligations. In addition, a significant proportion of the mentally ill people are living alone, and there is no family member that could be involved in their care.

Thus, in most settings the requirements for community psychiatric care (as originally designed and as currently understood by many decision-makers and health workers) are not satisfied, and it is necessary and urgent to redefine them. Among the changes of its definition will have to be (a) much more emphasis on help to carers or foster carers, with appropriate financial support, and with a public recognition of the work that they are doing (e.g. by counting the years spent in looking after a severely mentally ill person as years of work when calculating an old age pension); (b) a change in the education of health personnel to ensure that they learn about ways of providing care in the community; (c) a change in the distribution of tasks among members of the mental health team; and possibly others. The community care plank of the mental health platform as currently defined is no longer useful. It will have to be reviewed and revised.

Task shifting

There are far too few psychiatrists in the world. Even in highly developed countries, health services report that they are lacking psychiatrists and other mental health personnel. The projections for the developing countries indicate that the disproportion between those who need care and highly trained specialists is so large that it will take a long time – maybe several decades or even longer – before the numbers of specialists working in the country reach an adequate number. The achievement of such a goal requires a substantial additional investment to improve psychiatric education and to make mental health facilities attractive and effective so as to make students interested in entering the discipline. Neither of these two requirements is likely to be met in the near future. The stigma of mental illness and the poor image of psychiatry (seen at best as an inefficient and at worst as a corrupt and dangerous branch of medicine) conspire to keep the priority of psychiatry low in developing countries and a likely subject for substantial budgetary cuts in the industrialised world.

It therefore seemed logical to suggest that the tasks which mental health specialists were doing should be passed on to non-specialised health workers, for example, general practitioners or to specialists in other disciplines – for example, that of internal medicine who often encounter patients who suffer from common mental disorders. The official blessing of this idea came with the recommendations of an Expert Committee convened by the World Health Organization (WHO) in 1973 and by subsequent statements in WHO's governing bodies, which are composed of top health officials in the 190 member states of the WHO [4]. A study of the feasibility of extending mental health care by training general health-care workers in developing countries followed and demonstrated that simply trained health workers – if given short-lasting additional training – can deal with common mental disorders and learn whom to refer for specialised care or advice [5].

It thus seemed logical that countries will take on the task of training their general health workers about the recognition and treatment of common mental disorders and of re-organising the service to make it possible for them to provide care to people with mental health problems who come to them for help. This did happen in some places and for some mental disorders, but the change was not a sufficiently convincing demonstration that mental health care can be provided differently, without continuous and exclusive reliance on mental hospitals, and thus did not lead to revolutionary all-embracing reform of mental health care as it should have done.

The reasons for this were many. First, while in the studies that were proving that it is feasible to make general health workers take on mental health tasks there was a powerful incentive of participating in a major international undertaking (or national studies), subsequent work lacked external incentives.

Some of the general health-care staff liked dealing with mental health problems but most of them did not, possibly because their competence to provide adequate care (and be encouraged by its success) was limited. The undergraduate training of medical students and students of other health professions in most countries of the world did not change. The training in psychiatry continued to be given too late in the curriculum. Lectures continued to be the main form of instruction. Education concentrated on the most severe and rare forms of mental disorders, with little or no time given to common mental disorders. Postgraduate training in psychiatry continued to focus on the recognition and treatment of severe and therapy-resistant forms of mental disorders: training in skills of teaching others and of conveying knowledge about mental illness to the general public continued to be a rarity. The instructions about the treatment of mental disorders remained arcane, often unaffected by results of recent research.

Gradually, it became obvious that policies, proclamations about task shifting and the delegation of treatment of mental disorders to general health-care staff and specialists in disciplines other than psychiatry do not suffice and that there are several other interventions that are necessary to make the general health-care staff take on the lion's part of mental health care.[1]

These will include a revision of the manner of inservice training which should become a regular feature of health plans and which should focus on the management of common mental disorders. The training about these matters is best delivered by experienced general health-care staff who are knowledgeable about mental illness, possibly in the presence of a psychiatrist as a resource person (and not as the main teacher). Rather than training all health-care staff, it will be wiser to concentrate on those who are aware of the frequency and severity of mental health problems and who are interested in learning about ways which could help them to manage such problems. Instructions about the recognition and treatment of mental disorders – which are nowadays often complex and contain a lot of that is not necessary – will have to be written in a manner that will make it easy to understand and follow. The training will have to concentrate on disorders that are commonly seen in their practice (not on all psychiatric disorders) and can be treated by means that are available to the general health-care worker. A structure of incentives for an active engagement in mental health care would be useful, particularly while introducing changes. Regular supply of medications that can be used in the treatment of mental disorders is also important, at least as important as that of other medications. A system of referral would be useful and should be put in place, giving it priority over other changes of the mental health system. All of these suggestions refer to obvious needs: yet, in most countries of the world, few if any of them are being realised at present. Task shifting can, therefore, be seen as a worthwhile goal that will have to be prepared, rather than as a measure that can help the system of health care for the mentally ill in the immediate future.

Mental health care can be provided at a low cost

One of the most popular arguments presented to the public and to decision-makers when proposing a mental health programme is that the cost of such an undertaking will be low. A person with a severe mental illness can be provided treatment, the economic argument goes, for a few dollars per month; once recovered, such persons will be able to work again and make their full contribution to society.

This sounds good, but several parts of this argument are wrong. First, arguing that something should be introduced because it is cheap is not convincing. If an army has to be vaccinated against some disease which may prevail in the part of the world to which it is sent, the argument is not that the vaccines are cheap but that they are necessary because they will make soldiers able to fulfill their mission. Second, the words 'cheap', 'low cost', and 'expensive' refer to the value that the object that is to be obtained has. People with mental illness are considered by many – including most decision-makers – as being without any value to society. They are, in their opinion, incurable and in addition usually lazy, sometimes dangerous and usually unpleasant to be with. In this frame of mind, no matter how little the medications or other treatment for mental illness might cost, they will always be considered too expensive – simply because they are an expenditure concerning people without any value. It is perfectly true, for example, that many mental disorders can be successfully treated in primary health care and that this is much less expensive than treatment by specialists in institutions, but the power of that argument should be based on the improvement of health, better quality of life, enhanced competence of general practitioners and similar gains rather than on the argument that it is cheaper.

The second part of the argument, that the indirect cost of mental illness will be eliminated once they are recovered and that persons with mental illness will be able to contribute to society by working, is also wrong. In most parts of the world, 'working' is equated with employment. In current conditions of high unemployment rates, it is very unlikely that persons who had recovered from a severe mental illness will be employed if they admit that they had a mental illness. Even when the conditions of the labour market are better and when there are jobs, the stigma of mental illness makes re-employment after a period of being mentally ill improbable.

It is thus necessary to build the argument for the introduction of mental health programmes or for an increased investment in mental health care on different arguments. Psychiatrists and other mental health specialists are not particularly skillful when presenting the successes of their discipline. They have not marshalled the arguments that would convince decision-makers about the usefulness of investment in mental health care. Perhaps, for the time being, it might be better to build a case for mental health care by predicting scandals in case care is not provided: the fear of scandals is a powerful motive for action by politicians who hope for re-elections. Perhaps it would be wise to consider whether fighting for an improvement of mental health care should be postponed and all effort placed on action that will diminish stigmatisation by mental illness. An analysis of what worked and why it did is a necessary step in defining a strategy that will lead to a higher priority for mental health programmes: the low cost argument has certainly not been useful in the past and should not be used in the future.

Coda

I selected four of the elements of currently used strategies to improve mental health programmes as examples of reasons why mental health programmes remain feeble although the need for them grows. They have obvious shortcomings, and their continuing use is not likely to make mental health services better or stronger. I could have selected some other elements – planks in the platform for mental health care – and could have demonstrated their weaknesses. The point that this chapter makes is that it is high time to critically examine the premises on which we are to build mental health programmes and that it is necessary to have the courage to replace them by components that are valid at present and might be useful now and for some time; after a while, they will also have to be examined and possibly replaced by better ones.

Note

1 In many instances, the general practitioners and other general health-care staff did deal with common mental disorders without realising that they were doing this. Thus, for example, people who came forward with a multitude of somatic complaints (for which it was impossible to find an organic basis) did receive reassurance, tranquilisers and advice which seemed to be useful in such cases without the recognition that these problems might be due to a depressive illness.

References

[1] World Health Organization. (2011) *Mental Health Atlas 2011*. Geneva: WHO.
[2] Goldstein JL, Godemont MML. (2003) The legend and lessons of Geel. *Community Mental Health Journal* **39**: 441–458.
[3] Scull A. (2005) *Madhouse. A Tragic Tale of Megalomania and Modern Medicine*. New Haven/London: Yale University Press.
[4] World Health Organization. (1975) *Organization of Mental Health Services in Developing Countries*. Technical Report Series 564. Geneva: WHO.
[5] World Health Organization. (1984) *Mental Health Care in Developing Countries: A Critical Appraisal of Research Findings*. Technical Report Series 698. Geneva: WHO.

CHAPTER 25

Treatment gaps and knowledge gaps in mental health: Schizophrenia as a global challenge

Assen Jablensky

School of Psychiatry and Clinical Neurosciences, The University of Western Australia, Australia

Introduction: Schizophrenia in the global burden of disease

In the 1990s, the World Health Organization (WHO) initiated the Global Burden of Disease (GBD) study which introduced a novel unit of measurement, the disability-adjusted life year (DALY). As a 'health gap' measure, the DALY quantifies the years of healthy life lost in a given population due to the joint effects of mortality and disability [1]. A surprising outcome of the first GBD assessment for the year 2000, and of the updated projections from 2002 to 2030 [2], was that several psychiatric conditions, including unipolar depressive disorders, bipolar affective disorder, schizophrenia and self-inflicted injuries were among the top ten conditions worldwide accounting for the largest proportions of DALYs in age groups 15–44 years among 135 diseases or health conditions. Schizophrenia ranked eighth, accounting for 2.8% of the total, and in terms of years lost to disability it was third, accounting for 4.9% of the total. With the caveat that countries' annual statistical reports, which provide the basic data for the DALY model, may under-report psychiatric disorders, the findings on schizophrenia are likely to reflect broadly the burden of morbidity and disability that the disorder inflicts on individuals, families and communities the world over, including, as a minimum, 33 million people in developing countries [3]. However, such estimates are in need of a qualification since the concept of schizophrenia as a monolithic disease entity has been open to questions from the time of its inception and into the present [4].

Improving Mental Health Care: The Global Challenge, First Edition.
Edited by Graham Thornicroft, Mirella Ruggeri and David Goldberg.
© 2013 John Wiley & Sons, Ltd. Published 2013 by John Wiley & Sons, Ltd.

Origins and metamorphoses of the concept of schizophrenia

By the mid-nineteenth century, European psychiatrists began singling out from the bulk of 'insanity' a particular disorder of unknown causes which tended to affect young people and often progressed to chronic deterioration [5]. In France, Morel [6] labelled such cases as *démence précoce*, and in Scotland, Clouston [7] coined the term 'adolescent insanity'. Kahlbaum [8], in Germany, delineated the catatonic syndrome, and Hecker [9] described hebephrenia. By 1896, Kraepelin [10] integrated those varied clinical pictures into a single nosological entity of *dementia praecox*, claiming that 'we meet everywhere the same fundamental disorders...in very varied conjunctions, even though the clinical picture may appear at first sight ever so divergent'. In 1911, Bleuler renamed the disorder as *schizophrenia* but at the same time stated that 'it is not a disease in the strict sense, but appears to be a group of diseases' [11]. During the decades that followed, a bewildering number of clinical subentities and variants have been proposed, including schizoaffective disorder [12], schizophreniform psychoses [13], process–non-process [14] and systematic–unsystematic schizophrenia [15]. Though often based on discerning clinical observation, such refinements did not mend the inherent weaknesses of the disease concept of schizophrenia, namely, that most of its diagnostic descriptors were symptom-based, relying on the clinician's interpretation of patients' reported subjective experiences, and that the whole concept was predicated on the assumption of an underlying but still unknown disease process for which objective biological markers are still unavailable.

Uses and abuses of the concept of schizophrenia

By the mid-twentieth century, nearly one-third of all hospital beds in the industrialised countries were psychiatric beds, and the majority of hospitalised patients had been diagnosed with schizophrenia. The under-stimulating routine of the mental hospital tended to produce a secondary handicap of institutionalism or 'institutional neurosis' which was superimposed on the residual symptoms of the primary psychiatric illness [16]. To quote Laing [17], 'the standard psychiatric patient is a function of the standard psychiatrist, and of the standard mental hospital'. The 'active' treatments, as a rule used without patients' informed consent, ranged from metrazol shock and insulin coma therapy to electroconvulsive therapy and psychosurgery (during the 1940s and 1950s, the latter procedure has been administered to over 40 000 patients in the United States and to 10 365 patients in the United Kingdom [18]). But the darkest episode in the history of twentieth-century psychiatry was the extermination of some 180 000 psychiatric patients in Nazi Germany, including many suffering from chronic schizophrenia and regarded as 'incurable' [19]. In the 1960s, the stigmatising 'cuckoo's nest' subculture of the psychiatric hospital gave rise to critical investigations, such as Goffman's classic 'Asylums' [20], and to the counterculture movement of anti-psychiatry whose protagonists were psychiatrists and psychologists aiming to expose schizophrenia as a social construct in the service of deviance control [21]. The radical anti-psychiatrist Szasz [22] referred to schizophrenia as 'the sacred symbol of psychiatry' or *panchreston* (in ancient Greek, something that explains all, and therefore nothing).

Schizophrenia today: Advances in neuroscience and genetics

It is now widely accepted that schizophrenia is an extremely complex disorder with a major genetic contribution to its aetiology, involving multiple genes of small effect, individual assortments of rare mutations (copy number variation, CNV) and molecular pathways that are likely to be highly heterogeneous both within and across populations [23]. Environmental factors, ranging from neurodevelopmental insults to psychosocial adversity, interact with the genetic susceptibility to produce widespread phenotypic variation, including transmission of risk genotypes that may remain unexpressed as clinical disorder [24, 25]. The rapid advances of research technologies in service of molecular genetics, genomics and neuroscience provide at present unprecedented opportunities for an integrated approach in the search for the genetic underpinnings, neurodevelopmental trajectories and brain pathophysiological mechanisms of the disorder. Yet, the prevailing paradigm in any domain of schizophrenia research – genetics, neurophysiology or neuroimaging – is still based on the implicit assumption that schizophrenia is a single, uniform disorder, and that its diagnosis, based on DSM-IV or ICD-10 criteria, identifies a meaningful biological entity. Genetic heterogeneity, which is common in the complex diseases including schizophrenia, is likely to be a critical part of the explanation for the many non-replications of initially promising, significant findings of the genome-wide association studies (GWAS) conducted in recent years [26]. What makes schizophrenia refractory to the current methods for resolving heterogeneity is the confounding effect of the phenotype, defined solely by a set of clinically conspicuous symptoms and behaviours which may mask an unknown number of underlying brain disorders characterised by differing pathogenetic mechanisms and developmental trajectories. It is now accepted that no single symptom is absolutely necessary for diagnosing schizophrenia, and that any subset of symptoms from an agreed checklist, such as the DSM-IV criteria, can be sufficient for the diagnosis. In practice, this 'polythetic' method of diagnosing the disorder implies that patients can be allocated to the diagnostic category without having a single symptom in common.

A possible way of resolving this diagnostic conundrum is the use of *endopheno-types* (also termed intermediate phenotypes) as an alternative, or a complement, to clinical diagnosis [27]. Endophenotypes are heritable, objectively measurable biological traits which co-segregate with clinical illness in pedigrees and may also be expressed in unaffected members. They are stable, persist across clinical states and are likely to be more proximal to the primary biological defect and its genetic signal than the clinical phenotype. Proposed and actually used endophe-notypes include neuropsychological tests of cognitive functioning, electrophysi-ological measures (event-related brain potentials) and neuroimaging variables [28]. Measures of cognitive deficit, which may range from pervasive to focal or patchy, have been shown to be particularly sensitive to dysfunction that sets schizophrenia patients apart from healthy controls. The cognitive indicators with high to moderate effect sizes include memory and attention deficits, exec-utive dysfunction and sensory gating [29]. Their use in genetic analyses to date has been promising by tentatively identifying specific subtypes of schizophrenia with different underlying genetic underpinnings [30, 31]. A plausible conclusion is that clinical schizophrenia is not a unitary disease but a broad syndrome arising as a 'common final pathway' out of a spectrum of aetiologically and pathogenetically different subtypes that may eventually explain the remarkable variation in its cross-sectional presentation and prognosis.

Variations in the prevalence and incidence of schizophrenia

Prevalence

The prevalence of a disease is the estimated number of cases per 1000 persons at risk present in a population at a given time (point prevalence), or over the lifespan (lifetime prevalence or *proportion of survivors affected*, PSA). Since schizo-phrenia cases in remission are likely to be missed in point prevalence surveys, it will be useful to estimate the lifetime prevalence by supplementing the cross section of the present mental state with data about past episodes of the disorder. The majority of past studies have produced point prevalence estimates in the range of 2.4–6.7 per 1000 population at risk in developed countries, and in the range of 1.4–6.8 per 1000 population at risk in developing countries [32]. However, these figures are not standardised and should be compared with caution due to demographic differences between populations in terms of age-specific mortality and migration.

A systematic review of 188 studies in 46 countries, published between 1965 and 2002 [33], estimated the median value for point prevalence at 4.6 per 1000 persons and for lifetime prevalence at 7.2 per 1000. In a recent nationwide survey of psychotic disorders in Australia [34], 7955 current users of mental health services were screened as positive for psychotic symptoms during a census month, and 1825 of them, sampled randomly, were interviewed in 2010 using a standardised schedule linked to the OPCRIT computerised diagnostic algorithm [35]. The estimated one-month treated prevalence was 3.5 per 1000 – almost exactly the same as an earlier survey of a closely similar design in 1998 [36].

Incidence

The incidence rate is the estimated annual number of first-onset cases in a defined population per 1000 persons at risk. Incidence is of greater interest for risk-factor epidemiology than prevalence since it is temporally closer to the antecedents of the disease or its precipitating factors. Summing up the age- and sex-specific rates across the period of risk (usually age 15–54) provides an estimate of the *lifetime morbid risk* (LMR). Its estimation depends critically on the capacity to determine reliably the point of onset of the disorder – a requirement that is difficult to satisfy in schizophrenia, due to its long prodromal period and the fuzzy boundary between premorbid state and onset of psychosis. Since objective biomarkers of the disease process are still lacking, onset is often defined as the point in time when clinical manifestations become recognisable and can be diagnosed according to specified criteria. The first hospital admission, used as a proxy for disease onset in many studies, is not a robust indicator because of the variable time lag to admission in diverse psychiatric treatment facilities. A better approximation is provided by the time point of the person's first contact with any psychiatric, general medical or alternative 'helping' agency, for reasons likely related to emerging psychosis.

Clearly, both first-admission and first-contact studies share the limitation of only assessing 'treated' incidence and may omit cases that do not present for treatment. This limitation can be overcome by periodically repeated door-to-door surveys or by longitudinal cohort studies, though both are difficult to mount for reasons of cost and logistics. The widely cited WHO Ten-Country Study [37, 38] compared the incidence of both 'broadly' defined (ICD-9) and 'narrowly' defined schizophrenia (CATEGO S + computer algorithm; [39]) across 12 settings in ten developed and developing countries using standardised methods and instruments. Whether schizophrenia was defined broadly or narrowly, there was an approximately two- to threefold difference between the sites with the lowest (0.16 per 1000 in Aarhus, Denmark) and the highest (0.42 per 1000 in Chandigarh, India) incidence rates.

A systematic review of the literature on the incidence of schizophrenia [40] identified 158 studies in 32 countries and found a median incidence rate of 0.15 per 1000, with a range of variation from 0.43 to 0.70 per 1000. This range of variation is by far more restricted than the variation observed in the incidence of other complex diseases, such as diabetes Type 1, where the difference between the highest rates in Sardinia and Finland and the lowest rate in China was more than 350-fold in 1990 [41]. Whether the apparent similarity of the incidence rates of schizophrenia across populations is attributable to a widely shared genetic liability, to ubiquitous constellations of environmental factors interacting with genetic risk or to multiple rare genetic variants leading to similar phenotypic expression is an unresolved issue to be addressed in future research.

Small area variations

Since schizophrenia is a low-incidence disorder, geographical variations in its prevalence are prominent when rates are obtained from relatively small areas and communities. In a study of an ethnically and socioeconomically homogeneous rural region in Ireland [42], the overall point prevalence of schizophrenia at 3.9 per 1000 was well within the modal range, but analysis by small district electoral divisions revealed significant variation, ranging from 0.0 to 29.4 per 1000.

Local variation can be attributed to several factors, for example, spatial clustering of cases due to shared genetic vulnerability within extended pedigrees, differential mobility and mortality and, possibly, to differential exposure to risk factors influencing intrauterine growth and early neurodevelopment. Such and other effects, still to be discovered, may give rise to 'outlier' pockets of high or low incidence and prevalence which tend to cancel each other in larger population agglomerations. Their systematic study, though involving considerable methodological difficulties, can be quite informative regarding the search for specific risk factors.

Genetic isolates

Isolated populations are another source of incidence and prevalence variation. Isolates are defined by a common descent from a small number of founder ancestors, a degree of inbreeding and a restricted admixture of immigrants, due to geographical or cultural seclusion over many generations. Such populations vary considerably in size but are likely to be less heterogeneous with regard to their genetic make-up and environmental exposures than the outbred populations in the world at large. A number of isolated populations in different parts of the world, for example, Finland, Iceland and northern Sweden; the Pima Indians; the Bedouins; the people of the Central Valley of Costa Rica, the Caucasus, several areas in Quebec, as well as religious communities, such as the Old Order Amish, the Hutterites and the Mennonites, have been studied by epidemiologists and geneticists with a view to finding very large pedigrees, informative for diseases ranging from asthma and diabetes to schizophrenia and bipolar disorder.

High rates of psychoses (two to three times the national or regional rate) have been reported for population isolates in northern Sweden and several areas in Finland. Though the whole population of Finland shares some features of an old isolate, one particular subregion with a current population of 18 000 has been founded by 40 families at the end of the seventeenth century, that is, only 12 generations back. Genetic-epidemiological studies in this isolate estimate a lifetime prevalence of 15 per 1000 for schizophrenia spectrum psychotic disorders and LMR of schizophrenia at 2.2%, compared to 1.2% for the whole of Finland [43].

Possibly the highest ever lifetime prevalence estimate for schizophrenia (4.9%) has been reported from one highland subisolate (3000 members) in Daghestan, Northern Caucasus (Russian Federation) [44]. The population of the Palau islands (Micronesia), currently 20 470 people, has been geographically and ethnically isolated from other Pacific populations for nearly 2000 years. A genetic epidemiological study of treated cases determined the lifetime prevalence of schizophrenia at 2.8% in males and at 2.0% in females. All of the 160 Palau cases were concentrated in 59 families, each traceable to a single common founder, with 11 of them having 5–11 affected members each [45]. At the other extreme, the lowest known lifetime prevalence of schizophrenia of 1.1 per 1000 has been found among the Hutterites in South Dakota, a Protestant sect of European descent (founded in the sixteenth century) whose members live in closely knit, endogamous rural communities [46].

Migrant populations

The exceptionally high incidence rate of schizophrenia (about 6.0 per 1000) that has been found in the African-Caribbean population in the United Kingdom is a special case in schizophrenia epidemiology [47]. The excess morbidity is not restricted to recent immigrants and is actually higher in the second generation of migrants [48]. Similar findings of two- to fourfold excess of psychoses among migrants over the general population rate have been reported in Denmark [49] and in the Netherlands [50]. The causes of the phenomenon remain obscure. Incidence studies in countries of origin do not indicate any excess schizophrenia morbidity in the indigenous populations from which migrants are recruited [51], nor is there evidence for selective migration by people at increased risk for psychosis [52]. Explanations in terms of biological risk factors have found little support. A finding in need of replication is the significantly higher incidence of schizophrenia among the siblings of second-generation African-Caribbean schizophrenia patients compared with the incidence of the disorder in the siblings of white patients [53]. Hypothetically, such 'horizontal' increase in the morbid risk could result from an environmental factor, for example, demoralisation stress due to blocked opportunities for upward social mobility, driving the penetrance of predisposing genes within a pedigree beyond the threshold of gene expression. Psychosocial hypotheses involving acculturation stress, minority status and racial discrimination are being explored [54] but not yet definitively tested.

Variations in the course and outcome of schizophrenia

Untreated schizophrenia

Since the majority of schizophrenia patients are today receiving pharmacological treatment, one could assume that under current drug treatments, the longitudinal pattern of the disorder no longer reflects the 'natural history' of untreated schizophrenia. Several studies, in an area in Scotland [55] and in remote rural areas in India [56] and China [57], have assessed people with schizophrenia who had never been hospitalised. About half of the Scottish patients had been prescribed neuroleptics by their general practitioners, while the Indian and Chinese patients were virtually untreated. In all three settings, the long-term outcomes were heterogeneous, but they did not differ substantially from the outcomes in the treated groups. In a historical study of 70 Swedish patients with first admissions in 1925, lifetime records were retrieved and rediagnosed in accordance with DSM-III [58]. None of these patients had received neuroleptics. The final outcome was rated as 'good' in 33%, as 'profoundly deteriorated' in 43% and as 'intermediate' in 24%. In a rare recent study [59], a small sample of 64 patients with schizophrenia who had opted out of antipsychotic medication were followed up prospectively over 15 years, with the results pointing to prolonged periods of recovery and sustained global functioning, possibly associated with better premorbid characteristics within this group.

Secular trends

A meta-analysis of 320 studies on the course and outcome of schizophrenia (or *dementia praecox*), published from 1895 to 1992 and containing data on 51 800 subjects, provides a long-term perspective on the prognosis of the disorder over several generations [60]. Overall, about 40% of the patients have been described as 'improved' after an average length of follow-up of 5.6 years. A significant increase in the proportion of those 'improved' was observed during 1956–1985 as compared to 1895–1955. While the higher rate of improvement in the 1950s and thereafter was attributable to the introduction of neuroleptic treatment, a trend towards better outcomes with every successive decade had been present for much longer, suggesting that the transition to a less deteriorating course was associated with general improvements in patient care, progressive changes in hospital regime which occurred in a number of institutions since the 1930s and the expectation that psychosocial measures such as psychotherapy or rehabilitation could result in a remission of the disorder [61].

Concurrently with these trends in Europe and North America, studies based on relatively small clinical samples reported observations of high rates of recovery from schizophrenic psychoses in traditional societies such as Mauritius [62] and Sri Lanka [63]. Good outcome cases included patients who would be expected to have poor outcome, if 'Western' prognostic criteria had been applied [64]. As these studies were retrospective and based on hospital admissions only, selection or diagnostic bias could not be excluded. Furthermore, clinical improvement could have been confounded with the social adjustment many patients achieve in a comparatively undemanding environment. These caveats raised questions concerning the validity of the early observations of a better prognosis of schizophrenia in non-Western settings and pointed to the need for more systematic comparative studies.

The WHO studies on course and outcome of schizophrenia

The International Pilot Study of Schizophrenia (IPSS), 1965–1976 [65], employed a structured clinical interview and a computerised diagnostic algorithm in field studies which were conducted at nine research centres in developing and developed countries. A total of 1202 schizophrenia patients were assessed initially and followed up with reassessments at two and five years. The main finding was that higher proportions of patients in India, Nigeria and Colombia had better outcomes on most dimensions than their counterparts in the developed countries. Complete remissions of the initial psychotic episode had occurred within five years in as many as 42% of patients in India and 33% of patients in Nigeria, whereas the majority of patients in the developed countries had experienced persisting psychotic symptoms and disablement during the same period. However, since IPSS patients were recruited from hospitals, where admission policies could have led to over-inclusion of chronic cases in the developed countries, and of acute, recent-onset cases in the developing countries, selection bias could not be ruled out.

Such confounding factors were largely eliminated in the subsequent WHO Ten-Country Study [38], in which incidence cohorts of predominantly first-episode cases (a total of 1379 individuals) were uniformly assessed upon their first contact with community or hospital services in defined geographical areas. Diagnostic misclassification due to potential admixture of brief transient psychotic illnesses, or of psychoses due to acute physical illness, was ruled out, as such cases were excluded upon screening. The follow-up of these cohorts provided ample replication of the finding that the outcome of schizophrenia was generally better in developing than in developed countries. The better course and outcome in the developing country areas could not be attributed to any particular clinical subtype of the disorder. Analysis of the data revealed that the less disabling outcome in developing countries was mainly attributable to a significantly greater percentage of patients remaining in a prolonged clinical remission after a psychotic episode, rather than to milder or shorter psychotic episodes. This pattern was statistically predicted by the setting (developing vs developed country), type of onset, marital status and access to a supportive network of family or friends. The length of remission was unrelated to antipsychotic treatment, which generally was administered for shorter periods of time to patients in the developing countries.

A more recent long-term follow-up investigation, the International Study of Schizophrenia (ISoS), involving 18 research centres in 14 countries [66], traced about 75% of the cases that had been assessed in the earlier WHO studies, and included additional cohorts from China and India. Follow-up information was collected on a total of 1633 cases, and 890 patients were reinterviewed at either 15- or 25-year follow-up since their first assessment.

Several general conclusions were drawn from the WHO studies. The cumulative annual proportion of time during which patients experience psychotic episodes tends to remain stable or even decrease over time. At the end of the five-year follow-up, 57% of the patients had experienced a total of less than nine months of active psychosis; only 22% had been psychotic for 45–60 months. At 15- and 25-year follow-up, 43% and 41%, respectively, had been free of active psychotic symptoms for the last two years. Overall, most of the observed change in the clinical state and social functioning of patients between the two-year follow-up and the five-year follow-up had been towards improvement rather than deterioration. This was congruent with the findings at 15- and 25-year follow-up.

To sum up, the most striking finding from long-term follow-up studies is the high proportion of patients who eventually recover, completely or with mild residual abnormalities, after many years of severe illness. The proportion of good recovery tends to be higher in developing country settings. This is in contrast to the ingrained image of schizophrenia as an intractable, deteriorating illness that many clinicians tend to adopt, based on a limited follow-up horizon and selective case observations. It is unlikely that the high recovery rate in the long-term studies could be explained by diagnostic error, for example, affective illness or brief transient psychoses being misdiagnosed as schizophrenia. Similarly unlikely is the attribution of all the good outcomes to antipsychotic treatment, since comparable proportions of improvement or recovery have been reported for patients who never received neuroleptics. A tentative conclusion is that schizophrenia is not an invariably chronic deteriorating disorder. It should be noted, however, that some studies suggest a recent trend of worsening clinical and social outcomes in patients with schizophrenia, especially in developing countries [67]. People with schizophrenia are profoundly sensitive to their immediate social environment. Increasing social and economic stresses experienced by both rural and urban communities in many developing countries in the last two decades may be eroding the traditional support systems, thus resulting in worse outcomes.

The burden of comorbidity and mortality

Physical disease

Medical comorbidity in schizophrenia comprises mainly common diseases that affect schizophrenia patients more frequently than attributable to chance, as well as certain rare conditions or abnormalities which tend to co-occur with the disorder. Physical disease in schizophrenia patients tends to be seriously undetected and under-diagnosed [68]. Among the chronic non-communicable diseases, patients with schizophrenia have significantly higher than expected rates of ischaemic heart disease, cerebrovascular disease, diabetes and epilepsy [69]. In the recent Australian national survey of psychotic disorders [34], 53.5% of the participants in age groups 18–64 met the International Diabetes Federation criteria for metabolic syndrome, including at-risk levels for abdominal obesity (82.1%), high-density lipoproteins (49.7%), triglycerides (48.0%) and hypertension (48.8%). About one-quarter (24.0%) were at high risk for a cardiovascular event in the next five years based on the Framingham risk equation [34]. Obesity and the concomitant metabolic syndrome involving insulin resistance are becoming increasingly common problems in schizophrenia patients, likely to be attributed to a synergy of factors, including the metabolic side effects of some of the second-generation antipsychotic agents, poor diet, smoking and physical inactivity. Persons with schizophrenia, and especially those who are homeless or injection drug users, are at increased risk for potentially life-threatening communicable diseases, such as HIV/AIDS, hepatitis C and tuberculosis [70].

Substance abuse

Substance abuse is the most common associated health problem among patients with schizophrenia and may involve any drug of abuse or a poly-drug combination. The addictive use of cannabis, stimulants and nicotine is disproportionately high among schizophrenia patients and may be related to the underlying neurobiology of the disorder. In the Australian national survey of psychotic disorders [34], a diagnosis of harmful use or dependence on psychoactive substances was made in 63.2% of males and 41.7% of females with schizophrenia (compared to 12.0% and 5.8% in the general population). In addition to poorer prognosis of schizophrenia in patients with heavy cannabis use, a systematic review of published data on cannabis exposure and the onset of schizophrenia concluded that early use increased the risk of psychosis in a dose-related manner, especially in persons at high genetic risk of schizophrenia [71]. Heavy cannabis use can precipitate psychotic relapse in patients with schizophrenia who had previously achieved remission. Similarly, stimulants such as methamphetamine and cocaine tend to exacerbate acute psychotic symptoms in over 50% of schizophrenia patients. The prevalence of cigarette smoking among schizophrenia patients (71.1% in males and 58.8% in females according to the Australian survey) is, on the average, two to three times higher than in the general population.

Mortality

Schizophrenia is associated with excess mortality, well documented by epidemiological studies on large cohorts over extended periods. Population-based data from Norway, 1926–1941 and 1950–1974, indicate that, while the total mortality of psychiatric patients had been decreasing, the relative mortality of patients with schizophrenia remained unchanged at a level higher than twice that of the general population [72]. Similar findings have been reported from other European countries and North America, with *standardised mortality ratios* (SMR) of 2.6 or higher for patients with schizophrenia, which corresponds to about 20% reduction in life expectancy [73, 74]. A meta-analysis of 18 studies [75] estimated a crude mortality rate of 189 deaths per 10 000 population per year and a ten-year survival rate of 81%. Mortality was significantly higher in males than in females, and the difference was primarily due to a male excess in suicides and accidents.

Direct comparisons of mortality associated with schizophrenia in different populations and cultures are restricted by incomplete coverage and varying reporting practices. Yet cross-cultural follow-up studies of cohorts of cases assessed with similar methods, such as in the WHO ISoS [66], support the conclusion that excess mortality among schizophrenia patients is not limited to a particular type of setting. Whereas in the past the excess mortality among individuals with schizophrenia was due mainly to communicable diseases such as tuberculosis, the leading causes of premature death among patients with schizophrenia at present are cardiovascular and cerebrovascular disease, suicide and accidents. Suicide accounts for 28% of the excess mortality in schizophrenia patients, with aggregated SMR of 9.6 for males and 6.8 for females [76]. In China, the *relative risk* (RR) of suicide in individuals with schizophrenia, compared to those without the disorder, has been estimated at 23.8 [77]. Suicide in schizophrenia may occur at any stage of disorder, but the risk is particularly high in the first six months following the first psychotic episode, as well as after prolonged periods of frequent hospital admissions and discharge.

Several risk factors, relatively specific to schizophrenia, have been suggested: being young and male, experiencing multiple relapses and remissions, comorbid substance abuse, awareness of the deteriorating course of the condition and a sense of hopelessness with loss of faith in treatment [78]. Data from successive patient cohorts in Denmark, the United Kingdom and Australia suggest a trend of increasing mortality in the early stages of the disorder. In Denmark, the five-year cumulated SMR increased from 5.30 (males) and 2.27 (females) for the period 1971–1973 to 7.79 (males) and 4.52 (females) for the period 1980–1982 [79]. Particularly striking was the SMR of 16.4 for males in the first year after a diagnosis of schizophrenia. In an Australian study [80], the highest suicide risk was found to occur in the first seven days after discharge from inpatient care. Whether the increased suicide mortality is associated with the shift in the management of schizophrenia from hospital to community care remains to be established [81].

Social and economic costs of schizophrenia

The social and economic costs of schizophrenia are disproportionately high relative to its incidence and prevalence. Estimates by the WHO predict a greater than 50% increase in the disease burden attributable to schizophrenia in developing countries, that is, a burden approaching that of malaria and nutritional deficiency [1].

The social breakdown syndrome

Notwithstanding the variations in course and outcome, schizophrenia is associated with a greater burden of long-term disability than any other mental disorder. The onset is usually at a developmental stage of incomplete social maturation, educational attainment and acquisition of occupational skills. The intrusion of psychosis at this stage results in a severely truncated repertoire of social skills foretelling lifelong socioeconomic disadvantage. Both the positive and negative symptoms of the disease interfere with a person's capacity to cope with the expectations of daily living. Patients with schizophrenia experience particular cognitive difficulty in dealing with complex demands and environments, especially such that involve social interaction and decoding of social communication signals. These handicaps are exacerbated by the societal reaction to individuals manifesting behaviours associated with 'insanity', which generally involves stigma and social exclusion. These adverse factors interact with each other to cause the *social breakdown syndrome*, a term introduced by Gruenberg [82] to designate the cluster of secondary and tertiary impairments in schizophrenia resulting in a loss of social support networks and a greatly diminished quality of life.

Involvement in the criminal justice system

Offences committed by persons with schizophrenia tend to receive wide media coverage and to reinforce popular ideas about dangerousness associated with mental illness. However, carefully designed studies indicate that a relatively small proportion of patients with schizophrenia tend to be over-represented among the perpetrators of violent offences, including homicide. A meta-analysis of 20 published studies reporting on a total of 18 423 individuals with schizophrenia established odds ratios for violent offending in the range between 1 and 7, but most of the excess risk appeared to be mediated by comorbid substance abuse [83]. Thus, the *population-attributable fraction* of such offences committed by persons with schizophrenia is likely to be negligible compared with the total number of offences in the community. In contrast, people with schizophrenia are more likely to be victims of crime rather than perpetrators. A study in the United States [84] found that 46% of a cohort of 609 schizophrenia patients had some encounters with the criminal justice system over a period of a year; 67% of those encounters were related to being a victim of a crime. In the Australian national survey of psychotic disorders [34], the corresponding proportion was 38.6%. Nevertheless, the rates of arrest and incarceration tend to be high among patients with schizophrenia, especially because of offences related to public order. This contributes to the commonly perceived association between the disease and criminal behaviour and to the perpetuation of stigma. Issues of protecting patients' rights must therefore be an important part of anti-stigma campaigns in both developing and developed countries.

Direct and indirect economic costs

In developed countries, the direct costs of schizophrenia, incurred by hospital or community-based treatment, supervised accommodation and related services, amount to 1.4–2.8% of the national health-care expenditure and to up to one-fifth of the direct costs of all mental disorders [85]. Although estimates of the indirect costs of schizophrenia vary greatly depending on the method of analysis and the underlying assumptions, these costs are likely to be comparable in scale to the direct costs, considering lost productivity and employment, the economically devastating long-term impact of the illness on the patient's family, other caregivers' opportunity costs, the increased mortality of people with schizophrenia, the costs to the criminal justice system and other issues related to public concerns about safety. Estimates based on the Epidemiological Catchment Areas study in the United States [86] put the direct costs of schizophrenia at $17.3 billion and the indirect costs at $15.2 billion per annum. An important aspect of the economics of schizophrenia is the so-called funding imbalance effect: it is estimated that 97% of the total lifetime costs of schizophrenia are incurred by fewer than 50% of the patients diagnosed with the disorder. While this finding points to a hard-core subset of cases with severe chronic illness, multiple disabilities and excessive dependence on services and other support, it also suggests that in more than 50% of those with schizophrenia, the disorder is less disabling or treatment more effective.

Most of the available economic evidence on schizophrenia comes from studies conducted in Western societies. However, individual studies provide some insight into the likely economic impact of the disease in low-income settings in developing countries. Since both the direct and indirect costs of schizophrenia are context-bound, extrapolations even across countries at comparable levels of *gross domestic product* (GDP) per capita should be made with caution, given the diversity of cultures, social structures and health-care systems. Thus, although the generic cost-driving factors associated with schizophrenia are likely to be similar around the world, their relative weights and the structure of the direct and indirect costs of the illness are likely to vary considerably. Hospital or other residential care, which accounts for more than 75% of the direct costs of schizophrenia in high-income countries and up to 50% of the direct costs in some middle-income countries [87], may account for a much smaller fraction in low-income developing countries. A study in Nigeria [88] revealed that caregiver *opportunity costs* (e.g. family members' lost productivity or income) were comparable to those in the developed world. Yet, the aggregate family costs in developing countries may be substantially higher since a larger proportion of schizophrenia patients live with their families, as compared with patients in Western societies, and the family is likely to be the first line of treatment and management of psychotic episodes, including the purchase of prescribed antipsychotic medication which is usually borne by the family. Additional direct costs may be incurred by the necessity to travel, often long distances, to the nearest hospital or clinic, as well as by payment for the services of traditional healers [89]. In many traditional communities, the stigma associated with mental illness may affect the family as a whole and restrict, for instance, marital opportunities for younger family members. While lost educational opportunities are likely to be a problem, lost paid employment is more difficult to quantify, and therefore less likely to appear prominently in estimates of the indirect illness burden in developing countries. On the other hand, reintegration of a family member who has suffered a psychotic episode into the domestic economy may be easier to achieve than formal employment, and this may be one factor in the better and longer remissions of patients with schizophrenia observed in developing countries [90].

Conclusions and future directions

Closing the 'knowledge gap'

More than a century since the delineation of *dementia praecox* by Kraepelin, the aetiology, neuropathology and pathophysiology of schizophrenia remain elusive [28]. The availability of explicit guidelines and criteria allows today reliable diagnostic identification, but, essentially, ICD-10 and DSM-IV schizophrenia is a label for a broad clinical syndrome defined by variable sets of subjective symptoms, behavioural signs and patterns of course. Research has to date generated evidence for a large number of tentative biological indicators, such as neurocognitive dysfunction, structural and functional brain anomalies, neurochemical abnormalities and developmental markers, but none of them has been shown to have the sensitivity and specificity required for a diagnostic test. The results of recent GWAS of increasingly larger samples of cases and controls suggest that the total number of genetic variants underlying the risk of schizophrenia is of the order of thousands [23, 26, 91]. Genetic heterogeneity of the disorder is now a widely accepted proposition, pointing to the likely existence of many pathogenetic molecular pathways leading to the endpoint of clinical phenotype.

Important insights into the environmental risk factors contributing to schizophrenia have been gained from population-based studies. The syndrome of schizophrenia appears to be robust and identifiable reliably in diverse populations and cultures. At the level or large population aggregates, no major differences in incidence and morbid risk have to date been detected, though small geographical area variation exists, reflecting a mix of locally operating risk factors whose effects are attenuated in large, heterogeneous populations. Similarly, the study of 'atypical' populations, such as genetic isolates or minority groups, may be capable of detecting unusual variations in the incidence of schizophrenia that could provide novel clues to the pathogenesis of the disorder. Yet, at present, no single, or major, environmental risk factor influencing the incidence of schizophrenia has been conclusively demonstrated. Further studies using large samples are required to evaluate risk factors, antecedents and predictors, for which the present evidence is inconclusive.

Epidemiological research is increasingly making use of existing large databases, such as cumulative case registers or birth cohorts to test hypotheses about risk factors in case-control designs. Methods of genetic epidemiology are being integrated within population-based studies. These trends predict an important future role for epidemiology in the unravelling of gene–environment interactions that are likely to be the key to the understanding of the aetiology of schizophrenia. In this context, research into psychotic disorders in non-Western populations can provide valuable information on genetic heterogeneity, the impact of the environment and the course and outcome of schizophrenia.

Closing the 'treatment gap'

The vast majority of people whose lives are profoundly affected by schizophrenia reside in developing countries. The incidence and prevalence of schizophrenia in low-income countries are not very different from what is being found in the high- and middle-income countries, or may even be higher. Yet, it has been estimated that over 67% of all persons with schizophrenia in developing countries were not receiving any treatment [3]. Although a greater proportion of people with schizophrenia in developing countries experience longer periods of symptomatic recovery as compared with patients in the West, the burden of illness is severe and affects the productivity and quality of life of many families. The predicament of patients and families is likely to worsen as many of these countries are experiencing the pressures of economic restructuring, increasing income inequality, unemployment and cuts in public spending on health care. The traditional economic and psychosocial resources of the family, which in the past have been capable of absorbing much of the impact of severe mental illness, may quickly become eroded.

A common denominator in the great variety of situations and systems of care for people afflicted with psychotic illnesses in the developing world is that the modest successes achieved in some of these countries are vulnerable to the local repercussions of economic globalisation. In all societies, the stigma surrounding mental illness is likely to mean that people with severe mental disorders are among the first to be disadvantaged by shrinking government health expenditures. It is, therefore, imperative to initiate proactive measures on an international scale to forestall such developments. It is important that governments, development agencies and other sponsoring organisations should be made aware of the fact that schizophrenia is, in principle, a treatable condition, and that significant returns in terms of symptom control, containment of disablement, safeguarding the physical health – all leading to improvements in quality of life and reintegration into the community – can be achieved if increased funding and technical support is provided for local and regional programmes [92].

References

[1] Murray CJL, Lopez AD. (1996) *The Global Burden of Disease*. Boston: Harvard University Press.

[2] Mathers CD, Loncar D. (2006) Projections of global mortality and burden of disease from 2002 to 2030. *PLoS Medicine* **3**: 2011–2030.

[3] Institute of Medicine. (2001) *Neurological, Psychiatric and Developmental Disorders. Meeting the Challenge in the Developing World*. Washington, DC: National Academy Press, pp. 217–256.

[4] Jablensky A. (1999) The conflict of the nosologists: views on schizophrenia and manic-depressive illness in the early part of the 20th century. *Schizophrenia Research* **39**: 95–100.

[5] Jablensky A. (2010) The diagnostic concept of schizophrenia: its history, evolution, and future prospects. *Dialogues in Clinical Neuroscience* **12**: 271–287.

[6] Morel BA. (1860) *Traité des maladies mentales*. Paris: Masson.

[7] Clouston TS. (1904) *Clinical Lectures on Mental Disease*, 6th edn. London: Churchill.

[8] Kahlbaum KL. (1863) *Die Gruppierung der psychischen Krankheiten und die Einteilung der Seelenstörungen*. Danzig: Kafemann.

[9] Hecker E. (1871) Die Hebephrenie: ein Beitrag zur klinischen Psychiatrie. *Archiv für pathologische Anatomie und für klinische Medizin* **52**: 394–429.

[10] Kraepelin E. (1896) *Psychiatrie. Ein Lehrbuch für Studirende und Aerzte, fünfte Auflage*. Leipzig: Barth.

[11] Bleuler E. (1920) *Lehrbuch der Psychiatrie*. Berlin: Springer.

[12] Kasanin J. (1933) The acute schizoaffective psychosis. *American Journal of Psychiatry* **90**: 97–126.

[13] Langfeld G. (1939) *The Schizophrenic States: A Catamnestic Study Based on Individual Re-examinations*. Copenhagen: Munksgaard.

[14] Stephens JH, Astrup C. (1963) Prognosis in "process" and "non-process" schizophrenia. *American Journal of Psychiatry* **119**: 945–953.

[15] Leonhard K. (1999) *Classification of Endogenous Psychoses and Their Differentiated Etiology*, 2nd edn. Vienna: Springer.

[16] Wing JK, Brown GW. (1970) *Institutionalism and Schizophrenia*. London: Cambridge University Press.

[17] Laing RD. (1960) *The Divided Self: An Existential Study in Sanity and Madness*. Harmondsworth: Penguin.

[18] Rosenfeld JV, Lloyd JH. (1999) Contemporary psychosurgery. *Journal of Clinical Neuroscience* **6**: 106–112.

[19] Von Cranach M. (1990) *Die Psychiatrie in der Zeit des Nationalsozialismus*. Irrsee: Schwabenakademie.

[20] Goffman E. (1961) *Asylums. Essays on the Social Situation of Mental Patients and Other Inmates*. Harmondsworth: Penguin.

[21] Scheff TJ. (1966) *Being Mentally Ill: A Sociological Theory*. New Brunswick: Rutgers.

[22] Szasz TS. (1961) *The Myth of Mental Illness: Foundations of a Theory of Personal Conflict*. New York: Harper & Row.

[23] Sullivan PF, Daly MJ, O'Donovan M. (2012) Genetic architecture of psychiatric disorders: the emerging picture and its implications. *Nature Reviews Genetics* **13**: 537–551.

[24] Demjaha A, MacCabe JH, Murray RM. (2012) How genes and environmental factors determine the different neurodevelopmental trajectories of schizophrenia and bipolar disorder. *Schizophrenia Bulletin* **38**: 209–214.

[25] Gottesman II, Bertelsen A. (1989) Confirming unexpressed genotypes for schizophrenia: risks in the offspring of Fischer's Danish identical and fraternal discordant twins. *Archives of General Psychiatry* **46**: 867–872.

[26] Mowry BJ, Gratten J. (2013) The emerging spectrum of allelic variation in schizophrenia: current evidence and strategies for the identification and functional characterization of common and rare variants. *Molecular Psychiatry* **18**: 38–52.

[27] Gottesman II, Gould TD. (2003) The endophenotype concept in psychiatry: etymology and strategic intentions. *American Journal of Psychiatry* **160**: 636–645.

[28] Jablensky A. (2006) Subtyping schizophrenia: implications for genetic research. *Molecular Psychiatry* **11**: 815–836.

[29] Nuechterlein KH, Subotnik KL, Ventura J et al. (2012) The puzzle of schizophrenia: tracking the core role of cognitive deficits. *Development and Psychopathology* **24**: 529–536.

[30] Hallmayer JF, Kalaydjieva L, Badcock J et al. (2005) Genetic evidence for a distinct sub-type of schizophrenia characterized by pervasive cognitive deficit. *American Journal of Human Genetics* **77**: 468–476.

[31] Jablensky A, Angelicheva D, Donohoe GJ et al. (2012) Promoter polymorphisms in two overlapping *6p25* genes implicate mitochondrial proteins in cognitive deficit in schizo-phrenia. *Molecular Psychiatry* **17**: 1328–1339.

[32] Jablensky A, Kirkbride JB, Jones PB. (2011) Schizophrenia: the epidemiological horizon. In: Weinberger DR, Harrison PJ (eds.), *Schizophrenia*, 3rd edn. Chichester: Wiley-Blackwell, pp. 185–225.

[33] Saha S, Chant D, Welham J et al. (2005) A systematic review of the prevalence of schizo-phrenia. *PLoS Medicine* **2**: 413–433.

[34] Morgan VA, Waterreus A, Jablensky A et al. (2012) People living with psychotic illness in 2010: the second Australian national survey of psychosis. *Australian and New Zealand Journal of Psychiatry* **46**: 735–752.

[35] Castle DJ, Jablensky A, McGrath JJ et al. (2005) The diagnostic interview for psychoses (DIP): development, reliability and applications. *Psychological Medicine* **36**: 69–80.

[36] Jablensky A, McGrath J, Herrman H et al. (2000) Psychotic disorders in urban areas: an overview of the study on low prevalence disorders. *Australian and New Zealand Journal of Psychiatry* **34**: 221–236.

[37] Sartorius N, Jablensky A, Korten A et al. (1986) Early manifestations and first-contact incidence of schizophrenia in different cultures. *Psychological Medicine* **16**: 909–928.

[38] Jablensky A, Sartorius N, Ernberg G et al. (1992) Schizophrenia: manifestations, incidence and course in different cultures. A World Health Organization Ten-Country Study. *Psychological Medicine, Monograph Supplement* **20**: 1–97.

[39] Wing JK, Cooper JE, Sartorius N. (1974) *Measurement and Classification of Psychiatric Symptoms. An Instruction Manual for the PSE and Catego Program.* London: Cambridge University Press.

[40] McGrath J, Saha S, Welham J et al. (2004) A systematic review of the incidence of schizo-phrenia: the distribution of rates and the influence of sex, urbanicity, migrant status and methodology. *BMC Medicine* **2**: 1–22.

[41] Karvonen M, Viik-Kajander M, Moltchanova E et al. (2000) Incidence of childhood type 1 diabetes worldwide: Diabetes Mondiale (DiaMond) Project Group. *Diabetes Care* **10**: 1516–1526.

[42] Scully PJ, Quinn JF, Morgan MG et al. (2001) First-episode schizophrenia, bipolar disorder and other psychoses in a rural Irish catchment area: incidence and gender in the Cavan-Monaghan study at 5 years. *British Journal of Psychiatry* **181** (Suppl. 43): 3–9.

[43] Hovatta I, Terwilliger JD, Lichtermann D et al. (1997) Schizophrenia in the genetic isolate of Finland. *American Journal of Medical Genetics (Neuropsychiatric Genetics)* **74**: 353–360.

[44] Bulayeva KB, Leal SM, Pavlova TA et al. (2005) Mapping genes of complex psychiatric diseases in Daghestan genetic isolates. *American Journal of Medical Genetics Part B (Neuropsychiatric Genetics)* **132B**: 76–84.

[45] Myles-Worsley M, Coon H, Tiobech J et al. (1999) Genetic epidemiological study of schizophrenia in Palau, Micronesia: prevalence and familiality. *American Journal of Medical Genetics (Neuropsychiatric Genetics)* **88**: 4–10.

[46] Nimgaonkar VL, Fujiwara TM, Dutta M et al. (2000) Low prevalence of psychoses among the Hutterites, an isolated religious community. *American Journal of Psychiatry* **157**: 1065–1070.

[47] Fearon P, Kirkbride JB, Morgan C et al. (2006) Incidence of schizophrenia and other psychoses in ethnic minority groups: results from the MRC AESOP Study. *Psychological Medicine* **36**: 1541–1550.

[48] Bourque F, van der Ven E, Malla A. (2011) A meta-analysis of the risk for psychotic disorders among first- and second-generation immigrants. *Psychological Medicine* **41**: 897–910.

[49] Cantor-Graae E, Pedersen CB. (2007) Risk of schizophrenia in second-generation immigrants: a Danish population-based cohort study. *Psychological Medicine* **37**: 485–494.

[50] Veling W, Selten JP, Veen N et al. (2006) Incidence of schizophrenia among ethnic minorities in the Netherlands: a four-year first-contact study. *Schizophrenia Research* **86**: 189–193.

[51] Bhugra D, Hilwig M, Hossein B et al. (1996) First-contact incidence rates of schizophrenia in Trinidad and one-year follow-up. *British Journal of Psychiatry* **169**: 587–592.

[52] Selten JP, Cantor-Graae E, Slaets J et al. (2002) Ødegaard's selection hypothesis revisited: schizophrenia in Surinamese immigrants to the Netherlands. *American Journal of Psychiatry* **159**: 669–671.

[53] Hutchinson G, Takei N, Fahy TA et al. (1996) Morbid risk of schizophrenia in first-degree relatives of White and African-Caribbean patients with psychosis. *British Journal of Psychiatry* **169**: 776–780.

[54] Veling W, Hoek HW, Wiersma D et al. (2010) Ethnic identity and the risk of schizophrenia in ethnic minorities: a case-control study. *Schizophrenia Bulletin* **36**: 1149–1156.

[55] Geddes JR, Kendell RE. (1995) Schizophrenic subjects with no history of admission to hospital. *Psychological Medicine* **25**: 859–868.

[56] Padmavathi R, Rajkumar S, Srinivasan TH. (1998) Schizophrenic patients who were never treated – a study in an Indian urban community. *Psychological Medicine* **28**: 1113–1117.

[57] Ran M, Xiang M, Huang M et al. (2001) Natural course of schizophrenia: 2-year follow-up study in a rural Chinese community. *British Journal of Psychiatry* **178**: 154–158.

[58] Jonsson SAT, Jonsson H. (1992) Outcome in untreated schizophrenia: a search for symptoms and traits with prognostic meaning in patients admitted to a mental hospital in the preneuroleptic era. *Acta Psychiatrica Scandinavica* **85**: 313–320.

[59] Harrow M, Jobe TH. (2007) Factors involved in outcome and recovery in schizophrenia patients not on antipsychotic medications: a 15-year multifollow-up study. *Journal of Nervous and Mental Disease* **195**: 406–414.

[60] Hegarty JD, Baldessarini RJ, Tohen M et al. (1994) One hundred years of schizophrenia: a meta-analysis of the outcome literature. *American Journal of Psychiatry* **151**: 1409–1416.

[61] Ödegaard O. (1964) Patterns of discharge from Norwegian psychiatric hospitals before and after the introduction of psychotropic drugs. *American Journal of Psychiatry* **120**: 772–778.

[62] Murphy HBM, Raman AC. (1971) The chronicity of schizophrenia in indigenous tropical peoples. *British Journal of Psychiatry* **118**: 489–497.

[63] Waxler NE. (1979) Is the outcome for schizophrenia better in non-industrial societies? The case of Sri Lanka. *Journal of Nervous and Mental Disease* **167**: 144–158.

[64] Raman AC, Murphy HBM. (1972) Failure of traditional prognostic indicators in Afro-Asian psychotics: results of a long-term follow-up survey. *Journal of Nervous and Mental Disease* **154**: 238–247.

[65] World Health Organization. (1979) *Schizophrenia. An International Follow-Up Study*. Chichester: John Wiley & Sons, Ltd.

[66] Hopper K, Harrison G, Janca A et al. (eds.) (2007) *Recovery from Schizophrenia. An International Perspective.* Oxford: Oxford University Press.

[67] Kebede D, Alem A, Shibre T et al. (2003) Onset and clinical course of schizophrenia in Butajira-Ethiopia – a community-based study. *Social Psychiatry and Psychiatric Epidemiology* **38**: 625–631.

[68] Hatta K, Takahashi T, Nakamura H et al. (1999) Laboratory findings in acute schizophrenia. *General Hospital Psychiatry* **21**: 220–227.

[69] Saari KM, Lindeman SM, Viilo KM et al. (2005) A 4-fold risk of metabolic syndrome in patients with schizophrenia: the Northern Finland 1966 birth cohort study. *Journal of Clinical Psychiatry* **66**: 559–563.

[70] Sewell DD. (1996) Schizophrenia and HIV. *Schizophrenia Bulletin* **22**: 465–473.

[71] Galvez-Buccollini JA, Proal AC, Tomaselli V et al. (2012) Association between age at onset of psychosis and age at onset of cannabis use in non-affective psychosis. *Schizophrenia Research* **139**: 157–160.

[72] Ødegaard O. (1946) A statistical investigation of the incidence of mental disorder in Norway. *Psychiatric Quarterly* **20**: 381–401.

[73] Osborn DPJ, Levt G, Nazareth I et al. (2007) Relative risk of cardiovascular and cancer mortality in people with severe mental illness from the United Kingdom's General Practice Research Database. *Archives of General Psychiatry* **64**: 242–249.

[74] Chwostiak LA, Tek C. (2009) The unchanging mortality gap for people with schizophrenia. *Lancet* **374**: 590–592.

[75] Saha S, Chant DC, McGrath J. (2007) A systematic review of mortality in schizophrenia. *Archives of General Psychiatry* **64**: 1123–1131.

[76] Brown S. (1997) Excess mortality of schizophrenia. A meta-analysis. *British Journal of Psychiatry* **171**: 502–508.

[77] Phillips MR, Yang G, Li S et al. (2004) Suicide and the unique prevalence pattern of schizophrenia in mainland China: a retrospective observational study. *Lancet* **364**: 1062–1068.

[78] Hawton K, Sutton L, Haw C et al. (2005) Schizophrenia and suicide: systematic review of risk factors. *British Journal of Psychiatry* **187**: 9–10.

[79] Hiroeh U, Appleby L, Mortensen PB et al. (2001) Death by homicide, suicide, and other unnatural causes in people with mental illness: a population-based study. *Lancet* **358**: 2110–2112.

[80] Lawrence D, Jablensky AV, Holman CDJ et al. (2000) Mortality in Western Australian psychiatric patients. *Social Psychiatry and Psychiatric Epidemiology* **35**: 341–347.

[81] Heilä H, Haukka J, Suvisaari J et al. (2005) Mortality among patients with schizophrenia and reduced psychiatric hospital care. *Psychological Medicine* **35**: 725–732.

[82] Gruenberg EM. (1974) The epidemiology of schizophrenia. In: Arieti S (ed.), *American Handbook of Psychiatry*, vol. 2, 2nd edn. New York: Basic Books.

[83] Fazel S, Gulati G, Linsell L et al. (2009) Schizophrenia and violence: systematic review and meta-analysis. *PLoS Medicine* **6**: 1–15.

[84] Ascher-Svanum H, Nyhuis AW, Faries DE et al. (2010) Involvement in the US criminal justice system and cost implications for persons treated for schizophrenia. *BMC Psychiatry* **10**: 1–11.

[85] World Health Organization. (2001) *The World Health Report 2001. Mental Health: New Understanding, New Hope.* Geneva: World Health Organization.

[86] Keith SJ, Regier DA, Rae DS. (1991) Schizophrenic disorders. In: Robins LN, Regier DA (eds.), *Psychiatric Disorders in America. The Epidemiologic Catchment Area Study.* New York: Free Press.

[87] Phanthunane P, Whiteford H, Vos T et al. (2012) Economic burden of schizophrenia: empirical analyses from a survey in Thailand. *Journal of Mental Health Policy and Economics* **15**: 25–32.

[88] Igberase OO, Morakinyo O, Iawani AO et al. (2012) Burden of care among relatives of patients with schizophrenia in Midwestern Nigeria. *International Journal of Social Psychiatry* **58**: 131–137.

[89] Abbo C. (2011) Profiles and outcome of traditional healing practices for severe mental illnesses in two districts of Eastern Uganda. *Global Health Action* **4**..

[90] Jablensky A, Sartorius N. (2008) What did the WHO studies really find? *Schizophrenia Bulletin* **34**: 253–255.

[91] Wray NR, Visscher PM. (2010) Narrowing the boundaries of the genetic architecture of schizophrenia. *Schizophrenia Bulletin* **36**: 14–23.

[92] Chisholm D, Gureje O, Saldivia S et al. (2008) Schizophrenia treatment in the developing world: an interregional and multinational cost-effectiveness analysis. *Bulletin of the World Health Organization* **86**: 542–551.

Index

Note: Page numbers in *italics* refer to Figures; those in **bold** to Tables.

Improving Mental Health Care: The Global Challenge, First Edition.
Edited by Graham Thornicroft, Mirella Ruggeri and David Goldberg.
© 2013 John Wiley & Sons, Ltd. Published 2013 by John Wiley & Sons, Ltd.